T0136882

Contemporary Endocrinology

Series Editor

Leonid Poretsky
Division of Endocrinology
Lenox Hill Hospital
New York, NY, USA

More information about this series at http://www.springer.com/series/7680

Lynn Loriaux • Chaim Vanek

Editors

Endocrine Emergencies

Recognition and Treatment

Second Edition

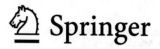

Springer

Editors
Lynn Loriaux
Department of Medicine
Oregon Health and Science University
Portland, OR
USA

Chaim Vanek
Department of Medicine
Oregon Health and Science University
Portland, OR
USA

ISSN 2523-3785   ISSN 2523-3793   (electronic)
Contemporary Endocrinology
ISBN 978-3-030-67457-1   ISBN 978-3-030-67455-7   (eBook)
https://doi.org/10.1007/978-3-030-67455-7

This Springer imprint is published by the registered company Springer Nature Switzerland AG
The registered company address is: Gewerbestrasse 11, 6330 Cham, Switzerland

Series Editor Foreword

Endocrine emergencies are too important to be left exclusively to endocrinologists. For this reason, the second edition, edited by Drs. Lynn Loriaux and Chaim Vanek, is of immense value for all practicing physicians regardless of their specialty. In this monograph, a stellar group of authors addresses in detail a variety of endocrine conditions that need to be recognized early and managed urgently.

The topics include not only the diagnoses that are traditionally considered to be endocrine emergencies (e.g., those of acute hormonal insufficiency or excess), but also a number of dangerous infectious complications that may afflict patients with endocrine disease, particularly with diabetes (e.g., necrotizing soft tissue infections, mucormycosis, emphysematous cholecystitis, and pyelonephritis).

In summary, this book authored by an outstanding multidisciplinary writing crew (in addition to endocrinologists—both adult and pediatric—the contributing authors include gynecologists, infectious disease specialists, and nephrologists) represents an invaluable tool for all students and practitioners of medicine.

New York, NY, USA   Leonid Poresky

Preface

Medical emergencies in the field of endocrinology encompass thyroid, adrenal, pituitary, and other hormonal systems. These "endocrine emergencies" require specific interventions, beyond normal resuscitation protocols, within 2 to 24 hours to successfully care for a patient. The purpose of this book is to detail the management of endocrine, diabetic, and metabolic emergencies by consensus of experts in the field. We believe that this book will bring the topic areas up to date, set a standard for diagnosis and treatment in each category, and comprehensively cover the area for the practicing clinician.

Each chapter begins with a Précis that presents, in concentrated form, what the physician needs to know to begin the evaluation and emergency treatment of known endocrine emergencies, such as facial pain in a patient with poorly controlled diabetes (mucormycosis), or the extreme urgency of a patient presenting with fever and generalized lymphadenopathy (adrenal insufficiency).

This is followed by an extended discussion of disease pathophysiology that can be read after initial treatment has begun. Extended discussions will reveal why David bested Goliath with a stone (pituitary apoplexy), explain paroxysms of palpitations and diaphoresis after consuming gruyere cheese with merlot (pheochromocytoma), and how to elicit "main d'accoucheur" sign for the assessment of acute hypocalcemia.

This revised edition has new updates in the evaluation and management of adrenal insufficiency, hypercalcemia, hyperchylomicronemia, and edits in the recognition/care of other endocrine emergencies.

Portland, OR, USA   Lynn Loriaux
                                                                            Chaim Vanek

Contents

Contributors

Karl E. Anderson, MD Preventive Medicine and Population Health, University of Texas Medical Branch, Galveston, TX, USA

Robert L. Barbieri, MD Department of Obstetrics and Gynecology, Brigham and Women's Hospital, Harvard Medical School, Boston, MA, USA

Glenn D. Braunstein, MD Medicine/Endocrinology, Cedars-Sinai Medical Center, Los Angeles, CA, USA

Kenneth Burman, MD Endocrine Sections, Georgetown University Medical Center/MedStar Washington Hospital Center, Washington, DC, USA

Philip E. Cryer, MD Barnes-Jewish Hospital, St. Louis, MO, USA

J. Stone Doggett, MD Division of Infectious Disease, Oregon Health and Science University, Portland, OR, USA

Ines Donangelo, MD Department of Medicine, David Geffen School of Medicine, University of California Los Angeles, Los Angeles, CA, USA

P. Barton Duell, MD Division of Endocrinology, Diabetes, and Clinical Nutrition, Oregon Health and Science University, Portland, OR, USA

David H. Ellison, MD Nephrology and Hypertension, Oregon Health and Science University, Portland, OR, USA

Pouyan Famini, MD Division of Endocrinology, Diabetes, and Metabolism, Cedars-Sinai Medical Center, Los Angeles, CA, USA

Silvio E. Inzucchi, MD Section of Endocrinology, Yale University School of Medicine, Yale-New Haven Hospital, New Haven, CT, USA

Vitaly Kantorovich, MD Division of Endocrinology and Metabolism, University of CT Health Center, Farmington, CT, USA

Robert Klein, MD Division of Endocrinology, Diabetes and Clinical Nutrition, Oregon Health and Science University, Portland, OR, USA

Lynn Loriaux, MD, PhD Department of Medicine, Oregon Health and Science University, Portland, OR, USA

Beatrice C. Lupsa, MD Section of Endocrinology, Yale University School of Medicine, Yale-New Haven Hospital, New Haven, CT, USA

Shlomo Melmed, MD Division of Endocrinology, Diabetes, and Metabolism, Cedars-Sinai Medical Center, Los Angeles, CA, USA

Walter L. Miller, MD Department of Pediatrics, Center for Reproductive Sciences, University of California, San Francisco, San Francisco, CA, USA

Akshata Moghe, MD, PhD University of Pittsburgh Medical Center, Pittsburgh, PA, USA

Karel Pacak, MD, PhD, Dsc Eunice Kennedy Shriver National Institute of Child Health and Human Development, National Institutes of Health, Bethesda, MD, USA

John J. Reyes-Castano, MD Section of Endocrine, Medstar Washington Hospital Center, Washington, DC, USA

Chaim Vanek, MD Division of Endocrinology, Diabetes and Clinical Nutrition, Oregon Health and Science University, Portland, OR, USA

Selma F. Witchel, MD Division of Pediatric Endocrinology, UPMC Children's Hospital of Pittsburgh, University of Pittsburgh, Pittsburgh, PA, USA

Brian Wong, MD Division of Infectious Disease, Oregon Health and Science University, Portland, OR, USA

Raghav Wusirika, MD Division of Nephrology, Oregon Health and Science University, Portland, OR, USA

Chapter 1
Acute Adrenal Insufficiency

Lynn Loriaux

Précis

1. Clinical setting: Shock resistant to volume and vasopressor resuscitation
2. Diagnosis:

    (a) History: Important complaints include weight loss, syncope, hypoglycemia, fatigue, and unexplained abdominal pain. Recent supraphysiological glucocorticoid steroid treatment or recent history of pituitary or hypothalamic disease. Adrenal surgery, abdominal trauma, unexplained flank pain associated with anticoagulation, and bleeding diathesis syndromes increase the likelihood of primary adrenal failure. Medications that interfere with glucocorticoid synthesis, secretion, and action are ketoconazole, etomidate, and mifepristone (RU-486).

    (b) Physical examination: Fever, orthostatic hypotension, hyperpigmentation of the skin, vitiligo, and lymphadenopathy. Calcification of auricular cartilage ("petrified ear") is a sign of adrenal insufficiency.

    (c) Laboratory values: A total plasma cortisol of less than 20 µg/dL, hyponatremia, hypoglycemia, relative lymphocytosis, eosinophilia, prerenal azotemia, and mild to moderate anion gap metabolic acidosis are common.

    (d) Imaging: Abnormalities of the hypothalamus/pituitary gland and abnormalities of adrenal size. Bilaterally small adrenal glands can be the result of autoimmune adrenal destruction or adrenal suppression. Large adrenal glands are caused by infection, infarction, infiltration, and hemorrhage.

3. Treatment: In addition to the standard treatment for shock, the treatment for acute adrenal insufficiency is an intravenous replacement of hydrocortisone in a

L. Loriaux (✉)
Department of Medicine, Oregon Health and Science University, Portland, OR, USA
e-mail: loriauxl@ohsu.edu

© Springer Nature Switzerland AG 2021
L. Loriaux, C. Vanek (eds.), *Endocrine Emergencies*, Contemporary Endocrinology,
https://doi.org/10.1007/978-3-030-67455-7_1

dose that replicates the plasma cortisol levels associated with critical illness. The standard dose is 50 mg hydrocortisone intravenously every 6 h until the crisis is past. If the pretreatment plasma cortisol is greater than 20 μg/dL, the cortisol administration can be discontinued when the crisis resolves. If the pretreatment cortisol level is less than 20 μg/dL, the intravenous dose of hydrocortisone should be reduced to an oral dose of 12–15 mg/m^2/day until the diagnosis of adrenal insufficiency can be confirmed or excluded. It can require 12 h following the first dose of hydrocortisone before the first therapeutic effects are clinically manifest.

Acute Adrenal Insufficiency

There are two forms of acute adrenal insufficiency. *Primary* (Addison's disease) adrenal insufficiency is associated with destruction of both adrenal glands. Autoimmunity, infection, infiltration, infarction, and hemorrhage are common etiologies. Both cortisol and aldosterone are deficient. *Secondary* acute adrenal insufficiency is associated with ACTH deficiency caused by hypothalamic or pituitary dysfunction. Only cortisol is deficient. Aldosterone secretion, regulated by the renin–angiotensin system, is normal in secondary adrenal insufficiency.

Thomas Addison (1790–1860) was born in Longbenton Village, 4 miles northeast of Newcastle upon Tyne, England. He went to medical school at the University of Edinburgh and graduated with a thesis on syphilis and "hydra guram" (G = hydraguros = "silver water" = mercury). He went to London, became an expert on sexually transmitted disease, was licensed by the London College of Physicians in 1819, and opened a practice. On March 15, 1849, at a meeting of the South London Medical Society, Addison presented his observations on a group of anemic patients with a unique hyperpigmentation of the skin:

"The discoloration pervades the whole surface of the body, but is most manifest on the face, neck, shoulders, and extremities." The condition was uniformly fatal. All patients that had postmortem examinations revealed destructive lesions of the adrenal glands [1–3].

The clinical syndrome defined by lack of cortisol and aldosterone was first described by Lipsett and Pearson:

"We have withdrawn cortisone from adrenalectomized patients in the attempt to maintain them without any steroid hormone administration. It soon became apparent that this was not possible. When cortisone was withdrawn, clinical collapse developed promptly. Within 24 h of cortisone withdrawal, the patient complained of malaise, lethargy, anorexia, and weakness. At 48 h, the patient noted giddiness in the upright position and such profound weakness that he was unwilling to leave the bed. At 72 h, the patient was usually unable to take food, and nausea, vomiting, diarrhea, and stupor frequently ensued. The blood pressure fell but not to shock levels as long as the patient remained horizontal. The patient developed a gaunt and ashen appearance, the skin was cold and gray, the pulse weak, and it appeared that death would soon follow. Administration of cortisone at this time brought about dramatic clinical improvement usually within 12 h, so that the patient was ready to eat and to ambulate, and he felt well" [4, 5] (Fig. 1.1).

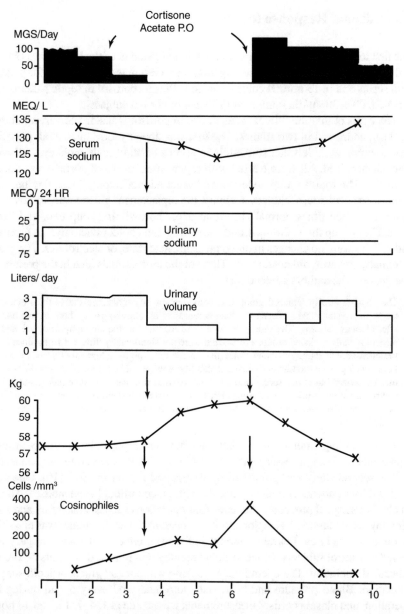

Fig. 1.1 The syndrome of acute glucocorticoid deficiency produced in an adrenalectomized person. (Reproduced from Pearson et al. [4], 543–544; 1956)

Adrenal crisis is characterized by cardiovascular collapse unresponsive to the administration of catecholamines. The catecholamine resistance is caused by the failure of catecholamine receptor biosynthesis [6, 7]. Without glucocorticoid, catecholamine receptor biosynthesis fails at transcription.

The Adrenal Response to Stress

The first to investigate the response of the adrenal gland to critical illness was Melby and Spink in 1958 [8]. These investigators measured plasma cortisol in 20 patients with sepsis and in 13 normal control subjects. Plasma cortisol in septic patients was elevated, 63 ± 30 µg/dL, compared to 13 ± 4 in normal subjects.

The concept that the "stress induced rise in cortisol is needed to survive stress" has been addressed in two studies. The first was done by Udelsman et al. [9] using rhesus monkeys. Udelsman studied three groups of adult male monkeys. All were adrenalectomized. All were treated with replacement doses of cortisol and fludrocortisone. The fourth group underwent a "sham adrenalectomy." One day before a planned surgical stress, cholecystectomy, the replacement glucocorticoid dose was changed to "ten times normal" in group one, "normal" in group two, and "1/10 normal" in group three. Group 4 underwent a "sham cholecystectomy." In groups 1 and 2, there were no changes in blood pressure, heart rate, or electrolytes. The group 3 animals, however, did not do well. Three of the nine animals died in the perioperative period. The authors contend that:

> The physiologically replaced group was hemodynamically indistinguishable from either the supraphysiological replaced or sham-adrenalectomy-placebo group, both before and after cholecystectomy. The mortality rates were identical in the supraphysiological and physiologically replaced groups (14 %) and were not significantly different from those in the sham-adrenalectomy-placebo group. In contrast, the sub-physiologically replaced monkeys developed marked hemodynamic instability, with significant reduction ($P<0.05$) in mean systemic blood pressure, cardiac index, systemic vascular resistance index, and left ventricular stroke work index. Surgical stress amplified this instability and resulted in a 30 % perioperative mortality rate ($P<0.05$) when compared with that in the sham-treated group).

These findings demonstrate that, at minimum, physiologic glucocorticoid replacement is both necessary and sufficient for primates to tolerate surgical stress.

The second study was published by Kehlet and Binder in 1973 [10]. One hundred and four patients chronically treated with glucocorticoid were studied. All had an elective surgical procedure. Seventy-four operations such as colectomy and splenectomy were classified as major surgical procedures. The remainder was classified as minor procedures. Fourteen normal individuals underwent minor surgery and served as control subjects. Glucocorticoid therapy was removed 36 hours before the scheduled operation. The operations were done without any glucocorticoid supplementation. Blood pressure and heart rate were measured every 5 min during the operation, and plasma cortisol measurements were made at 1, 4, 7, 12, and 14 hours

after the beginning of the surgical procedure. Glucocorticoid treatment was reiniti-
ated 72 hours after the procedures. In the major surgery group, 37 of 74 patients had
a subnormal cortisol response to surgery with hypotension in 18 of 74 patients, but
all recovered without an urgent need for glucocorticoids.

The lesson from these studies is that the most important thing the physician can
do to prevent acute adrenal insufficiency during stress in patients at risk for adrenal
insufficiency (known/presumed Addison's or secondary insufficiency from chronic
steroid usage) is to ensure that adequate glucocorticoid is "on board" 2 to 12 hours
before the stress is introduced. One hundred milligrams of hydrocortisone will suffice, and the patient should be returned to their regular hydrocortisone dose once in
stable postoperative recovery. The routine doubling or tripling of glucocorticoids
dosages for several days after surgical procedures is unnecessary.

The Cortrosyn® Stimulation Test

The diagnosis of adrenal insufficiency has rested upon the interpretation of the
Cortrosyn® (synthetic ACTH—adrenocorticotropic hormone) stimulation test.
Cortrosyn® is the first 24 of the 39 amino acids in the full ACTH peptide. A 250-µg
intravenous dose of Cortrosyn® is followed by plasma cortisol measurements at
fixed intervals of 30 and 60 min. The minimum normal Cortrosyn® stimulated
value is 18–20 µg/dL at 60 minutes [11]. An additional measure of normal response
has been the magnitude of the rise of plasma cortisol in response to Cortrosyn®. A
delta change between the basal and stimulated levels of less than 5–9 µg/dL, depending on the report, is considered an abnormal response to the Cortrosyn® stimulation
test. However, since the delta change is inversely related to the basal cortisol concentration [12, 13], this criterion is now rarely applied.

There are several clinical situations that can complicate the interpretation of the
Cortrosyn® test. The first is the acute loss of adrenocorticotropic hormone (ACTH)
secretion. For example, acute pituitary stalk resection from surgery or trauma will
not reliably result in abnormal values in the Cortrosyn® test for up to 12 days,
reflecting time for the adrenal glands to atrophy after ACTH hormone stimulation is
acutely withdrawn [14]. Second, circulating cortisol is bound to cortisol-binding
globulin (CBG) (70%) and albumin (20%). Ten percent of circulating cortisol is
free, i.e., not protein bound. At a total cortisol level of 20 µg/dL, 4 µg of cortisol is
bound to 4 g of albumin. If the plasma albumin level is reduced to 2 g/dL, only 2 µg
of cortisol will be albumin bound, and the total plasma cortisol level will fall by
2 µg/dL. This will alter the "cut-off" value [15] (Fig. 1.2). It is common for critically
ill patients to have reduced circulating albumin levels. The result is an increased
number of false-positive tests (failing to stimulate to 18–20 µg/dL) in the critically
ill. This same concept applies to changes in CBG concentrations which cause even
bigger changes in total plasma cortisol. A measurement of free cortisol levels is
helpful in this scenario.

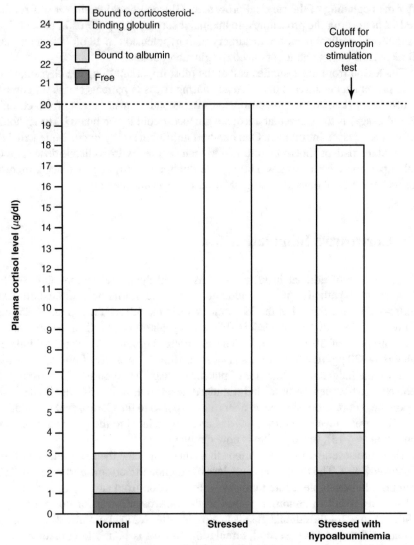

Circulating Plasma Cortisol Levels in a Normal Person, A
Stress Person, and a Stresses Person with Hypoalbuminemia.
Approximately 10 percent of cortisol is present in the free
(bioactive) state, unbound to protein; 20 percent is loosely
bound to albumin; and 70 percent is tightly bound to cortisol-
binding globulin. Binding to cortisol-binding globulin is nearly
saturated at plasma cortisol levels in the range of 15 to 18μg
per deciliter (413.8 to 496.6 nmol per liter). With stress and
hypoalbuminemia, the maximal total cortisol measurement will
fall below that in persons with a normal albumin concentration
and, often, below the traditional cutoff level for the cosyntropin stimulating test, even though the level of free,
bioactive cortisol is the same in these two groups and is
appropriate for the clinical situtation. To convert values to
nanomoles per liter, multiply by 27.6

Fig. 1.2 The effects of hypoalbuminemia on the Cortrosyn® stimulation tests. (Reprinted from
Loriaux [15])

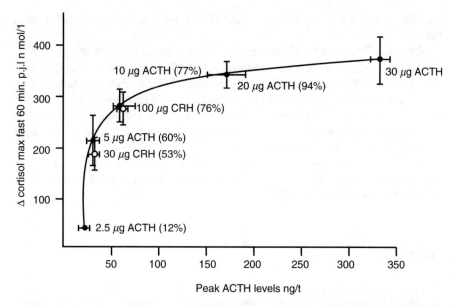

Fig. 1.3 The correlation between maximum serum cortisol and dose of human ACTH. Note the serum ACTH levels at the Vmax, plateaued portion of the curve

All of the baseline clinical data that we depend upon to interpret the Cortrosyn® stimulation test were determined with a Cortrosyn® dose of 250 μg. This is a maximally stimulating dose that is well out on the Vmax (maximum velocity), plateaued portion of the dose response curve (Fig. 1.3). If the Cortrosyn® dose is reduced so that it is on the rapidly rising part of the curve, the coefficient of variation of the test increases, and the results are less precise [16]. A 1-μg ACTH stimulation test has been proposed as better than the 250 μg test for identifying patients with what is thought to be a partially functioning pituitary gland [16]. However, this author strongly advises against the use of the 1-μg dose as it will lead to incorrectly identifying patients as having adrenal insufficiency. Furthermore, Cortrosyn® is approved by the US Food and Drug Administration (FDA) at *only* 250 μg dose for the evaluation of adrenal insufficiency.

Conclusion

The diagnosis of acute adrenal insufficiency is a clinical one: shock poorly responsive to volume and vasopressor therapy. All patients with this syndrome should be treated with 200 mg of hydrocortisone given in 50 mg intravenous boluses at 6-hour intervals. Treatment should be continued until the hypotension is resolved. Twelve hours after the initiation of glucocorticoids, the patient will have a vigorous diuresis of the fluids given at an initial resuscitation; serum osmolality must be closely monitored. Intravenous desmopressin (DDAVP) is useful to prevent excessive water loss [17].

When can the cortisol be discontinued? The most useful tool in making this decision is the total plasma cortisol measured before glucocorticoid treatment is initiated. Patients with values over 20 µg/dL can have the hydrocortisone discontinued over a few days. Those with total plasma cortisol levels less than 20 µg/dL should have the dose reduced over a period of several days to an oral replacement dose of 12–15 mg/m^2 and kept at that dose until primary or secondary adrenal insufficiency can be excluded with a Cortrosyn® test.

High-dose steroids for several days are used in serious infections to treat the inflammatory component of the immune response; this is a separate clinical situation from acute adrenal crisis [18].

References

1. Pearce JMS. Thomas Addison (1793 – 1860). J R Soc Med. 2004;97:297.
2. Addison T. Chronic suprarenal insufficiency, usually due to tuberculosis of suprarenal capsule. London Med Gazette. 1849;43:717–8.
3. Addison T. On the constitutional and local effects of disease of the supra-renal capsules. London: Samuel Highley; 1855.
4. Pearson OH, et al. Clinical and metabolic studies of bilateral adrenalectomy for advanced cancer in man. Surgery. 1953;34:543–56.
5. Lipsett MB, Pearson OH. Pathophysiology and treatment of adrenal crisis. N Engl J Med. 1956;254:511–4.
6. Davies AO, Lefkowitz RJ. Regulation of B-Adrenergic receptors by steroid hormones. Annu Rev Physiol. 1984;46:119–30.
7. Collins S, Bolanowski MA, Caron MG, Lefkowitz RJ. Genetic regulation of B-Adrenergic receptors. Annu Rev Physiol. 1989;51:203–15.
8. Melby JC, Spink WW. Comparative studies in adrenal cortisol function and cortisol metabolism in healthy adults and in patients with shock due to infection. J Clin Invest. 1958;37:1791–7.
9. Udelsman R, Loriaux DL, Chrousos GP. Reevaluation of the role of glucocorticoids in surgical stress. Surg Forum. 1985;36:18–20.
10. Kehlet H, Binder CH. Adrenocortical function and clinical course during and after surgery in glucocorticoid treated patients. Br J Anesth. 1973;45:1043–8.
11. Kehlet H, et al. Short ACTH test in assessing hypothalamic-pituitary-adrenocortical function. Br Med J. 1976;7:249–51.
12. May ME, Carey RM. Rapid adrenocorticotropic hormone test in practice. Am J Med. 1985;79:679–84.
13. Speckart PF, Nicolloff JT, Bethune JE. Screening for adrenocortical insufficiency with Cosyntropin® (synthetic ACTH). Arch Intern Med. 1971;128:761–3.
14. Hjortrup A, Kehlet H, Lindholm J, Stentaft P. Value of the 30-minute adrenocorticotropin (ACTH) test in demonstrating hypothalamic-pituitary-adrenocortical insufficiency after acute ACTH deprivation. J Clin Endocrinol Metab. 1983;57:668–70.
15. Loriaux L. Glucocorticoid therapy in the intensive care unit. N Engl J Med. 2004;350:1601.
16. Oelker W. Dose response aspects in the clinical assessment of the HPA axis, and the low-dose adrenocorticotropin tests. Eur J Endocrinol. 1998;135:27–33.
17. Thomson AE, Brownell EG, Cuming GR. Water diuresis in adrenal cortical insufficiency. Ann Intern Med. Original Research: 1960, May 1.
18. Sterne JA. Association between Administration of systemic corticosteroids and mortality among critically ill patients with COVID-19. A meta-analysis. JAMA. Published online September 2, 2020. https://doi.org/10.1001/jama.2020.17023.

Chapter 2
Diabetic Ketoacidosis and Hyperosmolar Hyperglycemic Syndrome

Beatrice C. Lupsa and Silvio E. Inzucchi

Précis

1. Clinical setting: Any altered state of well-being in the context of significant hyperglycemia in a patient with type 1 (DKA) or advanced type 2 diabetes mellitus (DKA or HHS), particularly during acute illness, may signify one of these diabetic emergencies.

2. Diagnosis:

    (a) History: Most patients with diabetic ketoacidosis (DKA) or with hyperosmolar hyperglycemic state (HHS) will have a history of diabetes and a history of altered insulin dose, infection, and significant medical "stress." Antecedent symptoms of polyuria and polydipsia, lassitude, blurred vision, and mental status changes may predominate the clinical picture. With DKA, abdominal pain and tachypnea are often present.

    (b) Physical examination usually reveals an altered sensorium, signs of volume contraction/dehydration (tachycardia, hypotension, dry mucous membranes, "tenting" of the skin), and, in DKA, the odor of acetone in the breath.

    (c) Laboratory evaluation: The diagnostic criteria for DKA include blood glucose above 250 mg/dL, arterial pH < 7.30, serum bicarbonate <15 mEq/l, and moderate degree of ketonemia and/or ketonuria. Patients with HHS present with extreme hyperglycemia (blood glucose >600 mg/dL), increased osmolality (>320 mOsm/kg), and profound dehydration/volume contraction. The laboratory evaluation of a patient with hyperglycemic emergency should include measurement of blood glucose and hemoglobin A1c, arterial blood gases, serum electrolytes, ketones and osmolality, renal function, and

B. C. Lupsa (✉) · S. E. Inzucchi
Section of Endocrinology, Yale University School of Medicine, Yale-New Haven Hospital, New Haven, CT, USA
e-mail: beatrice.lupsa@yale.edu

© Springer Nature Switzerland AG 2021
L. Loriaux, C. Vanek (eds.), *Endocrine Emergencies*, Contemporary Endocrinology,
https://doi.org/10.1007/978-3-030-67455-7_2

urinalysis. A workup for sepsis or other precipitating causes should be initiated if indicated.

3. Treatment

  (a) DKA

    1. Fluid: Estimated fluid deficit is 5–7 liters. Correct with normal saline, 2 L in the first 2 hours, the remainder over the next 22 hours.
    2. Insulin: IV bolus of 0.1 U/Kg regular insulin followed by an intravenous infusion of 0.1 U/kg/h. The goal is to reduce plasma glucose by 50–75 mg/dL/h. Initial target plasma glucose is 200–250 mg/dL. Once achieved, reduce insulin rate and provide dextrose to "clamp" the plasma glucose until the acidosis/anion gap is resolved.
    3. Acid/base: pH will climb with plasma expansion and insulin administration. Use small amounts of sodium bicarbonate only for severe acidemia (pH < 6.9).
    4. Electrolytes: Close monitoring and correction of serum potassium are critical. (If serum potassium <3.5, correct hypokalemia *before* any insulin is given.)
    5. Search for cause: Seek to determine underlying precipitant, such as treatment nonadherence, infection, and myocardial infarction.

  (b) HHS

    1. Fluid: Estimated fluid deficits typically larger than in DKA (7–9 liters or 100–200 ml/kg). Correction/maintenance of plasma volume with normal saline is critical in older patients. Correct rate depends on blood pressure, other signs of volume contraction, and any history of underlying cardiovascular disease, especially heart failure.
    2. Insulin: Should be initiated *after* initial saline plasma expansion. IV bolus of 0.1 U/Kg regular insulin followed by an intravenous infusion of 0.1 U/kg/h. The goal is to reduce plasma glucose by 50–75 mg/dL/h. Target plasma glucose is 250–300 mg/dL.
    3. Acid/base: By definition, no major deficits related to HHS itself.
    4. Electrolytes: Derangements not as common as in DKA, but monitoring is still required.
    5. Serum osmolality correction should not exceed 3 mOsm/Kg/hr.

Introduction

Diabetic ketoacidosis (DKA) and hyperosmolar hyperglycemic syndrome (HHS) are two acute and life-threatening complications of diabetes requiring prompt recognition and aggressive therapy to optimize clinical outcomes. Although they share certain features, DKA and HHS differ clinically according to the degree of

Table 2.1 Diagnostic criteria for diabetic ketoacidosis (DKA) and hyperosmolar state (HHS)

	DKA			HHS
	Mild	Moderate	Severe	
Plasma glucose (mg/dL)	>250	>250	>250	>600
Arterial pH	7.25–7.30	7.00–7.24	<7.00	>7.30
Serum bicarbonate (mEq/L)	15–18	10 to <15	<10	>18
Urine ketones[a]	Positive	Positive	Positive	None (small)
Serum ketones[a]	Positive	Positive	Positive	None (small)
Effective serum osmolality (mOsm/kg water)[b]	Variable	Variable	Variable	>320
Anion gap[c]	>10	>12	>12	Variable but usually normal
Mental status	Alert	Alert/drowsy	Stupor/coma	Stupor/coma

Adapted from Kitabchi et al., *Diabetes Care*, 2001 [1]
[a]Nitroprusside reaction method
[b]Calculation: 2 [measured Na (mEq/L)] + glucose (mg/dL)/18
[c]Calculation: $Na + - (Cl- + HCO_3 -)$, in mEq/L

hyperglycemia and the presence of ketoacidosis. The fundamental difference between the two conditions is that a small residual amount of insulin prevents significant ketosis and acidosis in HHS. Descriptive definitions of DKA and HHS and the criteria for classification of the severity of the former are shown in Table 2.1.

Patients with DKA present with hyperglycemia, ketonemia, and metabolic acidosis secondary to absolute or profound relative insulin deficiency. HHS is characterized by a greater severity of plasma glucose elevation, marked increase of plasma osmolality, absent or mild ketosis, and altered mental status. In HHS, residual insulin secretion minimizes ketone body production but is not able to control hyperglycemia. The older terms "hyperglycemic hyperosmolar nonketotic coma" and "hyperglycemic hyperosmolar nonketotic state" have been replaced with the term "hyperglycemic hyperosmolar syndrome (or state)" to reflect the fact that different levels of mentation and ketosis may indeed be present.

Most patients with DKA have type 1 diabetes, which is associated with absolute insulin deficiency. Patients with advanced or severe type 2 diabetes can also be at risk during acute illnesses. HHS occurs almost exclusively in type 2 diabetes patients, who continue to demonstrate some degree of insulin secretion.

Pathogenesis

The events leading to DKA and HHS are shown in Fig. 2.1. In DKA, absent or severely reduced insulin concentrations, increased insulin-counterregulatory hormones (cortisol, glucagon, growth hormone, and catecholamines), and peripheral

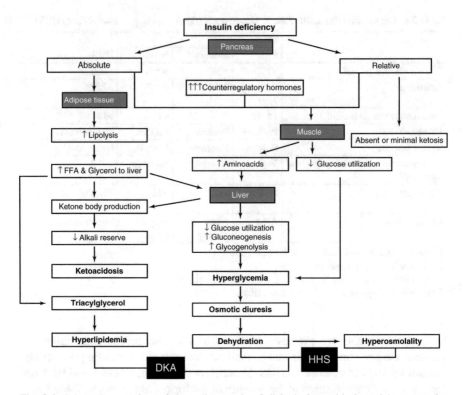

Fig. 2.1 Schematic overview of the pathogenesis of diabetic ketoacidosis and hyperosmolar hyperglycemic syndrome. (Adapted from Kitabchi et al., Diabetes Care, 2001 [1]). *DKA* diabetic ketoacidosis, *FFA* free fatty acids, *HHS* hyperosmolar hyperglycemic syndrome

insulin resistance result in hyperglycemia and ketosis. Hyperglycemia evolves through decreased glucose utilization by peripheral tissues and accelerated hepatic gluconeogenesis and glycogenolysis [1–4]. Due to increased lipolysis and decreased lipogenesis, abundant circulating free fatty acids are converted to ketone bodies (beta-hydroxybutyrate, acetoacetate, and acetone) by the liver. Beta-hydroxybutyrate and acetoacetate are two relatively strong acids. At a physiological pH, these two ketoacids dissociate completely, and the excess hydrogen ions bind bicarbonate, resulting in decreased serum [HCO$_3$ −] concentrations. Ketones thus circulate in the anionic form, leading to the development of the anion gap metabolic acidosis that characterizes DKA. Hyperglycemia-induced osmotic diuresis also leads to dehydration, hyperosmolality, electrolyte losses, and subsequent decreased plasma volume and glomerular filtration. With decline in renal function, glycosuria and ketonuria are attenuated, further exacerbating hyperglycemia, hyperosmolality, and ketoacidosis. Activation of the sympathoadrenal system further counteracts insulin action, heightening all of these features.

HHS is also caused by a reduction in the net effective action of circulating insulin and an increase in counterregulatory hormones, leading to hyperglycemia and hyperosmolality. The key difference between HHS and DKA is that insulin levels in HHS are inadequate to control hyperglycemia but generally sufficient to prevent significant ketosis and, as a result, acidosis.

Recent studies have shown that patients in hyperglycemic crisis also exhibit a severe proinflammatory state characterized by elevated cytokine (tumor necrosis factor-α (alpha), interleukin-β (beta), −6, and −8), C-reactive protein, reactive oxygen species, lipid peroxidation, and plasminogen activator inhibitor-1 [5].

New-onset type 1 diabetes (and, in some circumstances, type 2) can present with DKA. The most common precipitating factors are omission of insulin or inadequate insulin coverage especially during some other acute illnesses (e.g., gastroenteritis, influenza), severe infections, myocardial infarction, stroke, pancreatitis, or major surgery. Insulin pump malfunction, psychiatric illness, eating disorders, and drug abuse can also be associated with DKA. Administration of medications such as corticosteroids, conventional and atypical antipsychotic drugs, thiazide diuretics, and beta-blockers has also been reported to promote the development of DKA.

HHS is seen exclusively in type 2 diabetes and can sometimes be its initial presentation. Infection is the major precipitating factor (pneumonia, pyelonephritis, etc.) occurring in about 50% of the patients. Other acute illnesses such as myocardial infarction and stroke, which cause the release of counterregulatory hormones, and intra-abdominal processes, including acute pancreatitis, can be the stimulus for HHS. Medications associated with DKA also have been associated with HHS. Nonetheless, in about 20% of patients presenting with hyperglycemic crisis, there is no obvious cause—likely due to an abrupt increased insulin requirement for some unidentifiable reason, with superimposed effects of gluco-toxicity, which describes the phenomenon of worsening beta-cell secretion of insulin caused by hyperglycemia itself.

Diagnosis

History and Physical Examination

DKA and HHS are medical emergencies that require urgent recognition and treatment. The initial approach to these patients should include a rapid but thorough history and physical examination with special focus on patency of airways, mental status, state of hydration, cardiovascular and renal integrity, and potential sources of infection.

The development of DKA is usually relatively acute, occurring in less than 24–48 h, whereas HHS usually evolves over several days to weeks. The typical symptoms of unrestrained hyperglycemia in both syndromes include polyuria, polydipsia, blurred vision, fatigue, weakness, and weight loss. DKA patients usually present with vomiting and abdominal pain probably due to delayed gastric emptying and ileus caused by electrolyte abnormalities and/or acidosis.

Physical findings include poor skin turgor, tachycardia, and hypotension. In DKA, there may be a fruity odor to the breath (from ketosis) as well as rapid, regular, and deep respirations (Kussmaul breathing), the latter representing an effort to mitigate the impact of metabolic acidosis by inducing a compensatory respiratory alkalosis. Patients with HHS can present with focal neurological signs (hemiparesis, hemianopsia) and seizures. Mental status can vary from alertness to lethargy and coma. Serum osmolality is the most important determinant of mental status in HHS. In particular, obtundation and coma may be seen when the effective osmolality exceeds 330 mOsm/kg [6].

Even though infection is a common precipitating factor for hyperglycemic crises, the body temperature can be misleadingly normal or low due to peripheral vasodilation.

Laboratory Findings

The easiest and most urgent laboratory tests are determination of blood glucose by finger stick and urinalysis with reagent strips for ketones and glucose allowing for the detection or at least the strong suspicion of these hyperglycemic crises before the patient is seen. These can be done by the patient at home.

The initial laboratory evaluation of a patient with DKA or HHS should include measurement of blood glucose, arterial blood gases, renal function, serum electrolytes, ketones, serum osmolality, complete blood count with differential, and urinalysis. A workup for sepsis should be initiated by obtaining blood and urine cultures and a chest X-ray if clinically indicated. Additional tests include EKG and determination of the hemoglobin A1c level, the latter to assess for chronicity and degree of hyperglycemia (Table 2.2).

Table 2.2 Initial laboratory evaluation for DKA and HHS

Metabolic evaluation	Infectious disease evaluation[a]	Others[a]
Glucose	CBC with differential	Electrocardiogram
Serum ketones	Chest X-ray	Urine toxicology panel
Electrolytes (monovalent and divalent: Na^+, K^+, Cl^-, HCO_3^-, Ca^{2+}, PO_4^{3-}, Mg^{2+})	Urine culture	Pregnancy test
Serum osmolality	Blood cultures	
Blood urea nitrogen (BUN) and creatinine	Viral nasal swab	
Arterial blood gases (ABG)		
Liver function tests		
Amylase and lipase		
Hemoglobin A1c		
Urinalysis		

[a]If clinically indicated

The diagnostic criteria for DKA include blood glucose above 250 mg/dL, arterial pH < 7.30, serum bicarbonate <15 mEq/L, and moderate degree of ketonemia and/ or ketonuria (Table 2.1) [1]. Hyperglycemia is a key diagnostic criteria of DKA; however, 10% of DKA patients will have a glucose level below 250 mg/dL [7], sometimes due to insulin administration before getting to the hospital decreased nutritional intake and decreased gluconeogenesis due to recent ethanol consumption or advanced liver disease [8, 9].

Accumulation of ketones results in an anion gap metabolic acidosis. The anion gap is calculated by subtracting the major measured anions (chloride and bicarbonate) from the major measured cation (sodium). In the older literature, a level above 14–15 mEq/L was thought to be consistent with an increased anion gap metabolic acidosis. However, most laboratories currently measure sodium and chloride using ion-specific electrodes. The plasma chloride level measured by this method is usually 2–6 mEq/L higher than with prior analytical methods. Therefore, using the ion-specific technique, an anion gap of >10–12 mEq/L would suggest the presence of an anion gap acidosis [10, 11]. Arterial blood gases support the diagnosis with the presence of acidemia.

Important laboratory features of DKA are ketonemia and ketonuria. The ratio between the two main ketoacids, beta-hydroxybutyrate and acetoacetate, depends on the prevailing redox state. In high redox states, such as DKA (as well as lactic acidosis), beta-hydroxybutyrate predominates. Assessment of ketone status is usually performed with the nitroprusside reaction, which provides a semiquantitative measurement of acetoacetate and acetone. However, the nitroprusside reaction does not detect beta-hydroxybutyrate, thus underestimating the severity of ketoacidosis. If available, direct measurement of serum beta-hydroxybutyrate can be helpful in establishing the diagnosis.

Patients with HHS present with extreme hyperglycemia (blood glucose >600 mg/ dL), increased osmolality (>320 mOsm/kg), and profound dehydration/volume contraction. The effective serum osmolality is calculated as follows: 2 [measured Na (mEq/L)] + glucose (mg/dL)/18, with normal value being 290 ± 5 mOsm/kg (blood urea nitrogen, which enters the equation for total serum osmolality, is not included here as it is freely diffusible across cell membranes and is therefore not considered an "effective osmole"). Usually in HHS, the anion gap is normal, and serum bicarbonate level is over 20 mEq/L. However, some patients can present with mild acidosis, due to the accumulation of ketone bodies in low concentration and/or lactate resulting from generalized hypoperfusion.

Both DKA and HHS are associated with large fluid and electrolyte deficits (Table 2.3). The development of dehydration and electrolyte depletion is the result of hyperglycemia, insulin deficiency, and, in DKA, keto-anion excretion.

Hyperglycemia causes an osmotic diuresis. During severe hyperglycemia the renal threshold of glucose and ketones is exceeded. The osmotic effect of glycosuria results in impaired water and sodium chloride reabsorption in the proximal tubule and loop of Henle [12]. Insulin deficiency itself may further contribute to fluid and electrolyte losses because insulin stimulates salt and water resorption in the proximal and distal nephron and phosphate reabsorption in the proximal tubule. Ketoacid

Table 2.3 Typical deficits of water and electrolytes in DKA and HHS

	DKA	HHS
Total water (L)	6	8
Water (mL/kg)[a]	100	100–200
Na^+ (mEq/kg)	7–10	5–13
$Cl-$ (mEq/kg)	3–5	5–15
K^+ (mEq/kg)	3–5	4–6
$PO_4{}^{3-}$ (mmol/kg)	5–7	3–7
Mg^{2+} (mEq/kg)	1–2	1–2
Ca^{2+} (mEq/kg)	1–2	1–2

Adapted from Kitabchi et al., Diabetes Care, 2006 [29]
[a]Per kilogram of body weight

excretion exacerbates solute diuresis by causing urinary cation excretion in the form of sodium, potassium, and ammonium salts.

The severity of dehydration is greater in HHS than in DKA likely due to more gradual and longer duration of metabolic decompensation and decreased fluid intake. Also, nausea and vomiting (in DKA) and fever, when present, can further contribute to dehydration.

Serum sodium concentration is markedly decreased because of intracellular water shifting to the extracellular compartment in order to equilibrate hyperosmolality. Usually the admission sodium is factitiously low because of the hyperglycemia and hyperlipidemia. The corrected sodium can be calculated by adding 1.6 mEq to the reported sodium value for every 100 mg of glucose over 100 mg/dL. As a result, a normal or high-measured serum sodium in this setting actually indicates a severe state of dehydration, as is often the case in patients presenting with HHS.

The patient's serum potassium may be initially elevated due to an extracellular shift of potassium caused by insulin deficiency, acidemia, and hypertonicity, which is *falsely reassuring* as the total body potassium stores are probably depleted. A low or low-normal potassium level suggests severe total body potassium depletion.

Patients with uncontrolled hyperglycemia are usually in a negative phosphate balance because of phosphaturia caused by osmotic diuresis and the shift of phosphate out of the cell in the setting of acidosis.

Leukocytosis around 10,000–15,000 mm^3 is a common finding in DKA and may not be the result of an infection. This is attributed to stress and elevation in stress hormones. However, leukocytosis above 25,000 mm^3 suggests a septic process and should trigger further evaluation.

Hyperamylasemia has been reported in patients with DKA. It is not always associated with pancreatitis. The origin of amylase in DKA is usually a non-pancreatic tissue such as the salivary glands. Measuring a lipase level can be useful in the differential diagnosis; however, lipase also can be elevated in the absence of pancreatitis [13]. The mechanisms of increased amylase and lipase levels in DKA are not well defined.

Moderate hypertriglyceridemia is common during episodes of DKA [14]. The deficiency of insulin activates lipolysis in adipose tissue releasing increased free fatty acids, which accelerates the formation of very-low-density lipoprotein (VLDL) in the liver. In addition, reduced activity of lipoprotein lipase in peripheral tissue decreases the removal of VLDL from the plasma, resulting in hypertriglyceridemia. Severe hypertriglyceridemia and hypertriglyceridemia-induced pancreatitis leading to DKA or HHS are well recognized [15]. Severe hypertriglyceridemia may falsely lower serum glucose (pseudo-normoglycemia) [16] and serum sodium (pseudohyponatremia) [17] in laboratories using volumetric testing and dilution samples with ion-specific electrodes.

Differential Diagnosis

DKA must be differentiated from other conditions that present with ketoacidosis and anion gap metabolic acidosis. Starvation and alcoholic ketoacidosis are not typically associated with hyperglycemia above 200 mg/dL, and, usually, the bicarbonate level is greater than 18 mEq/L. Other causes of an anion gap metabolic acidosis include lactic acidosis, acute renal failure, and the ingestion of methanol, ethylene glycol, paraldehyde, and salicylate. The origin of the anion gap can usually be ascertained by assessing the ketone concentrations in the plasma. HHS is difficult to confuse with other conditions, given its narrowly defined diagnostic criteria. Overlap syndromes with features of both DKA and HHS, however, can be encountered in the clinical practice. These may occur in patients with a slower development of ketoacidosis and, as a result, more protracted urinary losses of free water, resulting in hyperosmolality.

Treatment

The therapeutic goals of DKA and HHS management include restoration of volume status, correction of hyperglycemia and ketoacidosis (in DKA), correction of electrolyte abnormalities, treatment of precipitating factors, and prevention of the complications of DKA and HHS. Adequate intravenous (IV) access is essential with two larger bore IV peripheral lines or a central line. A suggested protocol for the management of patients with DKA and HHS is summarized in Fig. 2.2.

Fluid Therapy

In the emergency room, fluid resuscitation is critical for intravascular, interstitial, and intracellular volume and restoration of renal perfusion. The average fluid loss is approximately 5–7 L in DKA and 7–9 L in HHS (Table 2.3). The IV fluid administration replaces the fluid and electrolyte deficiencies while simultaneously reducing plasma glucose concentrations and counterregulatory hormones, partially through

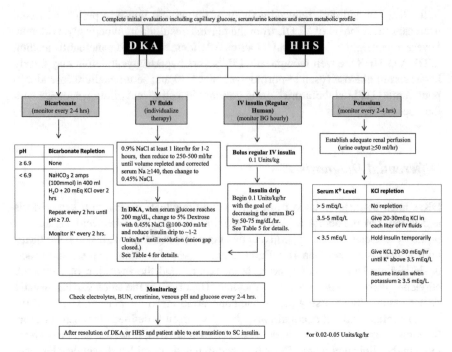

Fig. 2.2 Suggested protocol for management of adult patients with diabetic ketoacidosis and hyperosmolar hyperglycemic syndrome. (Adapted from Kitabchi et al., Diabetes Care, 2009 [18]). *BG* blood glucose, *DKA* diabetic ketoacidosis, *HHS* hyperosmolar hyperglycemic syndrome, *hr* hour, H_2O water, *IV* intravenously, *KCl* potassium chloride, *NaCl* sodium chloride, *mEq/L* milliequivalents per liter, *SC* subcutaneous

dilution but also through volume expansion and resultant expansion of plasma volume. IV fluids should be administered *before* starting insulin in HHS, especially in older patients with tenuous cardiovascular status, in order to preserve vascular volume (see below).

Normal saline is generally given in the first hour at a rate of 15–20 mL/kg body weight/h or 1–1.5 L in the first hour, although care is required in older patients with underlying cardiovascular disease. After initial stabilization, if the corrected serum sodium is normal or elevated, normal saline can be changed to half-normal saline at a rate of ~250–500 mL/h. If the corrected sodium is low, normal saline can be continued at a similar rate. Fluid replacement should correct the estimated deficit in the first 24 h, with 50% of fluid resuscitation in the first 8–12 h. In patients with HHS, the change in serum osmolality should not exceed 3 mOsm/kg water/h.

The response to fluid resuscitation is judged by monitoring hemodynamic parameters (blood pressure and heart rate), clinical exam, urinary output, and laboratory values. In patients with renal or cardiac compromise, fluid resuscitation should be conducted with caution to avoid fluid overload.

Once the serum glucose is 200–250 mg/dL in DKA, the insulin infusion rate should be reduced to 1–2 U/h, and 5% dextrose should be added to the IV fluids

Table 2.4 Suggested algorithm for clamping the blood glucose using dextrose-containing IV fluids and IV insulin in DKA

Serum glucose	IV fluid	Insulin infusion
200–250 mg/dL in DKA	Change to D$_5$0.45%NS 100–200 mL/h[a,b] 100 mL/h 200 mL/h	Reduce insulin drip to 1–2 U/h[b,c] 1 U/h 2 U/h
If serum glucose increases	Do not reduce IV fluids	Minor increases in insulin infusion rate (~0.5–1 U/h)[d]
If serum glucose decreases	Increase IV fluids	Do not decrease insulin infusion rate

[a]Provides 5–10 g of carbohydrates per hour
[b]Alternative is 0.02–0.05 U/kg/h
[c]Give insulin IV 1 U/h for every 5 g of dextrose IV/h
[d]Highly insulin-resistant patients who require large amounts of IV insulin may need as much as 5–10 U of insulin/h. Accordingly, insulin dose adjustments may need to be more aggressive. The insulin dose can likely be reduced gradually as hyperglycemia improves

(this is termed the "glucose-insulin clamp" by some authorities). This technique will prevent hypoglycemia but will allow continuation of insulin administration sufficient in amount to resolve the ketoacidosis in DKA (i.e., to close the anion gap). A proposed algorithm for clamping the serum glucose using dextrose-containing IV fluids and IV insulin is outlined in Table 2.4.

Due to concerns that lowering the serum glucose too fast in HHS might promote the development of cerebral edema, some authorities recommend adding 5% dextrose to the IV fluids when the serum glucose is 250–300 mg/dL until the patient is mentally alert [18]. In the majority of HHS cases, serum osmolality and mental status are normalized by the time the hyperglycemia is corrected; thus the "glucose clamp" will not often be necessary. Indeed, a simple lowering of the insulin infusion rate without the addition of dextrose can be sufficient, even in cases where the mental status remains abnormal.

Insulin Therapy

The only contraindication to insulin therapy is a current serum potassium below 3.5 mEq/L as insulin will worsen the hypokalemia by shifting the potassium into the cells.

The administration of continuous intravenous infusion of regular insulin is the preferred route as it has short half-life, is easy to titrate, and has a rapid onset and short duration of action. The insulin dose is similar in DKA and HHS. However, as mentioned before, initial volume expansion with crystalloid is recommended (at least 1 L) in the more profoundly dehydrated and older HHS patients. This recommendation is to protect the plasma volume; once insulin is administered, the consequent fall in circulating glucose concentrations will lead to an intracellular shift of

Table 2.5 Suggested algorithm for adjusting the IV insulin infusion during treatment of the hyperglycemic phase of DKA and HHS

Hourly change in blood glucose (BG)	Action
BG↑	Rebolus (0.1 U/kg) and double insulin rate
BG ↓ by 0–49 mg/dL/h	↑Insulin drip by 25–50%
BG ↓ by 50–75 mg/dL/h	No change in insulin drip
BG ↓ by >75 mg/dL/h	Hold insulin drip × 30 min and restart at 50% of most recent rate

water from the plasma compartment which can result in a precipitous drop in systemic blood pressure. Insulin treatment usually starts with an IV bolus of 0.1 U/kg body weight followed by a 0.1 U/kg body weight/hour continuous infusion. The goal of insulin therapy is to decrease serum glucose by 50–75 mg/dL/h. Overly aggressive reduction of glucose may result in brain edema. A suggested algorithm for adjusting the IV insulin drip during DKA and HHS treatment can be found in Table 2.5. Glucose levels should be monitored every 1 h initially and, once stabilized, every 2–3 h.

Treatment of patient with mild to moderate DKA with subcutaneous rapid-acting analogs (lispro, aspart) every 1–2 h in non-intensive care unit has been shown to be effective in several studies [19, 20]; however, until these studies are confirmed outside the research setting, the vast majority of patients with DKA and HHS should be treated with intravenous regular insulin. Preferably, patients with these hyperglycemic emergencies should be managed in an intensive care setting, mainly due to the requirements to continuous patient monitoring, frequent blood testing and reporting, and rapid titration of therapy that may be required.

Potassium Replacement

Potassium replacement is critical in managing patients with DKA and HHS. Renal and gastrointestinal losses contribute to a marked potassium deficit in most patients. Despite the total body potassium deficit, the serum potassium concentration can be normal or elevated at presentation due to acidosis, insulin deficiency, and hyperosmolality, all of which cause a potassium shift from the intracellular to the extracellular space. Administration of insulin results in a significant shift of potassium into the cells and a fall in the serum potassium level. To prevent hypokalemia, potassium chloride is usually added to the IV fluids if the serum potassium is below the upper level of normal for the particular lab (5.0–5.2 mEq/L) and there is a good urinary output (>50 mL/h). Careful monitoring of the serum potassium is a critical part in the management of all hyperglycemic emergencies. Ideally, the serum potassium should be measured every 2–4 h (along with other electrolytes) and maintained between 4 and 5 mEq/L. To avoid cardiac and respiratory complications, patients who are hypokalemic prior to the initiation of treatment should not receive insulin until the potassium level is above 3.5–4.0 mEq/L. Such patients should receive aggressive potassium replacement (20–30 mEq/h) until potassium level is above 3.5–4.0 mEq/L (see Fig. 2.2 for details).

Phosphate Replacement

At presentation, serum phosphate is often normal or high in spite of whole-body phosphate deficit due to movement of phosphate out of the cells. As with potassium balance, phosphate concentration decreases with insulin therapy. However, the fall in the serum phosphate level during DKA treatment is usually self-limited, is asymptomatic, and does not require treatment. Prospective randomized trials of patients with DKA failed to show any benefit associated with supplementation [21], and phosphate replacement can have adverse effects such as hypocalcemia and hypomagnesemia [22]. Thus, phosphate replacement is not routinely recommended; however, it should be considered in patients at risk for cardiac dysfunction, hemolytic anemia, and respiratory depression or when the phosphate concentration is below 1 mg/dL. When needed, potassium phosphate 20–30 mEq/L can be added to the replacement fluids. The rate of phosphate replacement should not exceed 4.5 mmol/h [23]. Because of the risk of hypocalcemia, serum calcium and phosphate levels should be monitored during phosphate infusion. No studies are available on the use of phosphate in treatment of HHS. Phosphate levels should be tested but less frequently than routine electrolytes, perhaps every 8–12 h.

Bicarbonate Therapy

Bicarbonate use in DKA remains controversial. Treatment with insulin inhibits lipolysis and ketoacid production and promotes keto-anion metabolism. Because protons are consumed during keto-anion metabolism, bicarbonate is regenerated leading to partial correction of metabolic acidosis with insulin therapy and volume expansion alone. However, severe acidosis can lead to impaired cardiac contractility, cerebral vasodilatation, and severe gastrointestinal complications. A randomized trial of 21 DKA patients with an admission arterial pH between 6.9 and 7.1 showed no difference in morbidity and mortality with bicarbonate use [24]. Not surprisingly, there are no prospective randomized trials on the use of bicarbonate in DKA patients with an arterial pH less than 6.9. Potential side effects of bicarbonate therapy include hypokalemia, worsening intracellular acidosis (as a result of increased carbon dioxide production), delayed keto-anion metabolism, and development of paradoxical central nervous system acidosis [25–27].

Nonetheless, because severe acidosis may result in significant adverse cardiovascular effects, it is recommended that patients with pH values <6.9 should receive 100 mmol of sodium bicarbonate (two ampules) in 400 mL sterile water with

20 mEq potassium chloride at a rate of 200 mL/h for 2 h until the pH is >7. If the pH is still <7, the bicarbonate infusion can be repeated every 2 h until the pH is >7. Hypokalemia, if present, must be corrected before any bicarbonate administration. Profound acidosis can require a continuous bicarbonate infusion.

Search for Precipitating Factors

Infection is a major precipitating factor for hyperglycemic emergencies. Hence, it is important to search for underlying infections. If indicated, chest X-ray and blood and tissue cultures should be obtained. Appropriate antibiotic treatment should be initiated if a bacterial infection is identified.

Resolution of DKA and HHS

Criteria for resolution of DKA includes a serum glucose <200 mg/dL and two out of the following criteria: serum bicarbonate ≥15 mEq/L, a venous pH > 7.3, and a calculated anion gap ≤12 mEq/L. Resolution of HHS includes normal serum osmolality (<315 mOsm/kg) and normal mental status [18]. Please note that the serum bicarbonate may still be low even after DKA resolution due to an "expansion" non-gap acidosis associated with aggressive IV crystalloid repletion. Thus, the anion gap is the best indicator of DKA resolution.

Transition to Subcutaneous Insulin

If the DKA or HHS has resolved but the patient is to remain NPO, IV insulin and fluid replacement should be continued. However, if the patient is able to eat, subcutaneous insulin can be started, although this may be most conveniently done in conjunction with the patient's next planned meal. As the IV insulin has a very short half-life, in order to prevent the recurrence of hyperglycemia and acidosis, it is important to overlap for 1–2 h the subcutaneous and IV insulin. If the patient has a history of type 1 diabetes mellitus, the patient's routine therapy can be resumed as long as an inadequate home regimen was not the reason for the hyperglycemic crisis. In newly diagnosed patients, a multidose insulin regimen should be started at a dose of 0.5–0.8 U/kg/day, the higher end of this range reserved for patients who have substantial degrees of insulin resistance as reflected by the insulin infusion requirements, prior history, body weight, and other physical features, such as acanthosis nigricans. Typically, however, the recent insulin infusion rates are not helpful in determining subcutaneous insulin doses, since they may be rapidly fluctuating, and with the resolution of gluco-toxicity, insulin requirements can be quite valuable.

A variety of subcutaneous insulin regimens are available from relatively straightforward (twice per day premixed insulins) to relatively complex (e.g., long-acting insulin in the evening and rapid-acting insulin with meals, the so-called *basal-bolus* strategy). The latter is likely to result in the best glycemic control, although it requires more understanding and participation by the patient. The use of insulin sliding scale alone should be discouraged, even as a transition, as it cannot provide the necessary insulin requirement in patients recovering from hyperglycemic crises. Fingerstick glucose measurements before each meal and at night should be done after discontinuing the IV insulin to correct for possible fluctuations in insulin needs while in the hospital.

Complications

Hypoglycemia and hypokalemia are the most common iatrogenic complications during the treatment of DKA and HHS. These can be prevented by very close monitoring (every 2–4 h) of the potassium level and appropriate supplementation, adjustment of insulin dose, and use of dextrose-containing IV fluids.

Hyperchloremic non-anion gap metabolic acidosis is commonly seen after the resolution of DKA. It is usually explained by the high dose of chloride administered in IV fluids. This acidosis is self-limited and has no adverse clinical effects. Patients usually require several days to recover as the kidneys readjust bicarbonate production and acid secretion. The persistently low bicarbonate level due to hyperchloremic metabolic acidosis can be distinguished from persistent DKA due to inadequate insulin treatment by following the anion gap.

Cerebral edema is an uncommon but very serious complication of DKA and HHS treatment, associated with high mortality. For unclear reasons, it is seen more commonly in children with DKA. Symptoms of cerebral edema include headache, lethargy, pupillary changes, seizures, bradycardia, and cardiac arrest. The underlying mechanisms are not completely understood. Rapid decline in plasma osmolality and brain ischemia have been proposed as contributing mechanisms. Prevention of cerebral edema may be achieved by avoiding overzealous hydration and by maintaining plasma glucose ~200 mg/dL in DKA until the anion gap is closed. Patients should be carefully monitored for changes in mental and neurologic status. Mannitol infusion and mechanical ventilation are suggested for treatment of cerebral edema [28].

Noncardiogenic pulmonary edema can develop in DKA patients from excessive fluid replacement, even in patients without renal or cardiac problems. Pulmonary rales and an increased alveolar-arterial gradient should prompt a decrease in IV fluid rate and initiation of continuous pulse oximetry.

Prevention

Many cases of DKA and HHS can be prevented by better access to medical care, proper patient education, and effective communication with healthcare providers during an intercurrent illness. Patients and their families should receive education about managing sick days. The use of urine ketone testing or combined home glucose-ketone meters can allow early recognition of impending ketoacidosis and possibly prevent hospitalization for DKA.

One of the most common precipitating factors for hyperglycemic crisis is discontinuation of insulin for economic reasons. This suggests that the current mode of providing health care has significant limitations. Thus, resources need to be directed toward funding better access to medical care and educational programs tailored to individual needs.

References

1. Kitabchi AE, Umpierrez GE, Murphy MB, et al. Management of hyperglycemic crises in patients with diabetes. Diabetes Care. 2001;24(1):131–53.
2. van de Werve G, Jeanrenaud B. Liver glycogen metabolism: an overview. Diabetes Metab Rev. 1987;3(1):47–78.
3. Felig P, Sherwin RS, Soman V, et al. Hormonal interactions in the regulation of blood glucose. Recent Prog Horm Res. 1979;35:501–32.
4. Barrett EJ, DeFronzo RA, Bevilacqua S, Ferrannini E. Insulin resistance in diabetic ketoacidosis. Diabetes. 1982;31(10):923–8.
5. Stentz FB, Umpierrez GE, Cuervo R, Kitabchi AE. Proinflammatory cytokines, markers of cardiovascular risks, oxidative stress, and lipid peroxidation in patients with hyperglycemic crises. Diabetes. 2004;53(8):2079–86.
6. Kitabchi AE, Nyenwe EA. Hyperglycemic crises in diabetes mellitus: diabetic ketoacidosis and hyperglycemic hyperosmolar state. Endocrinol Metab Clin N Am. 2006;35(4):725–51, viii.
7. Miles JM, Gerich JE. Glucose and ketone body kinetics in diabetic ketoacidosis. Clin Endocrinol Metab. 1983;12(2):303–19.
8. Munro JF, Campbell IW, McCuish AC, Duncan LJ. Euglycaemic diabetic ketoacidosis. Br Med J. 1973;2(5866):578–80.
9. Burge MR, Hardy KJ, Schade DS. Short-term fasting is a mechanism for the development of euglycemic ketoacidosis during periods of insulin deficiency. J Clin Endocrinol Metab. 1993;76(5):1192–8.
10. Winter SD, Pearson JR, Gabow PA, Schultz AL, Lepoff RB. The fall of the serum anion gap. Arch Intern Med. 1990;150(2):311–3.
11. Sadjadi SA. A new range for the anion gap. Ann Intern Med. 1995;123(10):807.
12. Hypernatremic and polyuric states. In: Selain A, Giebisch G, editors. The kidney: physiology and pathophysiology. New York: Raven; 1992. p. 1578.
13. Yadav D, Nair S, Norkus EP, Pitchumoni CS. Nonspecific hyperamylasemia and hyperlipasemia in diabetic ketoacidosis: incidence and correlation with biochemical abnormalities. Am J Gastroenterol. 2000;95(11):3123–8.
14. Fulop M, Eder HA. Plasma triglycerides and cholesterol in diabetic ketosis. Arch Intern Med. 1989;149(9):1997–2002.
15. Fulop M, Eder H. Severe hypertriglyceridemia in diabetic ketosis. Am J Med Sci. 1990;300(6):361–5.
16. Rumbak MJ, Hughes TA, Kitabchi AE. Pseudonormoglycemia in diabetic ketoacidosis with elevated triglycerides. Am J Emerg Med. 1991;9(1):61–3.
17. Kaminska ES, Pourmotabbed G. Spurious laboratory values in diabetic ketoacidosis and hyperlipidemia. Am J Emerg Med. 1993;11(1):77–80.
18. Kitabchi AE, Umpierrez GE, Miles JM, Fisher JN. Hyperglycemic crises in adult patients with diabetes. Diabetes Care. 2009;32(7):1335–43.

19. Umpierrez GE, Latif K, Stoever J, et al. Efficacy of subcutaneous insulin lispro versus continuous intravenous regular insulin for the treatment of patients with diabetic ketoacidosis. Am J Med. 2004;117(5):291–6.
20. Umpierrez GE, Cuervo R, Karabell A, Latif K, Freire AX, Kitabchi AE. Treatment of diabetic ketoacidosis with subcutaneous insulin aspart. Diabetes Care. 2004;27(8):1873–8.
21. Fisher JN, Kitabchi AE. A randomized study of phosphate therapy in the treatment of diabetic ketoacidosis. J Clin Endocrinol Metab. 1983;57(1):177–80.
22. Winter RJ, Harris CJ, Phillips LS, Green OC. Diabetic ketoacidosis. Induction of hypocalcemia and hypomagnesemia by phosphate therapy. Am J Med. 1979;67(5):897–900.
23. Miller DW, Slovis CM. Hypophosphatemia in the emergency department therapeutics. Am J Emerg Med. 2000;18(4):457–61.
24. Morris LR, Murphy MB, Kitabchi AE. Bicarbonate therapy in severe diabetic ketoacidosis. Ann Intern Med. 1986;105(6):836–40.
25. Narins RG, Cohen JJ. Bicarbonate therapy for organic acidosis: the case for its continued use. Ann Intern Med. 1987;106(4):615–8.
26. Okuda Y, Adrogue HJ, Field JB, Nohara H, Yamashita K. Counterproductive effects of sodium bicarbonate in diabetic ketoacidosis. J Clin Endocrinol Metab. 1996;81(1):314–20.
27. Hale PJ, Crase J, Nattrass M. Metabolic effects of bicarbonate in the treatment of diabetic ketoacidosis. Br Med J (Clin Res Ed). 1984;289(6451):1035–8.
28. Roberts MD, Slover RH, Chase HP. Diabetic ketoacidosis with intracerebral complications. Pediatr Diabetes. 2001;2(3):109–14.
29. Kitabchi AE, Umpierrez GE, Murphy MB, Kreisberg RA. Hyperglycemic crises in adult patients with diabetes: a consensus statement from the American Diabetes Association. Diabetes Care. 2006;29(12):2739–48.

Chapter 3
Hypoglycemia

Philip E. Cryer

Précis

1. Clinical setting: A patient with some combination of neurogenic symptoms (sweating, hunger, tremor, palpitations), neuroglycopenic manifestations (confusion, aberrant behavior, seizure, coma), and signs of sympathoadrenal activation (pallor, diaphoresis) [1, 2].
2. Diagnosis:

    (a) Important findings include a history of hypoglycemic or hyperglycemic episodes; a confirmed diagnosis of diabetes; medications used to treat hypoglycemia; alcohol abuse; liver, kidney, and pituitary disease; and a history of bariatric surgery.
    (b) Physical examination: Vital signs (tachycardia), mental status (delirium, obtundation), and the "gag" reflex should be assessed.
    (c) Laboratory findings: The key laboratory measurement is a capillary blood plasma glucose of less than 55 mg/dL.

3. Treatment:

    (a) In the medical setting (office or hospital): Intravenous glucose is the standard initial treatment regardless of cause. An initial dose of 25 g of glucose as an intravenous bolus is recommended [5]. This should be followed by an intravenous infusion of glucose at a rate of 20 mg/kg/min until hypoglycemia is corrected [8]. In sulfonylurea-induced hypoglycemia infusion of the somatostatin analogue, octreotide, can be used to suppress insulin secretion [9].

P. E. Cryer (✉)
Barnes-Jewish Hospital, St. Louis, MO, USA
e-mail: pcryer@wustl.edu

© Springer Nature Switzerland AG 2021
L. Loriaux, C. Vanek (eds.), *Endocrine Emergencies*, Contemporary Endocrinology,
https://doi.org/10.1007/978-3-030-67455-7_3

(b) In the home setting, most episodes of hypoglycemia can be treated with oral carbohydrate in the form of glucose tablets, juices, soft drinks, candy, or food. An initial dose of 20 g carbohydrate is recommended. The carbohydrate must be swallowed: Glucose applied to the buccal mucosa is not absorbed [6]. This dose of carbohydrate should be repeated if the plasma glucose is not increased 15–20 min after administration.

(c) If the patient cannot take oral carbohydrate, a subcutaneous or intramuscular injection of 1 mg glucagon is very effective [7]. Glucagon works by stimulating hepatic glycogenolysis, it will be less effective in type 2 compared to type 1 diabetes; and will be ineffective in glycogen-depleted individuals such as the aftermath of an alcoholic binge or in patients with end-stage liver disease. Nasal glucagon, FDA approved in July 2019, for hypoglycemia is given as a single actuation into a single nostril.

After successful treatment of an episode of hypoglycemia, measures that will prevent its recurrence are required. An understanding of the pathogenesis of the initial hypoglycemic episode and a rational approach to its treatment are essential components of successful management.

Frequency and Impact of Hypoglycemia

Hypoglycemia is the limiting factor in the glycemic management of diabetes [1]. Iatrogenic hypoglycemia—triggered by treatment with a sulfonylurea, a glinide, or insulin—causes recurrent morbidity in most people with type 1 diabetes and many with advanced type 2 diabetes and is sometimes fatal. Indeed, while early studies indicated that 2–4% of people with type 1 diabetes die from hypoglycemia [10–12], more recent data indicate hypoglycemic mortality rates of 6% [13], 7% [14], and 10% [15] in type 1 diabetes. Hypoglycemic deaths occur in type 2 diabetes, but the mortality rate is as yet unknown [16, 17]. In addition, hypoglycemia generally precludes maintenance of euglycemia over a lifetime of diabetes and, therefore, full realization of the vascular benefits of glycemic control [18–22]. Lastly, hypoglycemia impairs defenses against subsequent falling plasma glucose concentrations and thus causes a vicious cycle of recurrent hypoglycemia [1].

Most people with type 2 diabetes ultimately require treatment with insulin. The incidence of iatrogenic hypoglycemia in insulin-treated type 2 diabetes is about one-third of that in type 1 diabetes [23], but the frequency increases over time [24]. Because type 2 diabetes is about 20-fold more prevalent than type 1 diabetes, most episodes of hypoglycemia, including those of severe hypoglycemia, occur in people with type 2 diabetes.

In contrast, hypoglycemia is an uncommon clinical event in individuals without diabetes [2]. Nonetheless, there is a differential diagnosis of Whipple's triad documented hypoglycemia (Table 3.1). The leading cause of hypoglycemia in such individuals is drugs other than those used to treat diabetes [3, 4]. The latter include alcohol and several drugs that are used commonly and are occasionally associated

Table 3.1 Differential
diagnosis of hypoglycemia

Ill or mediated individual
1. Drugs
Sulfonylurea, glinide, or insulin to treat diabetes
Alcohol
Many others [3, 4]
2. Critical illness
Renal, hepatic, or cardiac failure
Sepsis
Inanition
3. Hormone deficiency
Cortisol deficiency
Growth hormone deficiency
Glucagon and epinephrine deficiency in insulin-deficient diabetes
4. Nonislet cell tumor
Seemingly well individual
5. Endogenous hyperinsulinism
Insulinoma
Noninsulinoma pancreatogenous hypoglycemia including post-gastric bypass hypoglycemia
Autoimmune hypoglycemias: antibody to insulin, antibody to insulin receptor
Insulin secretagogue
Others
6. Accidental, surreptitious, or malicious hypoglycemia

Source: From ref. [2]

with hypoglycemia. Those include angiotensin-converting enzyme inhibitors and angiotensin receptor antagonists, β-adrenergic antagonists, selective serotonin reuptake inhibitors, some anti-arrhythmics (e.g., disopyramide), some quinolone antibiotics, sulfonamides, quinine, and analgesics including salicylates, acetaminophen, and indomethacin, among many other drugs [3, 4]. Clearly, intentional, accidental, surreptitious, and even malicious drug use should be considered when the mechanism of hypoglycemic episodes is obscure.

Physiologic and Behavioral Defenses Against Hypoglycemia

The physiologic defenses that normally prevent, or rapidly correct, hypoglycemia are (1) a decrease in pancreatic islet β-cell insulin secretion, (2) an increase in pancreatic islet α-cell glucagon secretion, and (3) an increase in adrenomedullary epinephrine secretion [25] (Fig. 3.1). The behavioral defense is carbohydrate ingestion, prompted by symptoms and the resulting recognition of hypoglycemia [25] (Fig. 3.1).

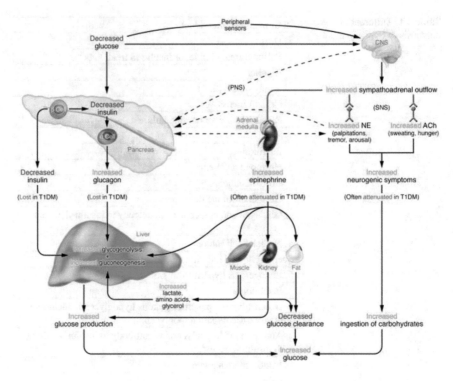

Fig. 3.1 The mechanisms of defense against falling plasma glucose concentrations. (*Source*: From Cryer [42] with permission of the American Society for Clinical Investigation)

Pathophysiology of Hypoglycemia

Hypoglycemia in diabetes is fundamentally iatrogenic, started by sulfonylurea, glinide, or insulin-induced increments in circulating insulin that are independent of the corresponding plasma glucose concentration. However, because of the effectiveness of the normal defenses against falling glucose levels, hypoglycemia rarely results from hyperinsulinemia per se. Rather, hypoglycemia in diabetes is typically the result of the interplay of therapeutic hyperinsulinemia and compromised physiological and behavioral defenses against falling plasma glucose concentrations [1] (Figs. 3.1 and 3.2). In type 1 diabetes, as glucose levels fall, those compromised defenses include (1) loss of the decrease in insulin and the result of β-cell failure; (2) loss of the increase in glucagon, which is also likely the result of β-cell failure since a decrease in β-cell insulin normally signals an increase in glucagon secretion during hypoglycemia [26]; and (3) an attenuated increase in sympathoadrenal activity. These abnormalities cause the clinical syndrome of defective glucose counterregulation which is associated with a 25-fold [27] or perhaps greater increased risk of severe hypoglycemia during aggressive therapy of type 1 diabetes [28]. The attenuated sympathoadrenal response, particularly the attenuated sympathetic

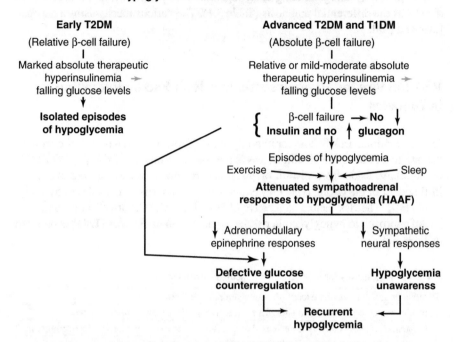

Fig. 3.2 Hypoglycemia-associated autonomic failure in diabetes. (*Source*: Modified from Cryer [43] with permission of the American Diabetes Association)

neural response [29, 30], causes the clinical syndrome of hypoglycemia unawareness (or impaired awareness of hypoglycemia) which is associated with a sixfold [31] or greater [32] increased risk of severe hypoglycemia during aggressive glycemic therapy of diabetes.

The concept of hypoglycemia-associated autonomic failure (HAAF) in diabetes posits that recent antecedent hypoglycemia, as well as sleep and prior exercise, causes both defective glucose counterregulation (by attenuating the epinephrine response to subsequent hypoglycemia in the setting of absent insulin and glucagon responses) and hypoglycemia unawareness (by attenuating the sympathoadrenal, sympathetic neural response to subsequent hypoglycemia). This can lead to a vicious cycle of recurrent hypoglycemia [1, 33]. Perhaps the most compelling support for the clinical relevance of HAAF is the finding, originally in three independent laboratories, that hypoglycemia unawareness, and to some extent the reduced epinephrine component of defective glucose counterregulation, is reversible in most affected patients [34–37].

The pathophysiology of glucose counterregulation is the same in type 2 diabetes and type 1 diabetes except that it develops more slowly as absolute β-cell failure develops more slowly in type 2 diabetes [1, 33, 38]. That explains why iatrogenic hypoglycemia becomes a major problem early in type 1 diabetes but only later in type 2 diabetes.

The pathophysiology leading to hypoglycemia in people without diabetes is as diverse as the differential diagnosis (Table 3.1). The various mechanisms have been reviewed [39].

Risk Factors for Hypoglycemia and Risk Factor Reduction in Diabetes

The conventional risk factors for hypoglycemia (Table 3.2) are based on the premise that relative or absolute insulin excess is the sole determinant of risk [1]. While this is important, aside from insulin or insulin secretagogue doses that are excessive, ill-timed, or of the wrong type, they explain only a minority of episodes of hypoglycemia [40]. The risk factors suggestive of HAAF (Table 3.2) are also relevant.

An approach to hypoglycemia risk factor reduction in diabetes [1, 41] is outlined in Table 3.3.

Table 3.2 Risk factors for hypoglycemia in people with diabetes

Relative or absolute insulin excess (the conventional risk factors):
1. Insulin or insulin secretagogue doses are excessive, ill-timed, or of the wrong type
2. Exogenous glucose delivery is decreased (e.g., after missed meals and during the overnight fast)
3. Endogenous glucose production is decreased (e.g., after alcohol ingestion)
4. Glucose utilization is increased (e.g., during and shortly after exercise)
5. Sensitivity to insulin is increased (e.g., after weight loss or improved glycemic control and in the middle of the night)
6. Insulin clearance is decreased (e.g., with renal failure)
Hypoglycemia-associated autonomic failure:
1. Absolute endogenous insulin deficiency
2. A history of severe hypoglycemia, hypoglycemia unawareness, or both as well as a relationship to recent antecedent hypoglycemia, prior exercise, or sleep
3. Aggressive glycemic therapy per se (lower A1C levels, lower glycemic goals)

Source: From ref. [1]

Table 3.3 Hypoglycemia risk factor reduction in diabetes

	Acknowledge the problem
	Apply the principles of aggressive glycemic therapy:
	1. Patient education and empowerment
	2. Frequent self-plasma glucose monitoring (or continuous glucose monitoring)
	3. Flexible and appropriate insulin (and other drug) regimens
	4. Individualized glycemic goals
	5. Ongoing professional guidance and support
	Consider the conventional risk factors
	Consider the risk factors indicative of hypoglycemic-associated autonomic failure

Source: From ref. [1]

Acknowledgments The author's original work cited was supported, in part, by the National Institutes of Health grants R37 DK27085, MO1 RR00036 (now UL1 RR24992), P60 DK20579, and T32 DK07120 and by a fellowship award from the American Diabetes Association. Ms. Janet Dedeke, the author's assistant, prepared this manuscript.

The author has served as a consultant to Novo Nordisk in the past year. He does not receive research funds from, hold stock in, or speak for any pharmaceutical or device firm.

References

1. Cryer PE. Hypoglycemia in diabetes. 3rd ed. Alexandria: American Diabetes Association; 2016.
2. Cryer PE, Axelrod L, Grossman AB, Heller SR, Montori VM, Seaquist ER, et al. Evaluation and management of adult hypoglycemic disorders: an Endocrine Society clinical practice guideline. J Clin Endocrinol Metab. 2009;94:709–28.
3. Murad MH, Coto-Yglesias F, Wang AT, Sheidaee N, Mullan RJ, Elamin MB, et al. Clinical review: drug-induced hypoglycemia: a systematic review. J Clin Endocrinol Metab. 2009;94:741–5.
4. Ben Salem C, Fathallah N, Hmouda H, Bouraoui K. Drug-induced hypoglycaemia: an update. Drug Saf. 2011;34:21–45.
5. Wiethop BV, Cryer PE. Alanine and terbutaline in treatment of hypoglycemia in IDDM. Diabetes Care. 1993;16:1131–6.
6. Gunning RR, Garber AJ. Bioactivity of instant glucose. Failure of absorption through oral mucosa. JAMA. 1978;240:1611–2.
7. Haymond MW, Schreiner B. Mini-dose glucagon rescue for hypoglycemia in children with type 1 diabetes. Diabetes Care. 2001;24:643–5.
8. Basu R, Basu A, Johnson CM, Schwenk WF, Rizza RA. Insulin dose–response curves for stimulation of splanchnic glucose uptake and suppression of endogenous glucose production differ in nondiabetic humans and are abnormal in people with type 2 diabetes. Diabetes. 2004;53:2042–50.
9. Boyle PJ, Justice K, Krentz AJ, Nagy RJ, Schade DS. Octreotide reverses hyperinsulinemia and prevents hypoglycemia induced by sulfonylurea overdoses. J Clin Endocrinol Metab. 1993;76:752–6.
10. Deckert T, Poulsen JE, Larsen M. Prognosis of diabetics with diabetes onset before the age of 31. I. Survival, causes of death, and complications. Diabetologia. 1978;14:363–70.
11. Tunbridge WMG. Factors contributing to deaths of diabetics under 50 years of age. Lancet. 1981;2:569–72.
12. Laing SP, Swerdlow AJ, Slater SD, Botha JL, Burden AC, Waugh NR, et al. The British Diabetic Association Cohort study. I: all-cause mortality in patients with insulin-treated diabetes mellitus. Diabet Med. 1999;16:459–65.
13. Diabetes Control and Complications Trial/Epidemiology of Diabetes Interventions and Complications Study Research Group, Jacobson AM, Musen G, Ryan CM, Silvers N, Cleary P, Waberski B, Burwood A, Weinger K, Bayless M, Dahms W, Harth J. Long-term effect of diabetes and its treatment on cognitive function. N Engl J Med. 2007;356:1842–52.
14. Feltbower RG, Bodansky HJ, Patterson CC, Parslow RC, Stephenson CR, Reynolds C, et al. Acute complications and drug misuse are important causes of death for children and young adults with type 1 diabetes: results from the Yorkshire Register of diabetes in children and young adults. Diabetes Care. 2008;31:922–6.
15. Skrivarhaug T, Bangstad H-J, Stene LC, Sandvik L, Hanssen KF, Joner G. Long-term mortality in a nationwide cohort of childhood-onset type 1 diabetic patients in Norway. Diabetologia. 2006;49:298–305.
16. Gerich JE. Oral hypoglycemic agents. N Engl J Med. 1989;321:1231–45.

17. Holstein A, Egberts EH. Risk of hypoglycaemia with oral antidiabetic agents in patients with Type 2 diabetes. Exp Clin Endocrinol Diabetes. 2003;111:405–14.
18. Control D, Group CTR. The effect of intensive treatment of diabetes on the development and progression of long-term complications in insulin-dependent diabetes mellitus. N Engl J Med. 1993;329:977–86.
19. Prospective UK. Diabetes Study (UKPDS) Group. Intensive blood-glucose control with sulphonylureas or insulin compared with conventional treatment and risk of complications in patients with type 2 diabetes (UKPDS 33). Lancet. 1998;352:837–53.
20. Prospective UK. Diabetes Study (UKPDS) Group. Effect of intensive blood-glucose control with metformin on complications in overweight patients with type 2 diabetes (UKPDS 34). Lancet. 1998;352:854–65.
21. Nathan DM, Cleary PA, Backlund JY, Genuth SM, Lachin JM, Orchard TJ, et al. Zinman B; Diabetes Control and Complications Trial/Epidemiology of Diabetes Interventions and Complications (DCCT/EDIC) Study Research Group. Intensive diabetes treatment and cardiovascular disease in patients with type 1 diabetes. N Engl J Med. 2005;353:2643–53.
22. Holman RR, Paul SK, Bethel MA, Matthews DR, Neil HA. 10-year follow-up of intensive glucose control in type 2 diabetes. N Engl J Med. 2008;359:1577–89.
23. Donnelly LA, Morris AD, Frier BM, Ellis JD, Donnan PT, Durrant R, et al. Frequency and predictors of hypoglycaemia in Type 1 and insulin-treated Type 2 diabetes: a population-based study. Diabet Med. 2005;22:749–55.
24. Hypoglycaemia Study Group UK. Risk of hypoglycaemia in types 1 and 2 diabetes: effects of treatment modalities and their duration. Diabetologia. 2007;50:1140–7.
25. Cryer PE. The prevention and correction of hypoglycemia. In: Jefferson LS, Cherrington AD, editors. Handbook of physiology, Section 7, The endocrine pancreas and regulation of metabolism, vol. II. New York: Oxford University Press; 2001. p. 1057–92.
26. Cooperberg BA, Cryer PE. Insulin reciprocally regulates glucagon secretion in humans. Diabetes. 2010;59:2936–40.
27. White NH, Skor DA, Cryer PE, Levandoski LA, Bier DM, Santiago JV. Identification of type I diabetic patients at increased risk for hypoglycemia during intensive therapy. N Engl J Med. 1983;308:485–91.
28. Bolli GB, De Feo P, De Cosmo S, Perriello G, Ventura MM, Benedetti MM, et al. A reliable and reproducible test for adequate glucose counterregulation in type I diabetes mellitus. Diabetes. 1984;33:732–7.
29. Towler DA, Havlin CE, Craft S, Cryer P. Mechanism of awareness of hypoglycemia. Perception of neurogenic (predominantly cholinergic) rather than neuroglycopenic symptoms. Diabetes. 1993;42:1791–8.
30. DeRosa MA, Cryer PE. Hypoglycemia and the sympathoadrenal system: neurogenic symptoms are largely the result of sympathetic neural, rather than adrenomedullary, activation. Am J Physiol Endocrinol Metab. 2004;287:E32–41.
31. Geddes J, Schopman JE, Zammitt NN, Frier BM. Prevalence of impaired awareness of hypoglycaemia in adults with Type 1 diabetes. Diabet Med. 2008;25:501–4.
32. Schopman JE, Geddes J, Frier BM. Prevalence of impaired awareness of hypoglycaemia and frequency of hypoglycaemia in insulin-treated type 2 diabetes. Diabetes Res Clin Pract. 2010;87:64–8.
33. Dagogo-Jack SE, Craft S, Cryer PE. Hypoglycemia-associated autonomic failure in insulin-dependent diabetes mellitus. J Clin Invest. 1993;91:819–28.
34. Fanelli CG, Epifano L, Rambotti AM, Pampanelli S, Di Vincenzo A, Modarelli F, et al. Meticulous prevention of hypoglycemia normalizes the glycemic thresholds and magnitude of most of neuroendocrine responses to, symptoms of, and cognitive function during hypoglycemia in intensively treated patients with short-term IDDM. Diabetes. 1993;42:1683–9.
35. Cranston I, Lomas J, Maran A, Macdonald I, Amiel SA. Restoration of hypoglycaemia awareness in patients with long-duration insulin-dependent diabetes. Lancet. 1994;344:283–7.

36. Fanelli C, Pampanelli S, Epifano L, Rambotti AM, Di Vincenzo A, Modarelli F, et al. Long-term recovery from unawareness, deficient counterregulation and lack of cognitive dysfunction during hypoglycaemia, following institution of rational, intensive insulin therapy in IDDM. Diabetologia. 1994;37:1265–76.

37. Dagogo-Jack S, Rattarasarn C, Cryer PE. Reversal of hypoglycemia unawareness, but not defective glucose counterregulation, in IDDM. Diabetes. 1994;43:1426–34.

38. Segel SA, Paramore DS, Cryer PE. Hypoglycemia-associated autonomic failure in advanced type 2 diabetes. Diabetes. 2002;51:724–33.

39. Cryer PE. Hypoglycemia. In: Melmed S, Polonsky KS, Larsen PR, Kronenberg HM, editors. Williams textbook of endocrinology. 12th ed. Philadelphia: Saunders; 2011. p. 1552–77.

40. Diabetes Control and Complications Trial Research Group. Epidemiology of severe hypoglycemia in the diabetes control and complications trial. Am J Med. 1991;90:450–9.

41. Cryer PE, Davis SN, Shamoon H. Hypoglycemia in diabetes. Diabetes Care. 2003;26:1902–12.

42. Cryer PE. Mechanisms of sympathoadrenal failure and hypoglycemia in diabetes. J Clin Invest. 2006;116:1470–3.

43. Cryer PE. The barrier of hypoglycemia in diabetes. Diabetes. 2008;57:3169–76.

Chapter 4
Necrotizing Soft Tissue Infections

J. Stone Doggett and Brian Wong

Précis

Necrotizing soft tissue infections:

1. Clinical setting: Up to 50% of patients that develop necrotizing soft tissue infections have diabetes mellitus, and are likely to present without the usual overt symptoms of necrotizing soft tissue disease.
2. Diagnosis:

   (a) History: Clinical findings include cellulitis that fails to respond to antibiotic treatment, pain out of proportion to the size of the lesion, the appearance of local anesthesia, bullous lesions, crepitus, inflammation, and edema beyond the margin of the skin findings. Fever and leukocytosis are almost always present.

   (b) Imaging: Radiologic studies lack the necessary specificity in this disease to be very useful. That said, the preferred test is a non-contrast CT because it can be performed quickly. CT findings include vessel thrombosis, fluid tracking, perifascial air, skin thickening, lymphadenopathy, muscle edema, and fat stranding.

3. Management: Once the diagnosis is clear, aggressive surgical debridement and broad-spectrum antibiotics must be initiated. Delayed "time to surgery" is consistently associated with increased morbidity and mortality. Without surgery, mortality approaches 100%. Multiple debridements are usually required.

   Empiric antibiotic therapy should cover gram-positive, gram-negative, and anaerobic bacteria. Empiric antibiotic therapy should include clindamycin plus

J. S. Doggett (✉) · B. Wong
Division of Infectious Disease, Oregon Health and Science University, Portland, OR, USA
e-mail: doggettj@ohsu.edu

© Springer Nature Switzerland AG 2021   37
L. Loriaux, C. Vanek (eds.), *Endocrine Emergencies*, Contemporary Endocrinology,
https://doi.org/10.1007/978-3-030-67455-7_4

piperacillin-tazobactam or a carbapenem or ceftriaxone and metronidazole plus vancomycin or other anti-MRSA antibiotics.

Necrotizing Soft Tissue Infection

Necrotizing soft tissue infections have been divided into different clinical entities based on the microbiology, location, and degree of tissue involvement. Despite different classifications, all necrotizing soft tissue infections are medical emergencies that require early diagnosis, parenteral antibiotics, and aggressive surgical debridement to achieve optimal outcomes.

The incidence of necrotizing soft tissue infection is estimated to be 0.04 cases per 1000 person-years in the USA and has ranged from 0.3 to 15.5 annual cases per 100,000 people in other regions of the world [1, 2]. Diabetics are more susceptible to skin and soft tissue infections in general, and in current studies, up to half of patients who develop necrotizing soft tissue infection have diabetes [3, 4]. Diabetics are also more likely to present without overt symptoms indicative of a necrotizing infection. Because of this, physicians should consider necrotizing soft tissue infection in diabetics who present with skin infection and systemic signs of illness or progressive infection despite antibiotics.

Necrotizing soft tissue infections are composed of necrotizing cellulitis and necrotizing fasciitis. Necrotizing cellulitis is characterized by gas formation in the skin, sparing the fascia and muscle. Necrotizing fasciitis spreads along the fascial plane, and overlying skin involvement may not be apparent. These infections may be mono-microbial or poly-microbial. Mono-microbial infections are most commonly due to *Streptococcus pyogenes* and *Clostridium* species, but *Staphylococcus aureus*, *Vibrio vulnificus*, anaerobic *Streptococci*, and *Aeromonas* species have been reported with some frequency. Up to half of the patients with poly-microbial necrotizing soft tissue infections have diabetes, whereas there is no clear association with diabetes and mono-microbial infections. An exception to this principle is infection caused by methicillin-resistant *Staphylococcus aureus* (MRSA), where up to one-fifth of patients have diabetes.

Necrotizing cellulitis and fasciitis are usually distinguished from one another by surgical exploration. Necrotizing infection may spread from a site of skin injury such as surgical wound, IV drug use, abscess, or in 20% of cases, no apparent lesion. No portal of entry is found in 50% of group A streptococcal necrotizing fasciitis [1]. Specific necrotizing soft tissue infection syndromes are denoted by the anatomic location. These include Fournier's gangrene, which is a necrotizing infection of the perineum, and cervical necrotizing fasciitis, which is located in the cervical area and typically follows odontogenic infection.

Clinical Presentation

Necrotizing fasciitis may be difficult to diagnose in its early stages when there is overlying cellulitis or a lack of distinguishing characteristics. Clinical features that suggest necrotizing fasciitis are failure to respond to antibiotics, pain out of proportion to appearance or anesthesia, signs of systemic illness, or altered mental status. Skin findings include bullous lesions, crepitus, necrosis, ecchymosis, or firm edema beyond the margin of skin findings. Patients typically have lab abnormalities consistent with systemic inflammation.

Diagnosis

Clinical prediction tools using laboratory data or CT findings have been proposed to distinguish between necrotizing and non-necrotizing soft tissue infections. The "laboratory risk indicator for necrotizing fasciitis score" created by Wong et al. assigns points for elevated C-reactive protein, leukocytosis, elevated creatinine, hyperglycemia, hyponatremia, and anemia [5]. Based on this score, patients are divided into low, intermediate, and high risk. In the retrospective validation cohort, 92.9% of patients with necrotizing fasciitis had an intermediate or high risk score. 91.6% of patients without necrotizing fasciitis had low risk scores. The authors recommend that patients with soft tissue infections who have intermediate or high risk scores undergo urgent evaluation for necrotizing fasciitis. This scoring system had limited sensitivity in some studies, one of which specifically evaluated infection with *Vibrio vulnificus*, and also in a study of children under 18 years old but was considered to be a useful clinical tool based on a systematic review of 16 studies in adults [6–11].

Radiographic studies lack the sensitivity required to detect necrotizing infection, and surgical evaluation should not be delayed for imaging. Of the imaging modalities, non-contrast CT is the most practical when it can be performed quickly. CT findings consist of vessel thrombosis, fluid tracking, perifascial air, skin thickening, lymphadenopathy, abscess, muscle edema, and fat stranding [12].

When evaluating diabetic patients with cellulitis, the signs and symptoms mentioned above should lead to surgical evaluation. If these clinical features are absent, suspicion for necrotizing infection should remain until the patient responds adequately to medical therapy. Currently, definitive diagnosis of necrotizing soft tissue infection requires surgical exploration. Surgical findings include necrotic tissue, lack of bleeding, vascular thrombosis, "dishwater" pus, non-contracting muscle, and a lack of resistance to blunt dissection of the fascial plane (Fig. 4.1) [13]. Tissue gram stain and cultures should be obtained during surgery to distinguish mono-microbial from poly-microbial infection and to detect drug-resistant organisms.

Fig. 4.1 A diagnostic incision was performed at the bedside in the left flank of a patient with necrotizing fasciitis. Necrotic fat is seen in the incision. The darkened discoloration of the skin is indicative of the loss of blood supply to the skin due to infection causing the thrombosis of blood vessels

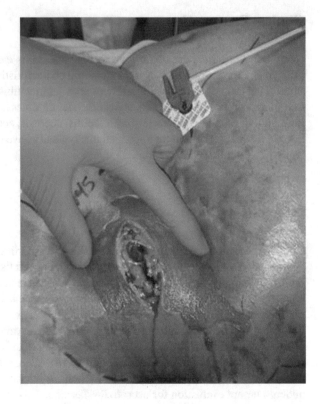

Treatment

Once the diagnosis of a necrotizing soft tissue infection is made, aggressive surgical debridement and broad-spectrum antibiotics must be initiated. Delayed time to surgery is consistently associated with increased morbidity and mortality. Mortality approaches 100% without surgery. After the initial debridement, patients should return to the operating room for further evaluation and may require multiple debridements. There are no clinical studies that have established a superior antibiotic regimen, and empiric coverage should be based on the patient's risk for drug-resistant infection and local bacterial drug-resistance patterns. That being said, empiric antibiotic therapy should cover gram-positive, gram-negative, and anaerobic bacteria. Suggested initial parenteral antibiotics include piperacillin-tazobactam or a carbapenem or the combination of ceftriaxone and metronidazole plus an anti-MRSA agent [14]. The treatment of Fournier's gangrene should include coverage of *Pseudomonas*. Clindamycin is often added based on in vitro studies that have demonstrated bacterial toxin suppression and mouse models of *Streptococcus pyogenes* myositis in which clindamycin had greater efficacy than penicillin [15, 16]. The efficacy of clindamycin is also supported by two small retrospective clinical studies that showed improved clinical responses with clindamycin in deep infection and in group A streptococcal necrotizing fasciitis [17, 18]. Once a microbiological diagnosis is made, antibiotics may be tailored for mono-microbial infections, but antibiotic coverage should remain broad for poly-microbial infection because all of the pathogens may not grow in culture. Group A streptococcal infection should be treated with intravenous penicillin G and clindamycin [19]. The great majority of necrotizing infections in diabetics are poly-microbial and require continued broad-spectrum antibiotics. Intravenous immunoglobulin and hyperbaric oxygen have been studied as adjunctive therapy, but there is not sufficient evidence to support their use.

Summary

Necrotizing soft tissue infections are one of the more common infectious emergencies in diabetics. While there are many distinct forms of necrotizing soft tissue infections, the management is similar. Patients typically present with acute, severe illness and prominent skin findings. However, a percentage of patients will present with subtle findings that may be difficult to delineate from cellulitis. Laboratory and radiographic scoring systems have been proposed to aid in the diagnosis of necrotizing soft tissue infections, but the role of these systems is evolving. Surgical evaluation remains the definitive means of diagnosis, and patients who are suspected of having necrotizing infection should be rapidly evaluated. Aggressive surgical debridement is essential to reduce morbidity and mortality and should be coupled with broad empiric antibiotic therapy. Recent studies have shown improvements in overall mortality to 12% or less [3, 4, 20]. When diabetics present with soft tissue infection, physicians should consider the possibility of underlying necrotizing infection and pursue surgical evaluation if there are signs of systemic illness, characteristic skin findings, failure to respond to antibiotics, or characteristic radiographic findings:

- Necrotizing soft tissue infections in diabetics are typically poly-microbial.
- Diagnosis of necrotizing soft tissue infection requires a high degree of clinical suspicion and is definitively diagnosed by surgical exploration.
- Necrotizing soft tissue infection should be treated empirically with broad-spectrum antibiotics and emergent surgical debridement.

References

1. Stevens DL, Bryant AE. Necrotizing soft-tissue infections. N Engl J Med. 2017; 377(23):2253–65.
2. Ellis Simonsen SM, van Orman ER, Hatch BE, et al. Cellulitis incidence in a defined population. Epidemiol Infect. 2006;134(2):293–9.
3. Bernal NP, Latenser BA, Born JM, Liao J. Trends in 393 necrotizing acute soft tissue infection patients 2000-2008. Burns. 2011;38:252.

4. Mills MK, Faraklas I, Davis C, Stoddard GJ, Saffle J. Outcomes from treatment of necrotizing soft-tissue infections: results from the National Surgical Quality Improvement Program database. Am J Surg. 2010;200(6):790–796; discussion 796-797.
5. Wong CH, Khin LW, Heng KS, Tan KC, Low CO. The LRINEC (Laboratory Risk Indicator for Necrotizing Fasciitis) score: a tool for distinguishing necrotizing fasciitis from other soft tissue infections. Crit Care Med. 2004;32(7):1535–41.
6. Corbin V, Vidal M, Beytout J, et al. Prognostic value of the LRINEC score (Laboratory Risk Indicator for Necrotizing Fasciitis) in soft tissue infections: a prospective study at Clermont-Ferrand University hospital. Ann Dermatol Venereol. 2010;137(1):5–11.
7. Wong CH. Tissue oxygen saturation monitoring in diagnosing necrotizing fasciitis of the lower limb: a valuable tool but only for a select few. Ann Emerg Med. 2005;45(4):461–462; author reply 462-463.
8. Holland MJ. Application of the Laboratory Risk Indicator in Necrotising Fasciitis (LRINEC) score to patients in a tropical tertiary referral centre. Anaesth Intensive Care. 2009;37(4):588–92.
9. Tsai YH, Hsu RW, Huang KC, Huang TJ. Laboratory indicators for early detection and surgical treatment of vibrio necrotizing fasciitis. Clin Orthop Relat Res. 2010;468(8):2230–7.
10. Bechar J, Sepehripour S, Hardwicke J, Filobbos G. Laboratory risk indicator for necrotising fasciitis (LRINEC) score for the assessment of early necrotising fasciitis: a systematic review of the literature. Ann R Coll Surg Engl. 2017;99(5):341–6.
11. Putnam LR, Richards MK, Sandvall BK, Hopper RA, Waldhausen JH, Harting MT. Laboratory evaluation for pediatric patients with suspected necrotizing soft tissue infections: a case-control study. J Pediatr Surg. 2016;51(6):1022–5.
12. McGillicuddy EA, Lischuk AW, Schuster KM, et al. Development of a computed tomography-based scoring system for necrotizing soft-tissue infections. J Trauma. 2011;70(4):894–9.
13. Anaya DA, Dellinger EP. Necrotizing soft-tissue infection: diagnosis and management. Clin Infect Dis. 2007;44(5):705–10.
14. Stevens DL, Bisno AL, Chambers HF, et al. Practice guidelines for the diagnosis and management of skin and soft tissue infections: 2014 update by the infectious diseases society of America. Clin Infect Dis. 2014;59(2):147–59.
15. Coyle EA, Cha R, Rybak MJ. Influences of linezolid, penicillin, and clindamycin, alone and in combination, on streptococcal pyrogenic exotoxin A release. Antimicrob Agents Chemother. 2003;47(5):1752–5.
16. Stevens DL, Gibbons AE, Bergstrom R, Winn V. The Eagle effect revisited: efficacy of clindamycin, erythromycin, and penicillin in the treatment of streptococcal myositis. J Infect Dis. 1988;158(1):23–8.
17. Mulla ZD, Leaverton PE, Wiersma ST. Invasive group A streptococcal infections in Florida. South Med J. 2003;96(10):968–73.
18. Zimbelman J, Palmer A, Todd J. Improved outcome of clindamycin compared with beta-lactam antibiotic treatment for invasive Streptococcus pyogenes infection. Pediatr Infect Dis J. 1999;18(12):1096–100.
19. Stevens DL, Bisno AL, Chambers HF, et al. Practice guidelines for the diagnosis and management of skin and soft-tissue infections. Clin Infect Dis. 2005;41(10):1373–406.
20. Huang KF, Hung MH, Lin YS, et al. Independent predictors of mortality for necrotizing fasciitis: a retrospective analysis in a single institution. J Trauma. 2011;71(2):467–473; discussion 473.

Chapter 5
Malignant (Necrotizing) Otitis Externa

J. Stone Doggett and Brian Wong

Précis

Malignant (necrotizing) otitis externa:

1. Clinical Setting: A patient with diabetes mellitus who has ear pain, often severe, and drainage from the external ear canal, often associated with headache or pain in the temporomandibular joint.
2. Diagnosis:

    (a) History: Almost all patients with malignant otitis externa are diabetics. Ear pain and otorrhea occur in 90% of patients. Systemic signs of infection such as fever and altered mental state are uncommon. The facial nerve is the most commonly affected, but other cranial nerves may be involved as well.
    (b) Imaging: Both CT and MRI are recommended. CT is better at detecting early cortical bone erosion, and MRI is better at detecting medullary changes in bone and thickening of the dura.
    (c) Biopsy: Biopsy is required to differentiate infection from malignancy in some cases.

3. Management: After biopsy has been taken, empiric therapy is started with an antibiotic that has antipseudomonal and anti-staphylococcal activity. Candidates include cefepime, piperacillin-tazobactam, or the antipseudomonal, carbapenem. Antibiotics can be narrowed in scope as specific organisms are identified.

    Surgical debridement is now reserved for cases in which there are abscesses or bony sequestration. Early surgical consultation for biopsy and to assess the need for debridement is mandatory.

J. S. Doggett (✉) · B. Wong
Division of Infectious Disease, Oregon Health and Science University, Portland, OR, USA
e-mail: doggettj@ohsu.edu

© Springer Nature Switzerland AG 2021
L. Loriaux, C. Vanek (eds.), *Endocrine Emergencies*, Contemporary Endocrinology,
https://doi.org/10.1007/978-3-030-67455-7_5

Malignant (Necrotizing) Otitis Externa

Malignant or necrotizing otitis externa is a rare, invasive infection that begins in the external ear canal and spreads to the adjacent tissue. Severe infection may extend to the base of the skull or intracranially. Medical knowledge of malignant otitis externa is primarily derived from retrospective case series. The majority of reported patients are elderly diabetics infected with *Pseudomonas aeruginosa*. Patients typically present with otalgia and otorrhea with little evidence of systemic illness. Diagnosis is based on clinical presentation, radiographic imaging with CT or MRI, and tissue histology and culture. Treatment requires prolonged systemic antibiotics, and surgery is not required for cure in most cases. Mortality for malignant otitis externa has improved since the disease was first characterized, but a significant number of patients have recurrent disease and require multiple courses of antibiotics. Clinicians should suspect malignant otitis externa in diabetic patients who present with symptoms of otitis externa.

Diabetic Susceptibility

Chandler coined the term "malignant external otitis" in 1968 when he described a series of 13 patients with severe invasive pseudomonal infection originating from the external ear canal [1]. Chandler's series, as well as a review of 262 cases 20 years later, found that 86–100% of patients had diabetes [2]. However, recent series have described greater variation in rates of diabetes (51–100%) as the number of malignant otitis externa patients with other immunosuppressive disorders, such as chronic prednisone use, AIDS, and hematologic malignancy has increased [3–5]. The majority of patients with diabetes are typically close to 70 years old, and poor glycemic control does not appear to be associated with malignant otitis externa [2]. This has led to speculation that increased susceptibility to invasive infection in diabetics is primarily due to diabetic microvascular disease.

Pathogenesis

Trauma and increased moisture in the external ear canal are thought to contribute to infection. Hearing aids and irrigation for cerumen disimpaction have been proposed as sources of trauma or increased moisture [6]. Moist conditions provide a favorable environment for *Pseudomonas aeruginosa*, a gram-negative aerobic bacterium that can colonize moist surfaces. Once infection crosses the epithelial surface of the ear canal, it may spread through various paths. Infection typically begins at the osseous-cartilaginous junction and spreads anteriorly-inferiorly through the fissures of Santorini to the mastoid and toward the parotid gland. It may also spread anteriorly to the temporomandibular joint or medially to the petrous apex of the temporal bone and the jugular foramen [7]. Rarely, infection may spread intracranially causing meningitis or abscess.

Pseudomonas aeruginosa is the most common pathogen and in early series made up close to 100% of cases [1, 2]. In recent series, *Pseudomonas* remains the most common pathogen but makes up a smaller percentage of cultures (27–69%) [3, 4, 7–10]. *Klebsiella* sp. and *Staphylococcus aureus* have been found in up to 20% of cultures in several recent studies. *Aspergillus* sp. and *Candida* sp. occur less frequently, but a small percentage have been seen in diabetics across multiple studies. A significant percentage of patients receive antibiotics prior to diagnosis, which results in negative cultures.

Clinical Presentation

Malignant otitis externa is typically a subacute progressive infection, and patients often present after several weeks of symptoms, though prodromes of several days are reported. Malignant otitis externa may be difficult to differentiate from otitis externa or otitis media, but the pain is often severe in malignant otitis externa. The most common symptoms, otalgia and otorrhea, are present in approximately 90% and 75% of cases, respectively. Pain is often worse at night, and severe pain should raise suspicion for deep infection. Pain may include headache or temporomandibular joint pain with palpation or mastication. Erythema or swelling of the external ear and canal may be present. However, many patients present after receiving empiric oral antibiotics for external otitis or otitis media and may not have visible signs of infection. Conductive hearing loss is often present secondary to soft tissue blocking the external canal.

Systemic signs of infection such as fever or altered mentation are uncommon. Granulation tissue on the floor of the external ear canal at the osseo-cartilaginous junction is found in over half of patients. The tympanic membrane and middle ear are typically spared. Twenty to forty percent of patients have cranial nerve palsies. The facial nerve is most frequently involved due to its proximity to the ear canal, but the glossopharyngeal, vagus, and spinal accessory nerve may be affected if infection spreads to the jugular foramen, causing dysphagia, dysphonia, or diminished shoulder elevation. Rarely, the trigeminal and abducens nerve may be affected when infection spreads to the petrous apex of the temporal bone. Laboratory values are frequently normal with the exception of elevations in erythrocyte sedimentation rate or C-reactive protein [3, 5].

Diagnosis

The diagnosis of malignant otitis externa should be suspected in older diabetic patients who present with otalgia. Diagnostic imaging with CT or MRI should be obtained if there is severe pain, granulation tissue, cranial nerve palsy, or failure to respond to therapy for otitis externa (Fig. 5.1). The diagnosis of malignant external otitis is based on imaging, tissue pathology, and culture. Carcinoma of the ear canal can have similar clinical and radiologic findings, and biopsy is required to distinguish infection from malignancy [5]. Various nuclear medicine studies have been used previously but are problematic for initial diagnosis because they lack sensitivity, specificity, and resolution, compared to CT and MRI. CT and MRI both have advantages as initial radiologic studies. CT is better than MRI at detecting early cortical bone erosion. However, MRI is better at detecting dural enhancement and changes in the medullary space of bones [7]. Overall, MRI is superior in fully defining the extent of infection in difficult cases [11]. As is the case with all forms of osteomyelitis, CT and MRI do not provide a reliable means for determining cure of infection and duration of treatment. However, response to therapy is supported by normalization of soft tissue and lack of further spread [6].

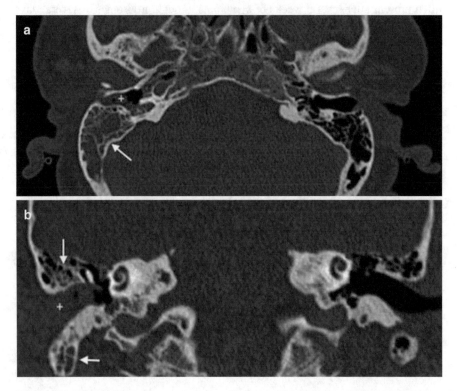

Fig. 5.1 Maxillofacial CT bone images of right-sided malignant otitis externa. Axial (**a**) and coronal (**b**) images show opacification of the right mastoid air cells (*arrows*) and occlusion of the right external auditory canal (+) with minimal involvement of the middle ear

Treatment

Malignant otitis externa is best treated with antimicrobial therapy based on tissue culture results. Prior series have demonstrated successful therapy with ciprofloxacin in treating *Pseudomonas* infection, and in some instances, ciprofloxacin has been used empirically. However, it is important to consider the diversity of pathogens in recent series and the emergence of fluoroquinolone-resistant *Pseudomonas* [4, 12]. These factors make tissue biopsy of greater importance and the choice of empiric antibiotic therapy more complex. After biopsy is obtained, or if the patient presents with severe infection, empiric therapy should be initiated with an agent that has antipseudomonal and anti-staphylococcal activity such as cefepime, piperacillin-tazobactam, or a carbapenem. When attempts to culture the pathogen are unsuccessful, empiric antibiotics should be continued, and the patient's response to therapy should be followed closely. If a pathogen is cultured, then antibiotics should be chosen according to the antimicrobial susceptibilities. In cases of ciprofloxacin-sensitive *Pseudomonas*, oral ciprofloxacin may be used for the full course of therapy. However, the development of resistance to ciprofloxacin during treatment has been reported [12]. The optimal duration of therapy is unknown, but given the high relapse rate when short courses of antibiotics have been used, the majority of patients should receive at least 6 weeks of culture-guided antibiotics. Topical antibiotics provide no benefit. In the case of *Aspergillus*, the majority of clinical experience in malignant otitis externa is with amphotericin B. However, voriconazole is a newer, orally available drug that is a promising alternative to amphotericin B. Voriconazole has been shown to be superior to amphotericin B in invasive pulmonary aspergillosis, is orally available, and has been used successfully in *Aspergillus* osteomyelitis and malignant otitis externa [13, 14].

Surgical debridement was once standard in all cases but is now reserved for cases in which there are abscesses or there is a need for debridement of granulation tissue or bony sequestration [1, 3]. Response to therapy should be monitored based on normalization of ESR or CRP and resolution of symptoms, appreciating that pain and cranial nerve palsies may resolve slowly. In many cases, cranial nerve palsies may not resolve or only recover partially [4].

Opinions regarding the use of imaging to evaluate response to therapy and resolution vary. Some authors suggest using nuclear medicine scans for diagnosis and monitoring response to therapy, while others use CT or MRI. Some authors use gallium 67 isotope scans to determine cure of infection, but cases of recurrence after normal gallium 67 scans have been reported [4, 6, 15]. The other approach commonly used is to follow clinical response combined with ESR or CRP to determine response to treatment. CT or MRI is then repeated several weeks after completion of 4–6 weeks of antibiotics as a baseline study, in case there are later concerns for recurrence [3, 6, 11, 16]. None of these approaches have been validated in controlled studies of malignant otitis externa, but the latter approach is similar to the general management of osteomyelitis. In cases where the pathogen is not identified and the patient is receiving empiric therapy, then imaging should be repeated during antimicrobial therapy to evaluate the initial response with the understanding that bony changes may not show improvement but soft tissue findings should be stable if not improved [11]. Tissue biopsy should be repeated if infection progresses despite treatment.

Prognosis

The mortality from malignant otitis externa has improved from 46% in Chandler's series in 1968 to 0–24% in more recent series [2, 3, 5, 8]. Improvements in mortality are likely related to better diagnostic imaging that allows earlier detection and improved antipseudomonal antibiotics, particularly ciprofloxacin. Despite improvements in treatment, recurrent infection remains an active concern in managing malignant otitis externa, with 15% to 20% of patients developing recurrent infection after completing antibiotics [3]. With this in mind, patients should be monitored after completion of therapy for recurrent symptoms.

Summary

Malignant otitis externa is a potentially devastating infection. Timely diagnosis requires a high degree of clinical suspicion when assessing diabetic patients with otalgia or with symptoms of persistent otitis. Diagnostic imaging with CT or MRI is required to detect invasive infection and to determine the extent of infection. Tissue biopsy for diagnosis and to guide therapy is imperative. Prolonged courses of antibiotics are required to cure infection. There are varying approaches to following response to therapy with imaging, but measuring ESR or CRP during therapy and monitoring patients after the completion of antibiotics are key elements of management. Outcomes of malignant otitis externa have improved, but the increasing frequency of drug-resistant bacteria could compromise successful treatment:

- Malignant otitis externa is an invasive infection of soft tissue and bone that begins in the external ear canal.
- Diagnosis is made by CT or magnetic resonance imaging (MRI).
- Treatment of malignant otitis externa consists of prolonged antibiotics that are based on tissue culture. In the case of negative culture, empiric antibiotics should include agents active against *Pseudomonas*.

References

1. Chandler JR. Malignant external otitis. Laryngoscope. 1968;78(8):1257–94.
2. Rubin J, Yu VL. Malignant external otitis: insights into pathogenesis, clinical manifestations, diagnosis, and therapy. Am J Med. 1988;85(3):391–8.

3. Ali T, Meade K, Anari S, ElBadawey MR, Zammit-Maempel I. Malignant otitis externa: case series. J Laryngol Otol. 2010;124(8):846–51.
4. Franco-Vidal V, Blanchet H, Bebear C, Dutronc H, Darrouzet V. Necrotizing external otitis: a report of 46 cases. Otol Neurotol. 2007;28(6):771–3.
5. Carfrae MJ, Kesser BW. Malignant otitis externa. Otolaryngol Clin N Am. 2008;41(3):537–549, viii–ix.
6. Rubin Grandis J, Branstetter BFT, Yu VL. The changing face of malignant (necrotising) external otitis: clinical, radiological, and anatomic correlations. Lancet Infect Dis. 2004;4(1):34–9.
7. Lee JE, Song JJ, Oh SH, Chang SO, Kim CH, Lee JH. Prognostic value of extension patterns on follow-up magnetic resonance imaging in patients with necrotizing otitis externa. Arch Otolaryngol Head Neck Surg. 2011;137(7):688–93.
8. Chen CN, Chen YS, Yeh TH, Hsu CJ, Tseng FY. Outcomes of malignant external otitis: survival vs mortality. Acta Otolaryngol. 2010;130(1):89–94.
9. Soudry E, Hamzany Y, Preis M, Joshua B, Hadar T, Nageris BI. Malignant external otitis: analysis of severe cases. Otolaryngol Head Neck Surg. 2011;144(5):758–62.
10. Hariga I, Mardassi A, Belhaj Younes F, et al. Necrotizing otitis externa: 19 cases' report. Eur Arch Otorhinolaryngol. 2010;267(8):1193–8.
11. Mehrotra P, Elbadawey MR, Zammit-Maempel I. Spectrum of radiological appearances of necrotising external otitis: a pictorial review. J Laryngol Otol. 2011;125(11):1109–15.
12. Carlton DA, Perez EE, Smouha EE. Malignant external otitis: the shifting treatment paradigm. Am J Otolaryngol. 2018;39(1):41–5.
13. Walsh TJ, Anaissie EJ, Denning DW, et al. Treatment of aspergillosis: clinical practice guidelines of the Infectious Diseases Society of America. Clin Infect Dis. 2008;46(3):327–60.
14. Hamzany Y, Soudry E, Preis M, et al. Fungal malignant external otitis. J Infect. 2011;62(3):226–31.
15. Amorosa L, Modugno GC, Pirodda A. Malignant external otitis: review and personal experience. Acta Otolaryngol Suppl. 1996;521:3–16.
16. Omran AA, El Garem HF, Al Alem RK. Recurrent malignant otitis externa: management and outcome. Eur Arch Otorhinolaryngol. 2011;269:807.

Chapter 6
Mucormycosis

J. Stone Doggett and Brian Wong

Précis

Mucormycosis:

1. Clinical setting: The diabetic patient usually has a history of moderate to poor control. A recent history of ketoacidosis is often present. The patient usually complains of rhinorrhea, headache, facial swelling, and pain.
2. Diagnosis: Diabetic patients presenting with the complaint of sinusitis associated with facial swelling, decreased vision, ophthalmoplegia, and other cranial nerve palsies associated with signs of infection that include necrosis and/or a black eschar in the nasal cavity or on the palate should prompt an urgent evaluation for mucormycosis:

   (a) Laboratory tests: The diagnosis of mucormycosis depends upon the demonstration of fungal elements in tissues. If the disease is suspected, urgent endoscopic sinus examination and biopsy are mandatory.
   (b) Imaging: The extent of disease should be determined by CT or MRI.

3. Treatment: Prompt and aggressive surgical debridement is essential. This should be associated with the administration of amphotericin B. The lipid formulations are currently preferred because they are less nephrotoxic. The standard initial dose is 5 mg/kg/day given intravenously over a 2-hour infusion at 2.5 mg/kg/hour. The dose and form of the amphotericin will be adjusted to optimize treatment as culture results become available.

J. S. Doggett (✉) · B. Wong
Division of Infectious Disease, Oregon Health and Science University, Portland, OR, USA
e-mail: doggettj@ohsu.edu

© Springer Nature Switzerland AG 2021   51
L. Loriaux, C. Vanek (eds.), *Endocrine Emergencies*, Contemporary Endocrinology,
https://doi.org/10.1007/978-3-030-67455-7_6

Mucormycosis

Most severe infections that disproportionately affect diabetics are caused by common bacterial pathogens. The fungal species in the order *Mucorales* that cause invasive mucormycosis are an exception. Mucormycosis is a rare infection that often starts in the sinuses of diabetics and may invade the orbit or cerebral structures leading to disfiguring or fatal outcomes. Early diagnosis and treatment are the primary means to limit the morbidity and mortality caused by mucormycosis.

Diabetic Susceptibility

Since the initial description of mucormycosis in 1885, diabetics have made up the largest percentage of patients described in reported cases and case series, but this distribution may be changing. In an extensive literature review of 929 cases and a systematic review of cases from 2000 to 2017, diabetes was the underlying condition in 36% and 40% of patients, respectively [1, 2]. Alternatively, mucormycosis also occurs in patients with immunosuppression due to bone marrow transplant, solid organ transplant, or hematologic malignancy. A prospective study of 230 European cases found that hematologic malignancy was the underlying condition in 41% of mucormycosis cases and diabetes was present in 9% of cases from 2005 to 2007 [3]. Mucormycosis also occurs in patients who receive iron chelation with deferoxamine, in injection drug users, and rarely in patients without an identifiable underlying condition.

Sinus-related infection that may involve the orbit or cerebral structures comprises two-thirds of reported cases in diabetics [1]. Rarely, diabetics may develop pulmonary or cutaneous infection. This differs from individuals with hematologic malignancy or transplant, who are more likely to have pulmonary infection, or immunocompetent patients, who most often develop cutaneous infection. In nondiabetic patients, mucormycosis may primarily involve the kidneys or gastrointestinal tract. Mucormycosis occurs in type 1 and type 2 diabetics. Diabetic ketoacidosis and poor glycemic control are frequently documented [4]. However, mucormycosis may also be the initial presentation of diabetes. Unlike other susceptible populations, it is very uncommon for diabetics to develop disseminated mucormycosis. Mucormycosis may present at any age, but average ages of 57 and 39 years have been described in an analysis of incidence based on hospital diagnostic codes and from literature review, respectively [1, 5].

Increased susceptibility to mucormycosis in diabetics is thought to be due to microvascular disease, impaired neutrophil function, and the increased availability of iron. The fungi that cause mucormycosis rely on iron chelators and iron permeases to obtain iron from the host. Diabetic ketoacidosis decreases the capacity of transferrin to bind iron, which increases the amount of iron that is available to fungi. Experiments have shown that *Rhizopus oryzae* growth is enhanced in the sera of patients with diabetic ketoacidosis. Similarly, growth is enhanced in nondiabetic sera when it is supplemented with iron and the pH is less than 7.4 [6]. The importance of iron is also supported by experiments that show reductions in expression of the high-affinity iron permease gene led to reduction in the virulence of *Rhizopus oryzae* in mice with diabetic ketoacidosis [7].

Pathogenesis and Microbiology

There are multiple pathogenic genera of the order *Mucorales* that cause mucormycosis. The most commonly reported are *Rhizopus*, *Mucor*, *Cunninghamella*, *Apophysomyces*, and *Absidia* [1]. *Rhizopus* species are the most frequent causes of sinus-related disease, whereas *Cunninghamella* is more often found in pulmonary disease [1]. These organisms are readily found in the soil and on decaying plant matter. Spores may be inhaled or introduced through skin trauma. Humans are frequently exposed to these fungi but very rarely develop infection. Calculations of incidence have varied from 0.43 to 1.7 cases per 1,000,000 people [5]. Although a significant percentage of cases have been reported in patients with no underlying immunocompromising condition, the majority of these reports were of cutaneous infection due to trauma. In diabetics, ketoacidosis contributes to susceptibility to infection by altering cellular immunity [8]. Once infection begins in the nasal turbinates or in alveoli, fungal hyphae invade vasculature causing thrombosis and tissue infarction. Invasive sinus infection then may spread to the face, to the orbit, or to the cerebrum. Intracranial extension may cause cavernous or sagittal sinus thrombosis and epidural and subdural abscesses, but meningitis is very rare.

Clinical Presentation

After mucormycosis develops in the nasal passages or sinuses, it usually progresses rapidly and often is advanced before infection is detected. Patients may present with rhinosinusitis, facial swelling, or erythema or with orbital or cerebral involvement (Figs. 6.1 and 6.2). Despite the severity of disease, patients may have minimal evidence of infection. In a literature review of 114 patients with sinus-related mucormycosis, there were few consistent overt clinical findings within the first 72 hours of presentation: fever (44%), nasal ulceration or necrosis (38%), periorbital or facial swelling (34%), decreased vision (30%), ophthalmoplegia (29%), sinusitis (26%), headache (25%), facial pain (22%), decreased mental status (22%), and increased white blood cell count (19%) [9]. Evidence of invasive disease includes necrosis or eschar of the nasal cavity, face, or palate, trigeminal or facial nerve palsies, diplopia, ophthalmoplegia, periorbital edema, proptosis, loss of vision, or decreased level of consciousness. These findings in a diabetic patient with poor glycemic control should prompt an urgent evaluation for mucormycosis.

Fig. 6.1 A 49-year-old man with diabetic ketoacidosis had rhino-orbital-cerebral mucormycosis, which was characterized by left-sided facial swelling and erythema, left-sided ophthalmoplegia, and left-sided facial numbness

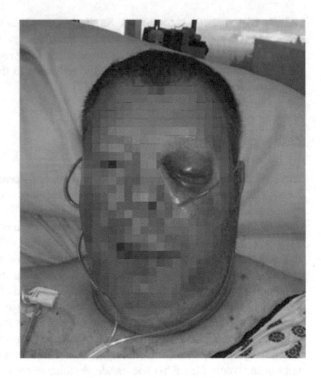

Diagnosis

Diagnosing mucormycosis before extensive tissue destruction occurs requires a high degree of suspicion. Physicians should consider this diagnosis in patients with diabetic ketoacidosis and the abovementioned features. However, it is noteworthy that mucormycosis occurs in diabetics without acidosis. The diagnosis of sinus-related mucormycosis relies on identification of fungal elements in the tissue. The fungal serum assays, 1,3-beta-D-glucan, and *Aspergillus* galactomannan do not detect mucormycosis. Early identification may be achieved by performing a potassium hydroxide (KOH) preparation and microscopy on tissue scrapings of mucosal ulcers. If mucormycosis is suspected, the diagnosis should be pursued through urgent endoscopic sinus examination and tissue biopsy. The characteristic histologic appearance of mucormycosis is broad hyphae that do not have septae and branch at right angles (Fig. 6.3). Tissue should be cultured for definitive identification, but culture may not be successful, and the diagnosis may rely on histology. The extent of disease should be determined with CT or MRI.

Treatment

The treatment of mucormycosis requires prompt aggressive surgical debridement and treatment with amphotericin B deoxycholate or with a lipid formulation of amphotericin B [9, 10]. Although there are few studies that compare amphotericin

Fig. 6.2 Axial T1 MRI images of the patient in Figure 6.1 (**a**) shows low signal edema in the premaxillary soft tissues, extending laterally (arrow) and near-complete opacification of the left maxillary sinus (+), and (**b**) left periorbital soft tissue thickening (arrow) as well as left orbital proptosis

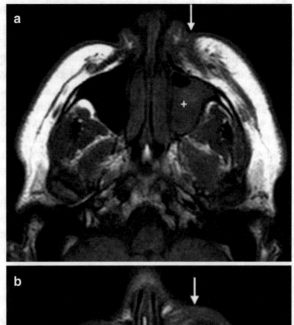

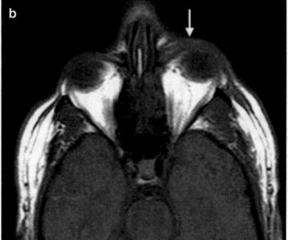

Fig. 6.3 Periodic acid-Schiff stain of mucormycosis at 400x that shows broad nonseptate hyphae that branch at right angles

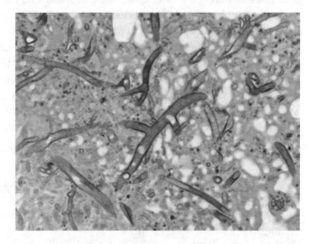

B deoxycholate to lipid preparations of amphotericin B, the majority of practitioners with access to lipid preparations prefer to use them out of concern for renal toxicity. Posaconazole and isavuconazole are antifungal agents that have been shown to be clinically effective in a retrospective study of salvage therapy and a non-randomized, open-label, single-arm study, respectively [11, 12]. These agents may be used in patients who fail or do not tolerate amphotericin B and as step-down therapy following amphotericin B. Echinocandins are sometimes used in combination with lipid preparations of amphotericin B based on improved outcomes in a retrospective study that compared 6 patients who received caspofungin in addition to amphotericin B lipid complex (5/6) or liposomal amphotericin B (1/6) to 31 patients who received amphotericin B or lipid formulations of amphotericin B alone [13]. Further studies are necessary to demonstrate the utility of adjunctive echinocandin therapy before its use can be routinely recommended. Timely intervention is essential and has been shown to decrease mortality and morbidity [9, 10, 14]. Acidosis, hyperglycemia, and immunosuppression should be corrected. Surgery is often disfiguring and multiple surgeries may be required.

Mortality

Despite improvements in the diagnosis and management of mucormycosis, overall mortality remains high at 47% [1, 3]. Although still high, mortality in diabetics is closer to 23% [9]. This is likely due to less severe immunosuppression conferred by diabetes and the greater percentage of sinus-related mucormycosis among diabetics.

Summary

Mucormycosis is a devastating infection in diabetics that has high mortality and requires prolonged treatment with amphotericin B and surgery. The majority of mucormycosis in diabetics is sinus-related disease that may spread to contiguous structures including the face, orbit, and cerebrum. Early diagnosis of mucormycosis is challenging because patients often present with subtle findings. Clinicians should have a high degree of suspicion in patients who present with diabetic ketoacidosis or poorly controlled diabetes and have findings suggestive of disease that involves the sinus, eyes, face, cranial nerves, or altered mental status. Diagnosis is made from tissue scrapings of lesions, tissue biopsy, endoscopic examination, fungal culture, and characteristic tissue histology. Tissue culture is definitive, but often does not grow. Urgent intervention with antibiotics and surgery improves clinical outcomes, but despite appropriate therapy, a significant number of patients will die or be disfigured:

- Mucormycosis, in diabetics, typically involves the sinuses and may spread to the orbit or brain.
- Diagnosis is made by demonstrating fungal elements of one of the *Mucorales* fungi on tissue scraping or tissue biopsy.
- Treatment of mucormycosis consists of aggressive surgical debridement and amphotericin B.

References

1. Roden MM, Zaoutis TE, Buchanan WL, et al. Epidemiology and outcome of zygomycosis: a review of 929 reported cases. Clin Infect Dis. 2005;41(5):634–53.
2. Jeong W, Keighley C, Wolfe R, et al. The epidemiology and clinical manifestations of mucormycosis: a systematic review and meta-analysis of case reports. Clin Microbiol Infect. 2019;25(1):26–34.
3. Skiada A, Pagano L, Groll A, et al. Zygomycosis in Europe: analysis of 230 cases accrued by the registry of the European Confederation of Medical Mycology (ECMM) Working Group on Zygomycosis between 2005 and 2007. Clin Microbiol Infect. 2011;17(12):1859–67.
4. Chakrabarti A, Das A, Mandal J, et al. The rising trend of invasive zygomycosis in patients with uncontrolled diabetes mellitus. Med Mycol. 2006;44(4):335–42.
5. Bitar D, Van Cauteren D, Lanternier F, et al. Increasing incidence of zygomycosis (mucormycosis), France, 1997-2006. Emerg Infect Dis. 2009;15(9):1395–401.
6. Kontoyiannis DP, Lewis RE, editors. Agents of Mucormycosis and Entomophthoramycosis. 7th ed. Philadelphia: Churchill Livingstone Elsevier; 2010. Mandell, Douglas, and Bennett's principles and practice of infectious diseases; No. 2
7. Ibrahim AS, Gebremariam T, Lin L, et al. The high affinity iron permease is a key virulence factor required for Rhizopus oryzae pathogenesis. Mol Microbiol. 2010;77(3):587–604.
8. Speert DP, Silva J Jr. Abnormalities of in vitro lymphocyte response to mitogens in diabetic children during acute ketoacidosis. Am J Dis Child. 1978;132(10):1014–7.
9. Yohai RA, Bullock JD, Aziz AA, Markert RJ. Survival factors in rhino-orbital-cerebral mucormycosis. Surv Ophthalmol. 1994;39(1):3–22.
10. Sun HY, Singh N. Mucormycosis: its contemporary face and management strategies. Lancet Infect Dis. 2011;11(4):301–11.
11. van Burik JA, Hare RS, Solomon HF, Corrado ML, Kontoyiannis DP. Posaconazole is effective as salvage therapy in zygomycosis: a retrospective summary of 91 cases. Clin Infect Dis. 2006;42(7):e61–5.
12. Marty FM, Ostrosky-Zeichner L, Cornely OA, et al. Isavuconazole treatment for mucormycosis: a single-arm open-label trial and case-control analysis. Lancet Infect Dis. 2016;16(7):828–37.
13. Reed C, Bryant R, Ibrahim AS, et al. Combination polyene-caspofungin treatment of rhino-orbital-cerebral mucormycosis. Clin Infect Dis. 2008;47(3):364–71.
14. Chamilos G, Lewis RE, Kontoyiannis DP. Delaying amphotericin B-based frontline therapy significantly increases mortality among patients with hematologic malignancy who have zygomycosis. Clin Infect Dis. 2008;47(4):503–9.

Chapter 7
Emphysematous Cholecystitis

J. Stone Doggett and Brian Wong

Précis

Emphysematous cholecystitis:

1. Clinical setting: The clinical picture of cholecystitis in a diabetic patient is usually a male over 50 years of age. Two-thirds of the patients have gallstones compared to 90% in typical cholecystitis. Crepitus of the abdominal wall over the gallbladder can occur. The most common symptoms are right upper quadrant pain, nausea, and vomiting. Fever is the rule.
2. Diagnosis: All diabetic patients with a problematic or confirmed diagnosis of cholecystitis must be suspected of having emphysematous disease:

    (a) History: The severity of the diabetes, history of control, and presence or absence of diabetic complications do not influence the probability of this condition in a diabetic patient.
    (b) Imaging: The diagnosis of emphysematous cholecystitis is made radiographically or at the time of surgery. Gas in the gallbladder wall, lumen, or pericholecystic space can be seen on plain film and ultrasonography. CT, however, is the test of choice in this setting.

3. Management: The recommended approach is parenteral antibiotics with surgical intervention within 48–72 hours.

    Empiric antibiotic therapy includes regimens for complicated acute cholecystitis such as piperacillin-tazobactam or cefepime plus metronidazole.

J. S. Doggett (✉) · B. Wong
Division of Infectious Disease, Oregon Health and Science University, Portland, OR, USA
e-mail: doggettj@ohsu.edu

© Springer Nature Switzerland AG 2021   59
L. Loriaux, C. Vanek (eds.), *Endocrine Emergencies*, Contemporary Endocrinology,
https://doi.org/10.1007/978-3-030-67455-7_7

Emphysematous Cholecystitis

Emphysematous cholecystitis is a rare, severe form of acute cholecystitis in which infection leads to gas formation in the gallbladder wall or pericholecystic space. The risk of gallbladder perforation in emphysematous cholecystitis is up to five times that of ordinary acute cholecystitis [1]. Timely recognition and treatment are crucial, and clinicians should be aware that ultrasound may fail to detect gas formation. Patients who develop emphysematous cholecystitis differ from typical cholecystitis patients as well: 38–50% are diabetics, males outnumber females 2:1, and the majority are 50 to 70 years old [2, 3]. It is thought that these patients have vascular disease and that the distinct characteristics of emphysematous cholecystitis result from vascular occlusion and ischemia.

Pathogenesis and Microbiology

The bacterial pathogens and gallbladder pathology found in emphysematous cholecystitis differ from typical cholecystitis. Gallstones are found in 40–70% of patients with emphysematous cholecystitis, as opposed to 90% of typical cholecystitis cases. The anaerobic bacterium *Clostridium perfringens* is the most frequently reported pathogen [1–4]. In a review of 109 cases, *Clostridium* species made up of 46% of positive cultures and *E. coli* which was present in 33%, often with *Clostridia, Klebsiella, Bacteroides, Staphylococcus, Streptococcus, Pseudomonas*, and *Salmonella*, have also been reported [1–4]. Examinations of gallbladder pathology frequently reveal occlusion of the cystic artery or pericholecystic abscess [1, 5].

Clinical Presentation

The clinical presentation of emphysematous cholecystitis is very similar to typical acute cholecystitis. However, crepitus in the abdominal wall over the gallbladder may rarely be detected and should raise suspicion for emphysematous infection. Otherwise, patients typically complain of right upper quadrant pain and fever. Half of patients report nausea and vomiting.

Diagnosis

The diagnosis of emphysematous cholecystitis is made at the time of surgery. The first preoperative diagnosis of emphysematous cholecystitis was made in 1931. This led to recognition of emphysematous cholecystitis as a distinct clinical entity [2]. The gallbladder lumen and pericholecystic space may be seen on plain films, ultrasound, or CT (Figs. 7.1 and 7.2). CT is the most sensitive and specific imaging modality. Ultrasonography can demonstrate highly echogenic reflections with

Fig. 7.1 Noncontrast axial CT image demonstrating a thick-walled gallbladder prolapsing into a large abdominal wall hernia. There is pericholecystic inflammation and three small locules of gas in the wall

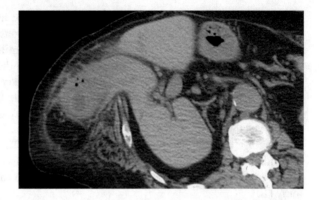

Fig. 7.2 Abdominal radiograph demonstrating mottled gas outlining the wall of the gallbladder as well as lucency within the gallbladder lumen also representing gas

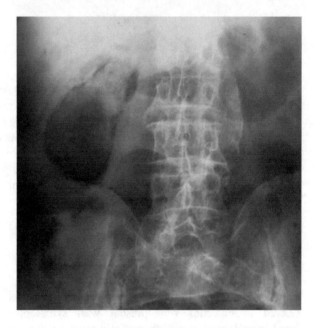

posterior shadowing and reverberation artifacts. The "champagne" sign shows bubbles rising up from the dependent portions of the gallbladder lumen, often misinterpreted as bowel gas [6–8]. Inability to visualize the gallbladder with ultrasound is an indication for CT scan.

Treatment

Traditionally, the recommended approach uses parenteral antibiotics and surgical intervention within 48 to 72 hours. Emphysematous cholecystitis can progress rapidly, as illustrated in the report of a patient who developed radiographic findings of emphysematous cholecystitis within 24 hours after a normal CT [9]. This is consistent with older reports of patients with gangrene and perforation who presented with fewer than 72 hours of symptoms [1]. In contrast, some authors argue that the use of CT has led to increased detection of a milder spectrum of disease. These authors report several patients who did well after delaying surgical intervention for 2–4 weeks, suggesting that delayed surgical intervention has a role in the management of emphysematous cholecystitis [7]. While there may be a subset of patients that do not require urgent surgery, the majority of the literature supports cholecystectomy within 48 to 72 hours. When surgery is contraindicated, percutaneous drainage with cholecystostomy tubes can be used. There is limited literature to determine whether open or laparoscopic cholecystectomy is superior. However, a recent small series has shown equivalent results with laparoscopic cholecystectomy [10].

Prognosis

Heightened awareness and timely diagnosis of emphysematous cholecystitis are important because of the need for urgent surgical evaluation. The mortality of emphysematous cholecystitis was 15% compared to 4% of acute cholecystitis in a large series in 1975 [1]. A more recent series in 1999 found a mortality rate of 25% in emphysematous cholecystitis [4]. Increased mortality is related to higher rates of perforation or complicated infection. In a review of 20 patients with emphysematous cholecystitis, seven patients had gallbladder perforation, nine had pericholecystic abscess, and three had bile peritonitis [4].

Summary

Emphysematous cholecystitis is a distinct form of cholecystitis that should be considered in diabetics who present with symptoms of typical cholecystitis. Emphysematous cholecystitis carries a greater risk of complication. The increased rates of complications are thought to be related to vascular occlusion and gallbladder ischemia. Treatment consists of parenteral antibiotics and cholecystectomy within 48 to 72 hours:

- Emphysematous cholecystitis may progress more quickly than typical cholecystitis and has higher rates of complication.
- CT is the preferred diagnostic test for emphysematous cholecystitis.
- Treatment of emphysematous cholecystitis consists of parenteral antibiotics and cholecystectomy within 48–72 hours.

References

1. Mentzer RM Jr, Golden GT, Chandler JG, Horsley JS 3rd. A comparative appraisal of emphysematous cholecystitis. Am J Surg. 1975;129(1):10–5.
2. Sarmiento RV. Emphysematous cholecystitis. Report of four cases and review of the literature. Arch Surg. 1966;93(6):1009–14.
3. Moanna A, Bajaj R, del Rio C. Emphysematous cholecystitis due to Salmonella derby. Lancet Infect Dis. 2006;6(2):118–20.
4. Garcia-Sancho Tellez L, Rodriguez-Montes JA. Fernandez de Lis S, Garcia-Sancho Martin L. Acute emphysematous cholecystitis. Report of twenty cases. Hepato-Gastroenterology. 1999;46(28):2144–8.
5. Edinburgh A, Geffen A. Acute emphysematous cholecystitis; a case report and review of the world literature. Am J Surg. 1958;96(1):66–75.
6. Grayson DE, Abbott RM, Levy AD, Sherman PM. Emphysematous infections of the abdomen and pelvis: a pictorial review. Radiographics. 2002;22(3):543–61.
7. Gill KS, Chapman AH, Weston MJ. The changing face of emphysematous cholecystitis. Br J Radiol. 1997;70(838):986–91.
8. Sunnapwar A, Raut AA, Nagar AM, Katre R. Emphysematous cholecystitis: imaging findings in nine patients. Indian J Radiol Imaging. 2011;21(2):142–6.
9. Seow VK, Lin CM, Wang TL, Chong CF, Lin IY. Acute emphysematous cholecystitis with initial normal radiological evaluation: a fatal diagnostic pitfall in the ED. Am J Emerg Med. 2007;25(4):488 e483-485.
10. Hazey JW, Brody FJ, Rosenblatt SM, Brodsky J, Malm J, Ponsky JL. Laparoscopic management and clinical outcome of emphysematous cholecystitis. Surg Endosc. 2001;15(10):1217–20.

Chapter 8
Emphysematous Pyelonephritis

J. Stone Doggett and Brian Wong

Précis

Emphysematous pyelonephritis:

1. Clinical setting: The typical picture is fever, flank or abdominal pain, nausea, and vomiting in a patient with diabetes. The commonest pathogens are *E. coli* (67%) and *Klebsiella* sp. (20%).
2. Diagnosis: All diabetic patients with the probable or confirmed diagnosis of pyelonephritis must be suspected of having emphysematous disease:

   (a) History: The severity of diabetes complications, the degree of control, and the duration of diabetes do not exclude the possibility of emphysematous disease.
   (b) Imaging: Emphysematous pyelonephritis is diagnosed by abdominal CT or MRI. Abdominal CT is the test of choice. Detection of gas in the parenchyma, collecting system, or perirenal space confirms the diagnosis.

3. Management: Initial management consists of prompt antibiotic treatment that will cover the multitude of organisms that are associated with emphysematous pyelonephritis. Second, a surgical consultation is essential. Some patients recover without surgical drainage or nephrectomy, but most do not. Surgical intervention is very likely, and it should be early rather than late.

   Empiric antibiotics for emphysematous pyelonephritis are the same as for severe pyelonephritis. A common regimen is piperacillin-tazobactam. The choice of antibiotic should be guided by local patterns of antimicrobial resistance, the patient's previous antibiotic exposure, and risk for drug-resistant bacteria.

J. S. Doggett (✉) · B. Wong
Division of Infectious Disease, Oregon Health and Science University, Portland, OR, USA
e-mail: doggettj@ohsu.edu

© Springer Nature Switzerland AG 2021
L. Loriaux, C. Vanek (eds.), *Endocrine Emergencies*, Contemporary Endocrinology,
https://doi.org/10.1007/978-3-030-67455-7_8

Antibiotic therapy should be modified based on urine and blood cultures. Drainage should be assessed with CT imaging; multiple drainage procedures can be required. Patients who fail to respond should undergo nephrectomy.

Infectious Emergencies in Diabetics

Emphysematous Pyelonephritis

Emphysematous pyelonephritis is a rare form of pyelonephritis that occurs more commonly in diabetics than in nondiabetics and requires urgent surgical intervention with percutaneous drainage or nephrectomy. This severe infection occurs predominantly in diabetics and other individuals with urinary obstruction due to strictures, calculi, or neoplasm. The underlying pathology that puts diabetic patients at increased risk for emphysematous infection is not known.

Diabetic women have an increased prevalence of bacteriuria and urinary tract infections compared to nondiabetic women. The prevalence of bacteriuria in diabetic women is 9–27% and increases with duration of diabetes; it is not related to glycemic control [1]. Although diabetic women with asymptomatic bacteriuria are not more likely to progress to urinary tract infection than those without bacteriuria, diabetic patients are diagnosed with urinary tract infections more frequently than nondiabetic patients [2]. Two large studies have found that diabetics had increased rates of urinary tract infections. In a prospective cohort of 7417 patients with type 1 and type 2 diabetes, the adjusted odds ratio for infection were 1.96 and 1.24, respectively [3]. Similarly, a retrospective cohort study of 513,749 diabetics found that risk ratios for hospitalization for cystitis and pyelonephritis were 1.39 and 1.95 for diabetic patients compared to nondiabetic patients [3].

The incidence of bacteriuria is directly related to the duration of diabetes. Since cellular immune defects have not been demonstrated in diabetics with urinary tract infections, it is thought that the increased prevalence of bacteriuria is related to autonomic neuropathy and urinary stasis [4]. This, as well as the increased incidence of urinary tract infections among diabetics, likely contributes to diabetic susceptibility to emphysematous pyelonephritis.

Diabetic Susceptibility to Emphysematous Pyelonephritis

More than 90% of patients with emphysematous pyelonephritis and 70% of patients with emphysematous cystitis have diabetes [5, 6]. The majority of diabetics with emphysematous pyelonephritis have poorly controlled diabetes. In one study, 76% of patients had hemoglobin A1c values greater than 7%, and in a separate study, 72% of patients had hemoglobin A1c values greater than 8% [6, 7]. While these two series indicate the importance of glycemic control, they also demonstrate that diabetics with well-controlled diabetes can develop emphysematous infection. The majority of nondiabetic patients have urinary obstruction. Women outnumber men 4:1, and the majority of patients are over 60 years old with a range of 24 to 83 [5].

Clinical Presentation

The clinical presentation of emphysematous disease is indistinguishable from severe pyelonephritis; fever (79%), flank pain or abdominal pain (71%), and nausea and vomiting (17%) [6]. Symptoms are usually acute but can develop over several weeks. The two most common pathogens are *Escherichia coli* (67%) or *Klebsiella* (20%) [5]. Other microbial species that have been reported infrequently are *Proteus, Pseudomonas, Enterobacter, Enterococcus, Staphylococcus, Clostridium, Pneumocystis, Candida*, and *Cryptococcus* [8, 9]. Bacteremia occurs in 26–54% of patients [6, 7]. The severity of the illness does not distinguish emphysematous pyelonephritis from typical pyelonephritis. A recent case series describes the frequency of signs of severe illness in emphysematous pyelonephritis that is consistent with older studies: hypotension (systolic blood pressure less than 90 mmHg) 28%, altered mental status 18%, leukocytosis (more than 14,000/uL) 46%, thrombocytopenia (less than 40,000/uL) 31%, and serum creatinine more than 2.5 mg/dL 46% [6, 7].

Diagnosis

The evidence regarding the importance of diagnosing emphysematous infection is limited to retrospective case series and is not definitive. However, emphysematous pyelonephritis should be considered in diabetic patients who present with symptoms of pyelonephritis. Suspicion should be heightened if there is not a response to medical therapy within the first 24 hours. Diagnosis of emphysematous pyelonephritis requires the demonstration of gas on abdominal imaging. Abdominal ultrasound, x-ray, or CT can detect gas in the renal or perirenal tissue, but CT is the preferred initial imaging study (Fig. 8.1) [10]. In a systematic review of 210 cases,

Fig. 8.1 Noncontrast axial CT image demonstrating gas in the right renal parenchyma (arrow), bilateral staghorn calculi, and perinephric inflammation

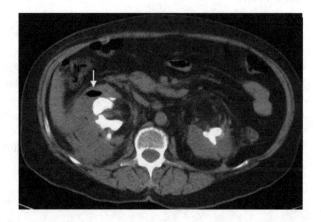

ultrasound and plain radiography were diagnostic in only 69% and 65% of cases, respectively, compared to CT [5]. Beyond the detection of gas, CT can sometimes identify the site of obstruction, the extent of infection, and prognostic findings.

Radiographic Classification

Several radiologic classification systems have been proposed for the prognosis and management of emphysematous pyelonephritis [6, 11, 12]. The two that are currently used are based on CT findings and have been retrospectively evaluated in subsequent studies. The classification system proposed by Wan et al. divides radiographic findings into two types. Images that show parenchymal destruction with either the absence of fluid collection or the presence of streaky or mottled gas are classified as type I. Type II is characterized by renal or perirenal fluid collections with bubbly or loculated gas or gas in the collecting system. Type I is associated with necrosis or hemorrhagic infarction and greater mortality [11, 13]. The system developed by Huang and Tseng divides images into five categories based on the involvement of gas in the collecting system (class 1), renal parenchyma (class 2), extension of gas or abscess into the perinephric space (class 3a), extension beyond the perinephric space (class 3b), or involvement of both kidneys or a solitary kidney (class 4). Despite inconsistencies between the original study and a subsequent study that evaluated this method of classification retrospectively, it can be concluded that patients with class 1 findings do well with antibiotics and percutaneous drainage and rarely require nephrectomy. Patients with findings of classes 2, 3, or 4 are more likely to fail management with percutaneous drainage and antibiotics, are more likely to undergo nephrectomy, and have higher mortality. Mortality and progression to nephrectomy in these classes are increased when there is more than one risk factor present (i.e., altered mental status, hypotension, thrombocytopenia, acute kidney injury) or parenchymal destruction of greater than 50% [6, 7].

Treatment

The optimal management of emphysematous pyelonephritis requires early recognition, parenteral antibiotics, and prompt surgical intervention based on the extent of infection or the presence of obstruction. Studies have suggested that patients treated with antibiotics alone or urgent nephrectomy have higher mortality [5]. However, these studies are limited in that they are retrospective and do not account for the severity of illness. The current literature supports a management strategy of supportive care, antibiotic therapy, early percutaneous drainage, and correction of any underlying urinary obstruction. Empiric antibiotic therapy should be initiated with a regimen for severe pyelonephritis, such as piperacillin-tazobactam, but the choice of initial antibiotic should ultimately be guided by local patterns of antimicrobial resistance and the patient's previous antibiotic exposure. Antibiotic therapy should subsequently be modified based on urine and blood cultures. Drainage should be assessed with imaging, and multiple drainage procedures may be required. Patients who fail to improve significantly should undergo nephrectomy [7, 9].

Prognosis

Mortality rates of up to 78% were reported until the late 1970s [9]. In contrast, a recent series of 39 patients found a mortality rate of 13% with a kidney salvage rate of 67% [7]. Changes in the reported mortality are likely due to increased detection of less severe infection with CT and earlier diagnosis and intervention. The preferred approach has shifted from urgent nephrectomy to that of percutaneous drainage, reserving nephrectomy for patients who do not improve clinically. Signs of poor prognosis that have been seen in multiple studies include the pattern or degree of gas formation on CT, infection of both kidneys, altered mental status, thrombocytopenia, acute kidney injury, and hypotension [6, 11–13]. Poorly controlled diabetes, age, and bacteremia were not associated with mortality [13].

Summary

Emphysematous pyelonephritis is a severe form of pyelonephritis that is found more frequently in diabetics and individuals with urinary tract obstruction. The majority of patients have poorly controlled diabetes, but a significant percentage of patients have well-controlled diabetes. The clinical presentation is similar to typical pyelonephritis, and abdominal imaging is required to diagnose emphysematous infection. CT scan is the preferred diagnostic imaging modality due to its capacity to detect gas and urinary obstruction. CT may also provide prognostic information by itself or in conjunction with clinical signs of severe illness. Treatment for emphysematous pyelonephritis consists of prompt antibiotics, correction of obstruction if present, and percutaneous drainage. In some cases of extensive infection, nephrectomy is necessary:

- Emphysematous pyelonephritis is clinically similar to typical pyelonephritis and should be suspected in diabetics who do not respond quickly to therapy.
- Computerized tomography (CT) is the preferred diagnostic test for emphysematous pyelonephritis.
- Successful treatment often requires percutaneous drainage or nephrectomy in addition to parenteral antibiotics.

References

1. Nicolle LE, Bradley S, Colgan R, Rice JC, Schaeffer A, Hooton TM. Infectious Diseases Society of America guidelines for the diagnosis and treatment of asymptomatic bacteriuria in adults. Clin Infect Dis. 2005;40(5):643–54.
2. Semetkowska-Jurkiewicz E, Horoszek-Maziarz S, Galinski J, Manitius A, Krupa-Wojciechowska B. The clinical course of untreated asymptomatic bacteriuria in diabetic patients--14-year follow-up. Mater Med Pol. 1995;27(3):91–5.
3. Shah BR, Hux JE. Quantifying the risk of infectious diseases for people with diabetes. Diabetes Care. 2003;26(2):510–3.
4. Balasoiu D, van Kessel KC, van Kats-Renaud HJ, Collet TJ, Hoepelman AI. Granulocyte function in women with diabetes and asymptomatic bacteriuria. Diabetes Care. 1997;20(3):392–5.
5. Somani BK, Nabi G, Thorpe P, Hussey J, Cook J, N'Dow J. Is percutaneous drainage the new gold standard in the management of emphysematous pyelonephritis? Evidence from a systematic review. J Urol. 2008;179(5):1844–9.
6. Huang JJ, Tseng CC. Emphysematous pyelonephritis: clinicoradiological classification, management, prognosis, and pathogenesis. Arch Intern Med. 2000;160(6):797–805.
7. Kapoor R, Muruganandham K, Gulia AK, et al. Predictive factors for mortality and need for nephrectomy in patients with emphysematous pyelonephritis. BJU Int. 2010;105(7):986–9.
8. Hildebrand TS, Nibbe L, Frei U, Schindler R. Bilateral emphysematous pyelonephritis caused by Candida infection. Am J Kidney Dis. 1999;33(2):E10.
9. Ubee SS, McGlynn L, Fordham M. Emphysematous pyelonephritis. BJU Int. 2011;107(9):1474–8.
10. Kawashima A, LeRoy AJ. Radiologic evaluation of patients with renal infections. Infect Dis Clin N Am. 2003;17(2):433–56.
11. Wan YL, Lee TY, Bullard MJ, Tsai CC. Acute gas-producing bacterial renal infection: correlation between imaging findings and clinical outcome. Radiology. 1996;198(2):433–8.
12. Michaeli J, Mogle P, Perlberg S, Heiman S, Caine M. Emphysematous pyelonephritis. J Urol. 1984;131(2):203–8.
13. Falagas ME, Alexiou VG, Giannopoulou KP, Siempos II. Risk factors for mortality in patients with emphysematous pyelonephritis: a meta-analysis. J Urol. 2007;178(3 Pt 1):880–885; quiz 1129.

Chapter 9
Thyrotoxic Crisis: Thyroid Storm

John J. Reyes-Castano and Kenneth Burman

Précis

1. Clinical setting: Patients presenting with goiter, tachycardia, signs of autonomic hyperactivity (i.e., loose stools, hyperreflexia), fever, excited delirium.
2. Diagnoses: Thyroid storm is an emergent type of severe hyperthyroidism. Diagnosis is based on clinical features and not on the severity of T4 nor T3 levels. The Burch and Wartofsky assessment indicates impending thyroid storm at point values above 25.
3. Management: These four principles should be enacted immediately upon diagnosis of thyroid storm:

    (a) Inhibit thyroid hormone synthesis and release with propylthiouracil (PTU) 400 mg by mouth every 6 hours.
    (b) Counteract the peripheral and biologic effects of thyroid hormones with propranolol 80 mg by mouth every 6 hours and hydrocortisone 100 mg IV every 8 hours.
    (c) Provide supportive therapy with IV fluids supplemented with thiamine.
    (d) Treat precipitating factors such as infection.

J. J. Reyes-Castano
Section of Endocrine, Medstar Washington Hospital Center, Washington, DC, USA

K. Burman (✉)
Endocrine Sections, Georgetown University Medical Center/MedStar Washington Hospital Center, Washington, DC, USA
e-mail: Kenneth.d.Burman@medstar.net

© Springer Nature Switzerland AG 2021
L. Loriaux, C. Vanek (eds.), *Endocrine Emergencies*, Contemporary Endocrinology,
https://doi.org/10.1007/978-3-030-67455-7_9

Pathogenesis

The pathogenesis of thyroid storm is still not fully understood as there is usually no difference in thyroid hormone levels between patients with "uncomplicated" thyrotoxicosis and those undergoing a thyrotoxic crisis [1, 2].

One hypothesis that may explain the pathogenesis of thyroid storm is a possible increase in target cell β (beta)-adrenergic receptor density or post-receptor modifications in signaling pathways [3–5] leading to an increased sensitivity to catecholamines.

Another theory to explain the cause of thyroid storm is an increase in the amount of free thyroid hormones. In one study comparing six subjects with thyroid storm to 15 subjects with more typical thyrotoxicosis, Brooks and colleagues [6] found that the mean free thyroxine (FT4) concentration was higher in subjects with thyroid storm, whereas the total thyroxine (TT4) concentration was similar in both groups.

Etiology (See Table 9.1)

Graves' disease remains the most common cause of thyrotoxic crisis/thyroid storm. Graves' disease is mediated by the thyrotropin (TSH) receptor antibodies that stimulate excess and uncontrolled synthesis and secretion of thyroid hormones (thyroxine (T4) or triiodothyronine (T3)). It is more frequent in young women but can occur in both genders and any age group.

Thyroid storm can also occur with a solitary toxic adenoma or toxic multinodular goiter. Rare causes of thyrotoxicosis that can lead to thyroid storm include hypersecretory thyroid carcinoma (specially follicular thyroid carcinoma), thyrotropin-secreting pituitary adenoma, struma ovarii/teratoma, and human chorionic gonadotropin-secreting hydatidiform mole. It is very rare for ingestion of excess exogenous T4 and/or T3 to be associated with thyroid storm.

Other causes include certain medications: interferon-α (alpha) (IFN-α) and interleukin-2 (IL-2) can cause thyrotoxicosis (via destructive thyroiditis) during treatment for viral hepatitis and HIV infection [7–10]. Of relevance is hyperthyroidism aggravated by iodine exposure, which can occur following the intravenous administration of radiocontrast dye or during or after amiodarone administration. Amiodarone contains 70–75 mg iodine per 200 mg tablet, and about 10% of it (7–7.5 mg) is released as free iodide during amiodarone metabolism (about a 35- to 50-fold increase when compared with the recommended optimal intake of 0.15–0.20 mg) [11].

A precipitating event usually causes the transition from thyrotoxicosis to thyroid storm. Triggering events include systemic insults such as surgery, trauma, myocardial infarction, pulmonary thromboembolism, diabetic ketoacidosis, parturition, or severe infection [7]. Thyroid storm has also been reported to be precipitated by the discontinuation of antithyroid drugs, excessive ingestion, intravenous administration of iodine (e.g., amiodarone, radiocontrast dyes), radioiodine therapy, and even pseudoephedrine and salicylate use (salicylates may increase free thyroid hormone levels disproportionately) [12].

Table 9.1 Etiology of thyrotoxicosis

Thyrotoxicosis with a normal or high radioiodine uptake[a]
Autoimmune thyroid disease (AITD)
Graves' disease (GD)
Hashitoxicosis
Autonomous thyroid tissue
Toxic adenoma (TA)
Toxic multinodular goiter (TMNG)
TSH-mediated
TSH-producing pituitary adenoma
Non-neoplastic TSH-mediated hyperthyroidism
Human chorionic gonadotropin-mediated
Hyperemesis gravidarum
Trophoblastic disease
Resistance to thyroid hormone (T3 receptor mutation)[b]
Thyrotoxicosis with a decreased or near-absent radioiodine uptake
Thyroiditis
Painless (silent, lymphocytic) thyroiditis
Subacute (de Quervain's, granulomatous) thyroiditis
Acute viral thyroiditis
Amiodarone-induced thyroiditis
Radiation thyroiditis
Palpation/Trauma thyroiditis
Exogenous thyroid hormone intake
Iatrogenic (improper thyroid hormone dosing) thyrotoxicosis
Factitious ingestion of thyroid hormone
Intentional levothyroxine suppressive therapy
Ectopic hyperthyroidism
Struma ovarii
Extensive metastasis from follicular thyroid carcinoma

Source: Adapted from: Bahn et al. [74]
[a]Uptake may be low if recent iodine load caused iodine-induced thyrotoxicosis
[b]Patients may not be hyperthyroid

The most common precipitating cause of thyroid storm currently seems to be infection, although it is difficult to know if published reports mirror actual frequencies [13].

Clinical Presentation

Thyroid storm is part of a continuum that begins with the development of decompensated thyrotoxicosis. The point at which thyrotoxicosis transforms to thyroid storm is not clear and is relatively subjective. In an effort to standardize and objectify thyroid storm, as compared with severe thyrotoxicosis, Burch and Wartofsky [3] have delineated a point system assessing degrees of dysfunction in various organ systems (see Table 9.2). Although this classification is helpful clinically, it is prudent, in most circumstances, to assume that someone with severe thyrotoxicosis has impending thyroid storm, and to treat them aggressively, rather than focus on specific definitions.

Table 9.3 summarizes the clinical manifestations of thyrotoxicosis.

Table 9.2 Point scale criteria for the diagnosis of thyroid storm

Criteria	Points
Thermoregulatory dysfunction	
Temperature (°F)/(°C)	
99.0–99.9/37.2–37.7	5
100.0–100.9/37.8–38.2	10
101.0–101.9/38.3–38.8	15
102.0–102.9/38.9–39.4	20
103.0–103.9/39.5–39.9	25
≥104.0/≥40.0	30
Cardiovascular	
Tachycardia (beats/min)	
100–109	5
110–119	10
120–129	15
130–139	20
≥140	25
Atrial fibrillation	
Absent	0
Present	10
Congestive heart failure	
Absent	0
Mild (pedal edema)	5
Moderate (bibasilar rales)	10
Severe (pulmonary edema)	20
Gastrointestinal-hepatic dysfunction	
Absent	0
Moderate (diarrhea, abdominal pain, nausea/vomit)	10
Severe (unexplained jaundice)	20
Central nervous system disturbance	
Absent	0
Mild (agitation)	10
Moderate (delirium, psychosis, extreme lethargy)	20
Severe (seizure, coma)	30
Precipitating history	
Absent	0
Present	10

Total score: ≥45, thyroid storm; 25–44, impending thyroid storm; <25, unlikely thyroid storm

Source: Adapted from: Burch and Wartofsky [3]

Table 9.3 Clinical manifestations of thyrotoxicosis

Constitutional [14]
Weight loss, despite having the same or greater caloric intake: due to the hypermetabolic state that results in an imbalance between energy production and use, resulting in increased heat production and elimination
The thermogenesis leads to increased perspiration and heat intolerance
Generalized weakness and fatigue
Neuropsychiatric [14, 16]
Emotional lability, restlessness, anxiety, agitation, confusion, psychosis, and even coma
Behavioral studies reveal poor performance in memory and concentration testing proportional to the degree of thyrotoxicosis
Muscle wasting, hyperreflexia, fine tremor, periodic paralysis
Gastrointestinal
Hyperdefecation due to increased peristalsis in the small bowel
Hepatic injury [69, 70]
Increase in the aspartate aminotransferase (AST) and alanine aminotransferase (ALT) was reported in 27% and 37% of patients, respectively. The majority of these patients showed no other clinical or biochemical features of liver impairment
The mechanism of injury appears to be relative hypoxia in the perivenular regions, due to an increase in hepatic oxygen demand without an appropriate increase in hepatic blood flow generally associated with the onset of heart failure (often precipitated by arrhythmias)
The clinical presentation of this type of injury is usually that of a self-limiting hepatitis; however, there are a few case reports of thyrotoxic patients presenting with fulminant hepatic failure
Cholestatic injury [71–73]
Elevated serum alkaline phosphatase (bone or liver origin) is seen in 64% of patients with thyrotoxicosis
Elevations in gamma-glutamyl transpeptidase (17%) and bilirubin (5%) as indicators of cholestasis
Jaundice is uncommon, but when it occurs, complications of thyrotoxicosis (heart failure/sepsis) or intrinsic liver disease need to be excluded
In the vast majority of cases, the hepatic abnormalities associated with hyperthyroidism are reversible, following the early recognition and treatment of the disorder
Reproductive symptoms [14]
Irregular menstrual cycle: oligomenorrhea and anovulation
In men: decreased libido, gynecomastia, and development of spider angiomas, perhaps related to an increase in sex hormone-binding globulin and a subsequent increase in estrogen activity
Cardiorespiratory [14]
Palpitations/tachycardia, hyperdynamic precordium, increased pulse pressure, and a strong apical impulse
Pleuropericardial rub may be heard
Congestive heart failure
Dyspnea on exertion. Dyspnea can be multifactorial in origin because of decreased lung compliance, engorged pulmonary capillary bed, or left ventricular failure
Chest pain similar to angina pectoris, owing to increased myocardial oxygen demand and coronary artery spasm. Coronary artery disease should be excluded as appropriate

(continued)

Table 9.3 (continued)

Thyroid [14, 15]
In Graves' disease, diffuse enlargement of the gland, and possibly a bruit, can be appreciated, due to increased vascularity and blood flow
With a toxic multinodular goiter, physical findings of the thyroid gland may include one or more nodules
With acute thyroiditis, a tender thyroid gland could be found
Dermatologic
Hair loss
Pretibial myxedema, palmar erythema, warm and moist skin
Ophthalmologic
Diplopia, eye irritation
Exophthalmos, ophthalmoplegia, conjunctival injection

Older individuals may not manifest the typical symptoms of thyrotoxicosis. They may present with "apathetic" thyrotoxicosis, with symptoms including weight loss, palpitations, weakness, dizziness, syncope, or memory loss, and physical findings of sinus tachycardia or atrial fibrillation [14].

Diagnosis

The distinction between severe thyrotoxicosis and life-threatening thyrotoxicosis or thyroid storm is a matter of clinical judgment. Objective means such as the point scale by Burch and Wartofsky (Table 9.2) can, and perhaps should, be used. However, it is most prudent to treat a patient suspected of having thyroid storm aggressively for his/her hyperthyroidism/thyrotoxicosis rather than excessively investigate whether this case really meets the criteria for thyroid storm. These patients require close clinical monitoring usually in an intensive care unit.

There is no arbitrary serum T4 or T3 cutoff that discriminates severe thyrotoxicosis from thyroid storm. Brooks et al. found no significant difference in the levels of serum triiodothyronine among patients with thyroid storm vs. uncomplicated thyrotoxicosis [2]. Also, systemically ill patients have decreased ability to convert T4 to T3. Therefore, a minimally elevated T3 or even a "normal" T3 may be considered inappropriately elevated in this context.

In thyroid storm, the pattern of elevated free T4 and free T3 with a depressed thyrotropin (TSH) (less than 0.05 mU/mL (in third-generation TSH assays)) can be comparable to the levels seen in "uncomplicated" thyrotoxicosis (the TSH is always undetectable).

The thyroid gland secretes all of the circulating T4. Approximately 80% of circulating T3 is derived from monodeiodination of T4 in peripheral tissues by types I (D1) and II (D2) deiodinases, whereas only about 20% comes from direct thyroidal secretion. Secreted T4 and T3 are bound to serum proteins: thyroxine-binding globulin (TBG), transthyretin, and albumin. Only a small fraction of the hormones, 0.025% of T4 and 0.35% of T3, are free and unbound [14, 15] and thus are available to the tissues to affect biologic action. Laboratory measurement of total T3 and total T4, but not free levels, may be affected by conditions that affect protein binding. Conditions that increase TBG (and as a result total T4 and T3) include infectious hepatitis, pregnancy, estrogens, and opiates. In addition, many drugs interfere with protein binding, including heparin, furosemide, phenytoin, carbamazepine, diazepam, salicylates, and nonsteroidal anti-inflammatory drugs. Therefore, free hormone concentrations are preferable in the diagnosis of thyrotoxicosis [12]. Serum total and free T3 concentrations are elevated in most patients who have thyrotoxicosis because of increased thyroidal T3 production and more enhanced extrathyroidal conversion of T4 to T3. In less than 5% of patients who have thyrotoxicosis, there can be an increase in serum-free T3 while having a "normal" free T4 ("T3 toxicosis") [14, 15]. The T3/T4 ratio may be helpful in distinguishing the etiology of thyrotoxicosis. With Graves' disease and toxic nodular goiter, as there tends to be a higher proportion of T3, the T3/T4 ratio is usually greater than 20. With thyrotoxicosis caused by thyroiditis, iodine exposure, or exogenous levothyroxine intake, there is generally a greater proportion of T4, with a T3/T4 ratio of less than 15 [15].

Other laboratory findings that may be associated with thyrotoxicosis include hyperglycemia (due to catecholamine-induced inhibition of insulin release and increased glycogenolysis), mild hypercalcemia (due to enhanced thyroid hormone-stimulated bone resorption), mildly elevated alkaline phosphatase (both form liver and bone origin), leukocytosis, and elevated liver enzymes (ALT, AST) [4, 12, 16, 17].

Adrenocortical function may also be affected by thyrotoxicosis. Thyrotoxicosis accelerates the metabolism of endogenous or exogenous cortisol by stimulating the rate-limiting step in the degradation of glucocorticoids (accomplished by the hepatic enzymes, D4,5 steroid reductases). Therefore, steroids, including cortisol, corticosterone, deoxycorticosterone, and aldosterone, are metabolized at an accelerated rate [18]. However, in thyrotoxicosis, both degradation and production of cortisol are accelerated, resulting in a normal to increased circulating cortisol level. Given the stressful condition of thyroid storm, a normal cortisol level may be interpreted as a relative adrenal insufficiency. Serum cortisol response to a corticotropin (ACTH) stimulation test should be normal. However, in long-standing, severe thyrotoxicosis, adrenocortical reserve can be diminished [18]. Tsatsoulis and colleagues [19] assessed adrenocortical reserve in ten subjects with severe, long-standing (4–6 months) thyrotoxicosis with a low-dose corticotropin (ACTH) stimulation test (0.1 μg/kg of ACTH given as IV bolus) and found that the cortisol response decreased significantly when subjects were thyrotoxic, compared with the cortisol response in the euthyroid state.

Cross-sectional imaging studies are not required to make the diagnosis of thyrotoxicosis or thyroid storm. However, in the evaluation of thyroid storm, a chest X-ray (or chest CT *without* iodinated contrast) would be helpful to determine a possible infectious source as a precipitant. The IV radiocontrast contains significant iodine and may aggravate the hyperthyroidism, especially in unblocked patients. Nuclear medicine imaging (radioactive iodine uptake and scan) is usually not performed initially given the urgency and clinical context. However, it can be helpful in determining the etiology of thyrotoxicosis [4] (see Table 9.1). A noninvasive readily available test is a thyroid ultrasound with Doppler flow to assess thyroid gland size, vascularity, and the presence of nodules. Typically, a thyroid gland secreting excessive hormones would be enlarged and have enhanced Doppler flow. On the other hand, in the setting of subacute, postpartum, or silent thyroiditis or exogenous causes of hyperthyroidism, the thyroid gland would be expected to be small, with decreased Doppler flow.

Electrocardiogram manifestations of thyrotoxicosis include sinus tachycardia (40%) and atrial fibrillation (10–20%), occurring more commonly in patients older than 60, who are more likely to have underlying structural heart disease or coronary artery disease [19].

Management

Medical treatment of thyroid storm is based on three principles: (1) inhibition of thyroid hormone synthesis and release; (2) counteracting the peripheral, biologic effects of thyroid hormones; and (3) treatment of systemic complications. These measures should bring about clinical improvement within 12–24 h [1].

Management of thyroid storm is outlined in Table 9.4.

Table 9.4 Management of thyroid storm

1. Inhibition of thyroid hormone synthesis (thionamides)[e]		
Methimazole	20–30 mg PO q6 h	
Propylthiouracil	200–400 mg PO q6–8 h	Decrease peripheral T4 → T3 conversion
2. Inhibition of thyroid hormone release from the thyroid gland[b,c]		
SSKI[d]	5 drops PO q6 h or	SSKI 1 g/mL contains 76.4% iodine, 20 drops/ mL = 764 mg iodine
	5–10 drops per rectum q6–8 h or	After antithyroid medications given
	8 drops sublingual q8 h	
Lugol's solution[d]	4–8 drops PO q6–8 h or 5–10 drops per rectum q6–8 h or 5–10 drops IV[d] q6–8 h	125 mg/mL of total iodine, 100 mL = 5 g of iodine and 10 g potassium iodide After antithyroid medications given
3. Counteraction of peripheral effects of thyroid hormone		
Beta-blockers[c]		
Propranolol	60–80 mg PO q4 h or 80–120 mg PO q6 h or 0.5–1 mg IV over 10–15 min every few hours as needed	At doses of >160 mg/day can have some effect on decreasing peripheral T4 → T3 conversion

Table 9.4 (continued)

Atenolol	50–200 mg PO qday (or divided bid)	
Metoprolol	100–200 mg PO qday (or divided bid)	
Nadolol	40–80 mg PO qday	
Esmolol	Loading dose of 250–500 µg/kg IV, then 50–100 µg/kg/min IV	Drip formulations useful for heart failure
Steroids[c]		
Hydrocortisone	100 mg IV q8 h	Treats presumed relative adrenal insufficiency
Dexamethasone	2 mg IV q6 h	
Betamethasone	0.5 mg IV or IM q6 h	
4. Supportive therapy		
Steroids	As above	Helps in vasomotor stability
Acetaminophen	325–650 mg PO/PR q4–6 h prn	Avoid salicylates (due to displacement of T4 from binding globulin, increasing free T4). Can be given as enema
Thiamine	100 mg IV	To prevent Wernicke's encephalopathy
Fluids D5%NS or D10%NS		
5. Treatment of systemic complications and precipitant factor		
Management of underlying disease/condition		
6. Alternative therapies: uncommonly used		
Lithium carbonate	300 mg PO q8 h	Suppresses thyroid function
Cholestyramine	4 g PO qday	Reduces enterohepatic circulation of thyroid hormone
Potassium perchlorate	1 g PO qday	Warning: aplastic anemia, nephrotic syndrome
Reserpine	2.5–5 mg IM q4 h	Anti-adrenergic
Guanethidine	30–40 mg PO q6 h	Anti-adrenergic

Source: Adapted from: Nayak and Burman [13]; Alfandhli and Gianoukakis [28]
[a]For non-oral formulations, please refer to Table 9.5
[b]Administer at least 1 h after thionamide
[c]Use one agent of each group as clinically indicated
[d]Routine pharmacologic sterility needed as indicated per local regulations

With regard to the use of thionamide (propylthiouracil and methimazole) therapy and iodine therapy, the order of therapy is important: Inhibition of thyroid gland synthesis of new thyroid hormone with a thionamide should be initiated *before* iodine therapy, to prevent the stimulation of new thyroid hormone synthesis that can occur when iodine is given initially [3, 7, 16]. The time delay between antithyroid medications and iodine administration is at least 60 minutes.

Antithyroid Medications (Thionamides)

The two specific antithyroid agent classes are thiouracils and imidazoles. Propylthiouracil (PTU) is a thiouracil, whereas methimazole (MMI) and carbimazole are imidazoles. Carbimazole is not available in the United States and is more commonly used in Europe. Carbimazole is metabolized rapidly to MMI [20, 21].

Thionamides interfere with the thyroperoxidase-catalyzed coupling process by which iodotyrosine residues are combined to form T4 and T3. Thionamides may also have an inhibitory effect on thyroid follicular cell function and growth [20]. PTU, but not MMI, also inhibits the peripheral conversion of T4 to T3. Thionamides may also have clinically relevant immunosuppressive effects, including decreasing antithyrotropin-receptor antibody titers over time and decreasing levels and activities of other immunologically important molecules, such as intracellular adhesion molecule 1 and soluble interleukin-2 (IL-2). Antithyroid drugs may also induce apoptosis of intrathyroidal lymphocytes and decrease HLA antigen class II expression [22].

MMI circulates free or unbound in the serum, whereas 80–90% of propylthiouracil is bound to albumin [20, 22]. Both agents are concentrated within the thyroid gland where they exert their major actions. It is believed that MMI has a longer duration of action as compared to PTU. The dosing of PTU in thyroid storm is 800 to 1200 mg daily in divided doses of 200 or 300 mg every 6 h. The dosing for MMI is 80 to 120 mg daily in divided doses of 20–30 mg every 6 h (once the patient is stable, the frequency of dosing can be decreased to once or twice daily, and the dose of these agents can be decreased) [16]. Typically, administration has been orally; however, both MMI and propylthiouracil can be administered rectally [23–27]. The rectal administration is most relevant to patients with severe GI issues in which they cannot take medication orally or if they have severe malabsorption.

MMI has shown to have similar pharmacokinetics for both oral and intravenous uses in normal subjects and in subjects with hyperthyroidism [28]. Although there are no commercially available parenteral formulations of the thionamides, there are case reports of MMI being administered intravenously when the oral and rectal routes could not be used [29, 30].

The rectal formulations of the antithyroid drugs have been prepared either as enemas or suppositories (Table 9.5).

Jongjaroenprasert et al. demonstrated that the enema form of PTU provided better bioavailability than the suppository form. However, both preparations proved to have comparable therapeutic effect [26].

Possible adverse effects of MMI and PTU include abnormal sense of taste, pruritus, urticaria, fever, and arthralgias. More rare but serious adverse effects include agranulocytosis, hepatotoxicity, and vasculitis.

A serious side effect is agranulocytosis. 0.37% of subjects receiving propylthiouracil and 0.35% of subjects receiving MMI develop severe agranulocytosis (<500/mm^3) in one study [31]. Most cases of agranulocytosis occur in the first 3 months of

Table 9.5 Non-oral formulations of antithyroid medications

Antithyroid medication	Quantity for formulation	Vehicle	Route	Dosage	References
Methimazole	1200 mg	12 mL water with 2 drops of polysorbate (span) 80, mixed with 52 mL of cocoa butter	Suppository	20–40 mg every 6–8 h	Nabil et al. [24]
Methimazole	500 mg powder	0.9% NaCl total volume of 50 mL (methimazole 10 mg/mL)	IV filtered through a 0.22 μm filter over 2 min, followed by saline flush[a]	20–40 mg every 6–8 h	Hodak et al. [30]
Propylthiouracil	600 mg	90 mL sterile water	Enema[b]	400–600 mg every 6 h	Yeung et al. [25]
Propylthiouracil	400 mg	60 mL fleet's mineral oil or 60 mL of Fleet's phospho-soda	Enema[b]	400–600 mg every 6 h	Walter et al. [26]
Propylthiouracil	400 mg	90 mL sterile water	Enema[b]	400–600 mg every 6 h	Jongjaroenprasert et al. [27]
Propylthiouracil	200 mg	Polyethylene glycol	Suppository	400–600 mg every 6 h	Jongjaroenprasert et al. [27]

[a]Routine pharmacologic sterility needed as indicated per local regulations
[b]For enema preparation, deliver by Foley catheter inserted into the rectum and inflate balloon to prevent leakage

treatment but can occur at any time. When MMI is the culprit, agranulocytosis tends to be dose-related, especially at doses more than 40 mg daily. However, agranulocytosis does not appear to be dose-related with propylthiouracil use [21, 22]. Nonetheless, agranulocytosis can occur at any time with either MMI or PTU, and close monitoring is mandatory. The use of granulocyte colony-stimulating factor (G-CSF) for treatment of agranulocytosis induced by antithyroid medications seems to be effective in shortening the recovery time if the granulocyte count was above 0.1×10^9/L [32, 33]. Another study, however, did not demonstrate this beneficial effect [34]. Therefore, the use of G-CSF can be recommended for treatment of antithyroid drug-induced agranulocytosis, with consideration of the individual context [22].

Hepatotoxicity can occur in 0.1–0.2% of patients using antithyroid drugs. PTU-induced hepatotoxicity tends to be an allergic hepatitis with evidence of hepatocellular injury, whereas MMI-induced hepatotoxicity tends to result in a cholestatic process [22].

Vasculitis is associated more commonly with propylthiouracil than with MMI, and is associated with serologic markers: perinuclear antineutrophil cytoplasmic antibodies (p-ANCA) and anti-myeloperoxidase (anti-MPO) antibodies. Antineutrophil cytoplasmic antibody (ANCA) positivity is associated with acute renal failure, arthritis, skin ulcerations, vasculitic rash, neurological changes, and possibly sinusitis or hemoptysis [22, 75].

MMI has become the most frequently prescribed thionamide for routine outpatient treatment of hyperthyroidism. As described above, the side effect profile favors MMI. Although agranulocytosis is a potential adverse effect of both thionamides, it is dose-related for MMI and less so for PTU. PTU is the cause of rare but potentially life-threatening hepatotoxicity, whereas severe hepatotoxic reactions related to MMI are extraordinarily rare. PTU is a far more common cause of ANCA-positive vasculitis than is MMI. Also, the more convenient dosing of MMI, translated into enhanced adherence, makes it preferable to PTU. And finally, MMI is more effective than PTU in controlling severe hyperthyroidism [35]. However PTU is the preferred treatment for hyperthyroidism in the first trimester of pregnancy. It is recommended that patients on MMI be switched to PTU if pregnancy is confirmed in the first trimester. Following the first trimester, consideration should be given to switching to MMI [36].

Iodine Therapy

Iodine therapy complements the effects of thionamide therapy by blocking the release of pre-stored thyroid hormone and decreasing iodide transport and oxidation in follicular cells. This decrease in organification due to increasing doses of inorganic iodide is known as the "Wolff-Chaikoff" effect. Over the short term of approximately 1–4 weeks, small increments in available iodide cause increased thyroid hormone synthesis; however, large amounts of exogenous iodide actually inhibit synthesis of thyroid hormone. However, despite maintenance of high doses of iodide, the thyroid gland eventually escapes this inhibition, approximately after 48–72 h, as the iodide transport system adapts to the higher concentration of iodide by modulating the activity of the sodium-iodide symporter [37] (this effect is termed "release from the Wolff-Chaikoff effect"). Although iodide is rapid and effective in reducing serum thyroid hormone levels, most patients escape the inhibition, returning to hyperthyroidism within 2–3 weeks. This increase in T4 and T3 synthesis and secretion can occur at variable time intervals and can also occur in patients being treated with PTU or MMI. As a result, the long-term use of exogenous iodine for hyperthyroidism is discouraged.

Administering iodine before thionamide therapy may influence treatment options for thyrotoxicosis in the short and longer term. In the acute setting, iodine therapy can stimulate new hormone synthesis if given prior to thionamide treatment. After the acute phase, when planning definitive therapy for thyrotoxicosis, the prior use of exogenous iodine can predispose a patient to increased surgical risk because of the enrichment of thyroid hormone stores. It can also cause postponement of radioiodine ablation until an adequate clearance of the iodine load occurs [3].

Oral formulations of inorganic iodine include Lugol's solution and saturated solution of potassium iodide (SSKI). The dosing for these preparations in thyroid storm is 0.2–2 g daily, with 4–8 drops of Lugol's solution (assuming 20 drops/mL and 6–8 mg iodine/drop) every 6–8 h and 5 drops of SSKI (with 20 drops/mL and 38 mg iodide/drop) every 6 h [3, 38].

β-Blockade

Propranolol is probably the most common β-blocker prescribed for management of thyroid storm. It is dosed usually at 60–80 mg orally every 4 h, with a maximum of 120 mg every 4 h. Large doses can be required in the setting of thyrotoxicosis because of the faster metabolism of the drug and possibly because of a greater quantity of cardiac β-adrenergic receptors [39]. The onset of action after oral dosing is approximately 1 h. Propranolol in large doses (greater than 160 mg daily) can decrease T3 levels by as much as 30% via the inhibition of 5′monodeiodinase, which is mediated slowly over 7–10 days.

Other oral β-blockers used alternatively in the management of thyroid storm include atenolol at 50–200 mg daily (divided once or twice daily) [21], metoprolol at 100–200 mg daily (divided once or twice daily), and nadolol at 40–80 mg daily [20]. Clinical response and titration must be done as appropriate.

β-Blockers can also be administered intravenously: propranolol at an initial bolus of 0.5–1 mg over 10 min followed by 1–3 mg over 10 min, every few hours [4, 40] and esmolol at 50–100 mg/kg/min (after an initial loading dose of 250–500 µg/kg) [20] (see Table 9.4). Intravenous administration of β-blockers should be performed in a monitored setting.

Moderate to severe congestive heart failure can be exacerbated in the acute setting by the administration of β-blockers. However, if the cause of the heart failure was considered to be underlying tachycardia, then β-blockade might be particularly useful. In situations in which the cause of the heart failure cannot be ascertained easily, β-blockade should only be administered with a short-acting drug (esmolol drip), under close hemodynamic monitoring [39].

In patients with reactive or obstructive airway disease, the use of cardio-selective β-blockers (metoprolol, atenolol) can be considered carefully [21].

Atrial fibrillation which occurs in 10–35% of thyroid storm cases [41] must be managed according to current guidelines.

Steroids

Glucocorticoids, mainly hydrocortisone and dexamethasone, have been used as adjuvant therapy in the treatment of thyroid storm, as they each have an inhibitory effect on peripheral conversion of T4 to T3, although the clinical relevance of this relatively minor effect is unknown. An added benefit for the use of steroids in thyroid storm is to treat possible relative adrenal insufficiency. Some studies have found improved survival in patients treated with glucocorticoids, as patients with thyroid storm may have inappropriately normal levels of serum cortisol [3, 42]. Therefore, treatment with glucocorticoids has become a standard practice in patients with thyroid storm because of the possibility of relative adrenal insufficiency or undiagnosed adrenal insufficiency [18]. Hydrocortisone is generally utilized at a dose of 100 mg intravenously every 8 h or dexamethasone at 2 mg intravenously every 6 h, with tapering and discontinuation as the patient improves clinically. When appropriate, relevant biochemical tests can be performed to assess underlying adrenal insufficiency.

Alternative Therapies (See Table 9.4)

Alternative or supplemental therapeutic options can be considered in the management of thyrotoxicosis crisis or thyroid storm when first-line therapies (thionamides, iodide, β-blockers, and glucocorticoids) are less effective than desired or cannot be used due to toxicity, allergy, or intolerance.

Lithium

Lithium appears to be actively concentrated in the thyroid follicular cell [43] and inhibits thyroid hormone release [44]. It can be used in combination with PTU or MMI [45]. Lithium decreases directly thyroid hormone secretion, thereby increasing intrathyroidal iodine content and inhibiting coupling of iodotyrosine residues that form iodothyronines (T4 and T3) [46–48]. Boehm et al. compared the relative therapeutic efficacy of iodine (I) and lithium (Li) in thyrotoxicosis and demonstrated that I and Li together displayed additive inhibition of thyroidal release only if I is administered initially, but the combination, if Li is used first, does not appear to be more effective than Li alone [45].

In thyroid storm, lithium can be used at a dose of 300 mg every 8 h [20]. Lithium levels should be monitored regularly (daily at first) to maintain a concentration of 0.6–1.0 mEq/L [16, 20]. As the patient becomes euthyroid, the lithium concentration may change.

Potassium Perchlorate

The perchlorate anion, ClO_4 −, is a competitive inhibitor of iodide transport [20]. However, historically due to possible side effects of aplastic anemia [49–51] and nephrotic syndrome, its use fell out of favor. The regimen of potassium perchlorate (1 g daily) and MMI (30–50 mg daily) has been found to normalize thyroid hormone levels successfully, with an average duration of treatment of 4 weeks. At this dose and duration, aplastic anemia and nephrotic syndrome did not occur in several studies [52–54].

Anti-adrenergic Agents

Reserpine is an alkaloid agent that depletes catecholamine stores in sympathetic nerve terminals and the central nervous system. Guanethidine also inhibits the release of catecholamines. Side effects of these medications include hypotension and diarrhea. Reserpine can also have central nervous system depressant effects. Guanethidine can be used in thyroid storm at 30–40 mg orally every 6 h and reserpine at 2.5–5 mg intramuscularly every 4 h [16]. These agents are used extremely rarely given the utility of β-blockers.

Cholestyramine

In states of thyrotoxicosis, there is increased enterohepatic circulation of thyroid hormones. Cholestyramine, an anion exchange resin, has also been used in the treatment of thyrotoxicosis, by decreasing the reabsorption of thyroid hormone from the enterohepatic circulation [55]. In several trials, cholestyramine therapy, in combination with MMI or propylthiouracil, caused a more rapid decline in thyroid hormone levels than standard therapy with thionamides alone. Solomon et al. evaluated 15 thyrotoxic patients in a double-blind placebo-controlled cross-over study and found that the cholestyramine-treated group had a more rapid decline in all thyroid hormone levels ($P < 0.01$) than the placebo group [55]. Cholestyramine has been dosed at 4 g orally every 6 h [55–58]. The effect of cholestyramine is generally minimal or moderate, and it should not be administered at the same time as other medications because it may inhibit their absorption. On the other hand, cholestyramine is generally not associated with significant adverse effects.

Plasmapheresis, Charcoal, and Resin Hemoperfusion

Removal of thyroid hormone from circulation must be considered when there is progressive clinical deterioration despite aggressive medical management. Plasmapheresis, charcoal hemoperfusion, resin hemoperfusion, and plasma exchange have been effective in rapidly reducing thyroid hormone levels in thyroid storm [59–62].

Plasmapheresis possibly works by removing thyroxine-binding globulin with bound thyroid hormones. The availability of unbound thyroxine-binding globulin can explain the lowering of free and bound hormone levels after plasmapheresis. In addition, removal of circulating autoantibodies against the thyroid gland could be a possible mechanism for decreased thyrotoxicosis. Plasmapheresis and hemoperfusion have been successfully used to diminish thyrotoxicosis due to thyroid medication overdose [63], iodinated radiocontrast-induced hyperthyroidism, amiodarone-induced hyperthyroidism, and thyrotoxicosis induced by molar pregnancy, as well as in cases of hepatotoxicity and coma induced by antithyroid drugs and in the preoperative and postoperative management of thyroid hormone in patients with severe thyrotoxicosis. Plasmapheresis has also been shown to yield rapid improvement of Graves' ophthalmopathy and pretibial myxedema, perhaps by removing circulating antibodies and immune complexes. It is important to realize, however, that the effect of plasmapheresis on thyrotoxicosis is transient and lasts for approximately 24–48 h. Hence, repeat therapy may be necessary until definitive therapy such as surgical intervention is performed [61].

Burman et al. [60] evaluated the ability of an extracorporeal hemoperfusion system employing neutral Amberlite® resin to bind thyroid hormone and to decrease circulating levels in dogs made thyrotoxic by the intramuscular administration of thyroid hormone. The mean serum T3, T4, and FT4 decreased during 2 h of resin hemoperfusion by 39%, 35%, and 46%, respectively.

Supportive Care/Treatment of Precipitating Cause

Hyperpyrexia is very common in patients with severe thyrotoxicosis. Antipyretics are indicated in this setting, and acetaminophen is the agent of choice. Salicylates should be avoided as they can decrease thyroid protein binding, causing an increase in free thyroid hormone levels [16, 40]. External cooling measures, such as alcohol sponging, ice packs, or a cooling blanket, can also be implemented as appropriate.

Fluid and electrolyte imbalance are also common in severe thyrotoxicosis. The fluid depletion can be secondary from the combination of fever, diaphoresis, vomiting, and diarrhea. Intravenous fluids with dextrose (isotonic saline with 5 or 10% dextrose) are the preferred solution to replenish glycogen stores [40].

Thiamine should be administered on admission to prevent Wernicke's encephalopathy, which could result from the administration of intravenous dextrose in the presence of thiamine deficiency [64, 76]. Thiamine deficiency occurs due to increased metabolic nutrient degradation from thyroid storm.

A fundamental tenet in the management of thyroid storm is assessment for and treatment of a precipitating cause. Given that the most common precipitant is thought to be infection, if a precipitating factor is not apparent, a search for an infectious source would be warranted in the febrile thyrotoxic patient (blood, urine, and sputum cultures and chest radiograph or *noncontrast* CT). However, empiric antibiotics are not recommended without an identified source of infection. Other possible precipitants include diabetic ketoacidosis, myocardial infarction, and pulmonary embolism. In those cases, appropriate management of the specific underlying condition must be started along with the treatment of thyrotoxicosis [3].

Perioperative Management

Preoperative management of the thyrotoxic patient can be divided into two categories: preparation for elective/nonurgent procedures and preparation for emergent procedures.

Elective/Nonurgent Procedures

The standard course of therapy in this setting would be to achieve euthyroidism before surgery. Thionamide therapy would be recommended and would generally achieve euthyroidism within several weeks [21]. The use of iodine as a method of decreasing thyroid vascularity and friability before thyroid surgery has been debated. Several studies have shown some evidence that iodine treatment decreases blood flow to the thyroid gland [65, 66]. However, one retrospective study that compared surgical outcomes in 42 hyperthyroid patients who underwent subtotal thyroidectomy with propranolol treatment alone, or propranolol and iodine treatment, revealed no benefit in terms of intraoperative blood loss [67]. Therefore, it seems reasonable to recommend that in the nonurgent setting, iodine use may be indicated only if thionamides cannot be tolerated.

Emergent Procedures

In this situation, rapid lowering of thyroid hormone levels, control of thyroid hormone release, and control of peripheral manifestations of thyroid hormone are needed. Table 9.6 outlines the management of rapid preparation of thyrotoxic patients for emergent surgery. In this context, emergency surgery could be for a thyroidectomy or for a non-thyroid cause.

Table 9.6 Rapid preparation of thyrotoxic patient for emergent surgery

Medication	Dosage	Postoperatively
Thionamide[a]		
Methimazole	20–30 mg PO q4 h	Stop after total or near-total thyroidectomy.
Propylthiouracil	200–400 mg PO q4 h	Continue after non-thyroidal surgery
Beta-blocker[a]		
Propranolol	60–80 mg PO q4 h or	Continue
	80–120 mg PO q6 h	
Esmolol	50–100 µg/kg/min IV	Change to oral agent
Steroids[a]		
Hydrocortisone	100 mg IV q8 h	Taper over 72 h or as clinically indicated
Dexamethasone	2 mg IV q6 h	
Betamethasone	0.5 mg PO, IM or IV q6 h	
Iodine[a]		
SSKI	5 drops PO q6 h	Stop
Lugol's solution	4–8 drops PO q6–8 h	

Source: Adapted from: Langley and Burch [22]
[a]Use one agent of each group as clinically indicated

In one study, thyroidectomy was performed on the 6th day after preoperative use of betamethasone, iopanoic acid (no longer available), and propranolol. Rapid lowering of thyroid hormone levels occurred with good surgical outcomes [68].

Following thyroidectomy in thyrotoxic patients, treatment with β-blockers may still be required for a short period of time because the half-life of T4 is 7–8 days. However, thionamide therapy usually can be stopped postoperatively, assuming that there is little thyroid tissue remaining.

Preoperative management of thyrotoxic patients aims to achieve a euthyroid status before surgery, hence decreasing significantly morbidity and mortality due to thyroid or non-thyroid surgery [21].

Definitive Therapy

Once the life-threatening aspects of thyroid storm are treated, an evaluation for definitive therapy of thyrotoxicosis must be considered. Thionamide therapy, at gradually decreasing doses, usually is required for weeks to months after thyroid storm, to attain euthyroidism. β-Adrenergic receptor blockade is also needed while the patient is still thyrotoxic. However, as the patient shows clinical improvement, some of the treatment modalities may be tapered and discontinued, as appropriate.

Radioactive iodine ablation may not be able to be used for weeks or months following treatment with inorganic iodine for thyroid storm. Thyroidectomy can be performed once the patient is euthyroid; it is preferable to allow the patient to be euthyroid for several weeks prior to surgery to decrease tissue stores of thyroid hormones. The goal of definitive therapy is to prevent a future recurrence of severe thyrotoxicosis/thyroid storm [3]. Usually radioactive iodine and thyroidectomy result in permanent hypothyroidism, and the patient will be placed on exogenous levothyroxine and have periodic monitoring.

References

1. Karger S. Thyroid storm—thyrotoxic crisis: an update. Dtsch Med Wochenschr. 2008;133(10):479–84.
2. Brooks MH, Waldstein SS, Bronsky D, Sterling K. Serum Triiodothyronine concentration in thyroid storm. J Clin Endocrinol Metab. 1975;40(2):339–41.
3. Burch HB, Wartofsky L. Life-threatening thyrotoxicosis. Thyroid storm. Endocrinol Metab Clin N Am. 1993;22:263–77.
4. Sarlis NJ, Gourgiotis L. Thyroid emergencies. Rev Endocr Metab Disord. 2003;4:129–36.
5. Silva JE, Landsberg L. Catecholamines and the sympathoadrenal system in thyrotoxicosis. In: Braverman LE, Utiger RD, editors. Werner's & Ingbar's the thyroid. 6th ed. Philadelphia: Lipincott, Williams & Wilkins; 1991. p. 816–27.
6. Brooks MH, Waldstein SS. Free thyroxine concentrations in thyroid storm. Ann Intern Med. 1980;93(5):694–7.
7. Goldberg PA, Inzucchi SE. Critical issues in endocrinology. Clin Chest Med. 2003;24:583–606.
8. Wong V, Fu AX, George J, Cheung NW. Thyrotoxicosis induced by alpha-interferon therapy in chronic viral hepatitis. Clin Endocrinol. 2002;56:793–8.
9. Lin YQ, Wang X, Murthy MS, Agarwala S. Life-threatening thyrotoxicosis induced by combination therapy with peg-interferon and ribavirin in chronic hepatitis C. Endocr Pract. 2005;11(2):135–9.
10. Jimenez C, Moran SA, Sereti I, et al. Graves' disease after Interleukin-2 therapy in a patient with Human Immunodeficiency Virus infection. Thyroid. 2004;14(12):1097–101.
11. Kurnik D, Loebstein R, Farfel Z, Ezra D, Halkin H, Olchovsky D. Complex drug-drug-disease interactions between amiodarone, warfarin, and the thyroid gland. Medicine. 2004;83:107–13.
12. Pimental L, Hansen K. Thyroid disease in the emergency department: a clinical and laboratory review. J Emerg Med. 2005;28:201–9.
13. Nayak B, Burman K. Thyrotoxicosis and thyroid storm. Endocrinol Metab Clin N Am. 2006;35:663–86.
14. Dabon-Almirante CL, Surks M. Clinical and laboratory diagnosis of thyrotoxicosis. Endocrinol Metab Clin N Am. 1998;27(1):25–35.
15. Ladenson P. Diagnosis of thyrotoxicosis. In: Braverman LE, Utiger RD, editors. Werner's & Ingbar's the thyroid. 9th ed. Philadelphia: Lipincott, Williams & Wilkins; 2005. p. 660–4.
16. Wartofsky L. Thyrotoxic storm. In: Braverman LE, Utiger RD, editors. Werner's & Ingbar's the thyroid. 9th ed. Philadelphia: Lipincott, Williams & Wilkins; 2005. p. 652–7.
17. Burman KD, Monchik JM, Earll JM, Wartofsky L. Ionized and total serum calcium and parathyroid hormone in hyperthyroidism. Ann Intern Med. 1976;84:668–71.
18. Dluhy RG. The adrenal cortex in thyrotoxicosis. In: Braverman LE, Utiger RD, editors. Werner's & Ingbar's the thyroid. 9th ed. Philadelphia: Lipincott, Williams & Wilkins; 2005. p. 602–3.
19. Tsatsoulis A, Johnson EO, Kalogera CH, Seferiadis K, Tsolas O. The effect of thyrotoxicosis on adrenocortical reserve. Eur J Endocrinol. 2000;142:231–5.
20. Wald D. ECG manifestations of selected metabolic and endocrine disorders. Emerg Med Clin North Am. 2006;24:145–57.
21. Cooper D. Treatment of thyrotoxicosis. In: Braverman LE, Utiger RD, editors. Werner's & Ingbar's the thyroid. 9th ed. Philadelphia: Lipincott, Williams & Wilkins; 2005. p. 665–94.

22. Langley RW, Burch HB. Perioperative management of the thyrotoxic patient. Endocrinol Metab Clin N Am. 2003;32:519–34.
23. Cooper DS. Antithyroid drugs. N Engl J Med. 2005;352:905–17.
24. Nabil N, Miner DJ, Amatruda JM. Methimazole: an alternative route of administration. J Clin Endocrinol Metab. 1982;54(1):180–1.
25. Yeung SC, Go R, Balasubramanyam A. Rectal administration of iodide and propylthiouracil in the treatment of thyroid storm. Thyroid. 1995;5(5):403–5.
26. Walter RM, Bartle WR. Rectal administration of propylthiouracil in the treatment of Graves' disease. Am J Med. 1990;88:69–70.
27. Jongjaroenprasert W, Akarawut W, Chantasart D, Chailurkit L, Rajatanavin R. Rectal administration of propylthiouracil in hyperthyroid patients: comparison of suspension enema and suppository form. Thyroid. 2002;12(7):627–31.
28. Alfandhli E, Gianoukakis A. Management of severe thyrotoxicosis when the gastrointestinal tract is compromised. Thyroid. 2011;21(3):215–20.
29. Okamura Y, Shigemusa C, Tatsuhara T. Pharmacokinetics of methimazole in normal subjects and hyperthyroid patients. Endocrinol Jpn. 1986;33:605–15.
30. Hodak SP, Huang C, Clarke D, Burman KD, Jonklaas J, Janicic-Kharic N. Intravenous methimazole in the treatment of refractory hyperthyroidism. Thyroid. 2006;16(7):691–5.
31. Sowinski J, Junik R, Gembicki M. Effectiveness of intravenous administration of methimazole in patients with thyroid crisis. Endokrynol Pol. 1988;39:67–73.
32. Tajiri J, Noguchi S. Antithyroid drug-induced agranulocytosis: special reference to normal white blood cell count agranulocytosis. Thyroid. 2004;14:459–62.
33. Tajiri J, Noguchi S. Antithyroid drug-induced agranulocytosis: how has granulocyte colonys-timulating factor changed therapy? Thyroid. 2005;15(3):292–7.
34. Tajiri J, Noguchi S, Okamura S, et al. Granulocyte colony-stimulating factor treatment of antithyroid drug-induced granulocytopenia. Arch Intern Med. 1993;153:509–14.
35. Fukata S, Kuma K, Sugawara M. Granulocyte colony-stimulating factor (G-CSF) does not improve recovery from antithyroid drug-induced agranulocytosis. Aprospective study. Thyroid. 1999;9:29–31.
36. Emiliano AB, Governale L, Parks M, Copper DS. Shifts in Propylthiouracil and Methimazole prescribing practices: antithyroid drug use in the United States from 1991–2008. J Clin Endocrinol Metab. 2010;95(5):2227–33.
37. Stagnaro-Green A, Abalovich M, Alexander E, et al. Guidelines of the American thyroid association for the diagnosis and management of thyroid disease during pregnancy and postpartum. Thyroid. 2011;21(10):1081–125.
38. Taurog A. Hormone synthesis: thyroid iodine metabolism. In: Braverman LE, Utiger RD, editors. Werner's & Ingbar's the thyroid. 6th ed. Philadelphia: Lipincott, Williams & Wilkins; 1991. p. 51–97.
39. Burman K. Hyperthyroidism. In: Becker K, editor. Principles and practice of endocrinology and metabolism. 2nd ed. Philadelphia: J.B. Lipincott Company; 1995. p. 367–85.
40. Klein I, Ojamaa K. Thyrotoxicosis and the heart. Endocrinol Metab Clin N Am. 1998;27(1):51–61.
41. McKeown NJ, Tews MC, Gossain V, Shah SM. Hyperthyroidism. Emerg Med Clin N Am. 2005;23:669–85.
42. Presti CE, Hart RG. Thyrotoxicosis, atrial fibrillation, and embolism, revisited. Am Heart J. 1989;117:976–7.
43. Mazzaferri EL, Skillman TG. Thyroid storm. A review of 22 episodes with special emphasis on the use of guanethidine. Arch Intern Med. 1969;124(6):684–90.
44. Berens SC, Wolff J, Murphy DL. Lithium concentration by the thyroid. Endocrinology. 1970;87(5):1085–7.
45. Barbesino G. Drugs affecting thyroid function. Thyroid. 2010;20(7):763–70.
46. Boehm TM, Burman KD, Barnes S, Wartofsky L. Lithium and iodine combination therapy for thyrotoxicosis. Acta Endocrinol. 1980;94:174–83.

47. Berens SC, Bernstein RS, Robbins J, Wolff J. Antithyroid effects of lithium. J Clin Invest. 1970;49(7):1357–67.
48. Burrow GN, Burke WR, Himmelhoch JM, Spencer RP, Hershman JM. Effect of lithium on thyroid function. J Clin Endocrinol Metab. 1971;32(5):647–52.
49. Spaulding SW, Burrow GN, Bermudez F, Himmelhoch JM. The inhibitory effect of lithium on thyroid hormone release in both euthyroid and thyrotoxic patients. J Clin Endocrinol Metab. 1972;35(6):905–11.
50. Barzilai D, Sheinfeld M. Fatal complications following use of potassium perchlorate in thyrotoxicosis. Report of two cases and a review of the literature. Isr J Med Sci. 1966;2(4):453–6.
51. Krevans JR, Asper SP Jr, Rienhoff WF Jr. Fatal aplastic anemia following use of potassium perchlorate. JAMA. 1962;181:162–4.
52. Johnson RS, Moore WG. Fatal aplastic anaemia after treatment of thyrotoxicosis with potassium perchlorate. Br Med J. 1961;1(5236):1369–71.
53. Erdogan MF, Gulec S, Tutar E, Başkal N, Erdogan G. A stepwise approach to the treatment of amiodarone-induced thyrotoxicosis. Thyroid. 2003;13(2):205–9.
54. Bartalena L, Brogioni S, Grasso L, Bogazzi F, Burelli A, Martino E. Treatment of amiodarone induced thyrotoxicosis, a difficult challenge: results of a prospective study. J Clin Endocrinol Metab. 1996;81(8):2930–3.
55. Martino E, Aghini-Lombardi F, Mariotti S, et al. Treatment of amiodarone associated thyrotoxicosis by simultaneous administration of potassium perchlorate and methimazole. J Endocrinol Investig. 1986;9:201–7.
56. Solomon BL, Wartofsky L, Burman KD. Adjunctive cholestyramine therapy for thyrotoxicosis. Clin Endocrinol. 1993;38:39–43.
57. Shakir KM, Michaels RD, Hays JH, Potter BB. The use of bile acid sequestrants to lower serum thyroid hormones in iatrogenic hyperthyroidism. Ann Intern Med. 1993;118(2):112–3.
58. Mercado M, Mendoza-Zubieta V, Bautista-Osorio R, Espinoza-de los Monteros AL. Treatment of hyperthyroidism with a combination of methimazole and cholestyramine. J Clin Endocrinol Metab. 1996;81(9):3191–3.
59. Tsai WC, Pei D, Wang T, et al. The effect of combination therapy with propylthiouracil and cholestyramine in the treatment of Graves' hyperthyroidism. Clin Endocrinol. 2005;62(5):521–4.
60. Burman KD, Yeager HC, Briggs WA, Earll JM, Wartofsky L. Resin hemoperfusion: a method of removing circulating thyroid hormones. J Clin Endocrinol Metab. 1976;42:70–8.
61. Ashkar F, Katims RB, Smoak WM III, Gilson L. Thyroid storm treatment with blood exchange and plasmapheresis. JAMA. 1970;214:1275–9.
62. Vyas AA, Vyas P, Fillipon NL, Vijayakrishnan R, Trivedi N. Successful treatment of thyroid storm with plasmapheresis in a patient with methimazole-induced agranulocytosis. Endocr Pract. 2010;16(4):673–6.
63. Tajiri J, Katsuya H, Kiyokawa T, Urata K, Okamoto K, Shimada T. Successful treatment of thyrotoxic crisis with plasma exchange. Crit Care Med. 1984;12(6):536–7.
64. Kreisner E, Lutzky M, Gross JL. Charcoal hemoperfusion in the treatment of levothyroxine intoxication. Thyroid. 2010;20:209–12.
65. Tietgens ST, Leinung MC. Thyroid storm. Med Clin North Am. 1995;79:169–84.
66. Marigold JH, Morgan AK, Earle DJ, Young AE, Croft DN. Lugol's iodine: its effect on thyroid blood flow in patients with thyrotoxicosis. Br J Surg. 1985;72:45–7.
67. Marmon L, Au FC. The preoperative use of iodine solution in thyrotoxic patients prepared with propranolol. Is it necessary? Am Surg. 1989;55:629–31.
68. Chang DC, Wheeler MH, Woodcock JP, et al. The effect of preoperative Lugol's iodine on thyroid blood flow in patients with Graves' hyperthyroidism. Surgery. 1987;102:1055–61.
69. Baeza A, Aguayo J, Barria M, Pineda G. Rapid preoperative preparation in hyperthyroidism. Clin Endocrinol. 1991;35(5):439–42.
70. Thompson P, Strum D, Boehm T, Wartofsky L. Abnormalities of liver function tests in tyrotoxicosis. Mil Med. 1978;143:548–51.
71. Choudhary AM, Roberts I. Thyroid storm presenting with liver failure. J Clin Gastroenterol. 1999;29:318–21.

72. Doran GR. Serum enzyme disturbances in thyrotoxicosis and myxoedema. J R Soc Med. 1978;71:189–94.
73. Fong TL, McHutchison JG, Reynolds TB. Hyperthyroidism and hepatic dysfunction: a case series analysis. J Clin Gastroenterol. 1992;14:240–4.
74. Bahn R, Burch H, Cooper D, et al. Hyperthyroidism and other causes of thyrotoxicosis: management guidelines of the American thyroid association and American association of clinical endocrinologist. Thyroid. 2011;21(6):593–646.
75. Vanek C, Samuels MH. CNS Vasculitis caused by Propylthiouracil. Thyroid. 2005;15(1):80–4.
76. Reuler JB, Girard DE, Cooney TG. Wernicke's encephalopathy. N Engl J Med. 1985;312:1035–9.

Chapter 10
Myxedema Coma

Ines Donangelo and Glenn D. Braunstein

Précis

1. Clinical setting: A patient with long-standing undiagnosed/untreated hypothyroidism who develops lethargy and hypothermia following a precipitating factor (intercurrent illness, surgery, use of sedatives or narcotics, or exposure to cold).
2. Diagnosis:

   (a) History: Important clues include history of hypothyroidism, thyroid surgery, and radioactive iodine treatment. A precipitating factor is often identified.
   (b) Physical exam: The presence of a thyroidectomy scar on examination. Features of severe hypothyroidism may be present (dry skin, scaly elbows and knees, yellowness of the skin without scleral icterus, coarse hair, puffiness of the face and hands, thinning of the lateral aspects of the eyebrows, macroglossia, hoarseness, delayed relaxation phase of deep tendon reflexes, and bradycardia), in a patient with decreased mental status and hypothermia (core body temperature <35 °C).
   (c) Laboratory values: Elevated TSH and low free T4 in primary hypothyroidism, while in central hypothyroidism, TSH is low normal to low. Cortisol levels should be obtained at the baseline, ideally following Cortrosyn stimulation.

3. Management: Treatment of myxedema coma is based on thyroid hormone replacement, glucocorticoids, supportive care, and management of coexisting illness such as infection. Thyroid hormone should be given as a venous loading

I. Donangelo
Department of Medicine, David Geffen School of Medicine, University of California Los Angeles, Los Angeles, CA, USA

G. D. Braunstein (✉)
Medicine/Endocrinology, Cedars-Sinai Medical Center, Los Angeles, CA, USA
e-mail: glenn.braunstein@cshs.org

© Springer Nature Switzerland AG 2021   93
L. Loriaux, C. Vanek (eds.), *Endocrine Emergencies*, Contemporary Endocrinology,
https://doi.org/10.1007/978-3-030-67455-7_10

dose followed by a daily maintenance dose of levothyroxine (200–500 μg IV loading, followed by 70–100 μg IV daily), liothyronine (10–20 μg IV loading, followed by 10 μg IV or by nasogastric tube every 4–6 h for days 2 to 3), or a combination of both (levothyroxine 200–300 μg IV followed by 100 μg IV 24 h later and 50 μg daily IV/PO/NG daily thereafter; liothyronine 10 μg IV and then 10 μg every 8–12 h until the patient is alert, at which time a switch to levothyroxine only regimen should be made). There are no prospective studies comparing outcomes with these different replacement regimens. Stress doses of hydrocortisone (50 mg IV every 6–8 h) should be given pending cortisol axis evaluation results due to the possibility of concomitant adrenal insufficiency, which occurs in 5–10% of cases. Supportive measures include early mechanical ventilation when indicated, passive rewarming for hypothermia, vasopressor agents for hemodynamic instability, and standard intensive care unit measures.

Introduction

"For the last few months my mother has been slowing down and today she stopped". (Son of an elderly woman presenting with myxedema coma as related to Dr. Braunstein.)

Myxedema coma is defined by severe and prolonged depletion of thyroid hormone leading to altered mental status, typically associated with hypothermia and other symptoms related to widespread organ system dysfunction. Although myxedema coma is currently a rare presentation of hypothyroidism given the widespread measurement of thyroid function with thyrotropin-secreting hormone (TSH) assays, its early recognition and treatment are crucial because of the high mortality associated with delays in the treatment of this medical emergency. The clinical presentation often follows prolonged symptoms of thyroid dysfunction, followed by a decrease in mental status related to an identifiable precipitating event. There may be a history of radioactive iodine treatment or prior thyroid surgery, or a thyroidectomy scar may be noted on physical exam. Initiation of treatment should be based on clinical suspicion and not delayed until the results of laboratory tests are available.

Historical Remarks

Adult patients with symptoms suggestive of severe hypothyroidism were not recognized until the nineteenth century, with the first reports of women who, though adults, looked like cretinous children. Dr. William M. Ord (1834–1902) described autopsy findings on such patients: "the skin in particular retained its oedematous condition even when cut up into small fragments, whereas the skin of dropsical patients collapses when so treated" and that it contained an excess of mucin as assessed by a crude gravimetric test. He gave it a specific name, myxedema ("mucinous edema"). He did find the thyroid follicles "mostly annihilated" but thought this—as everything else—was due to excess mucin. In 1888, the Committee to Investigate the Subject of Myxoedema presented their report at the Clinical Society of London. It included an analysis of clinical information on 109 patients with myxedema and the results on experimental animal models of thyroidectomy and concluded that: "While [myxoedema and endemic cretinism]…depend on, or… are associated with destruction or loss of the function of the thyroid gland, the ultimate cause of such destruction or loss is at present not evident." They noted that patients had "expressionless, apathetic, large-featured" physiognomy, intellectual slowness, "subnormal" body temperature, and often exhibited "watery dropsy." Worsening of symptoms culminating in death occurred in a subset of patients due to "pneumonia, exhaustion, coma, collapse, suffocation or increasing slowness of mind." At that time, there was no inkling of any treatment involving transplants or injection of thyroid tissue or thyroid extracts. Warmth, jaborandi (a plant containing alkaloids including pilocarpine), purified pilocarpine, and nitroglycerine were favored as treatment options.

Myxoedema (spelled myxedema after a while) is now recognized as a manifestation of hypothyroidism rather than being a specific separate disease. Much of the abnormal physical appearance of patients with myxedema is due to the excessive production of glycosaminoglycans, the present-day equivalent of "mucin," in the absence of adequate quantities of thyroid hormone. The term myxedema coma has remained to indicate extreme presentation of untreated or inadequately treated hypothyroidism [1].

Pathogenesis

Myxedema coma can result from the usual causes of hypothyroidism such as chronic autoimmune thyroiditis and post-ablative hypothyroidism (Table 10.1 [2–5]). The progression from long-standing untreated hypothyroidism to myxedema coma can

Table 10.1 Disorders that can result in hypothyroidism and myxedema coma	
	Chronic autoimmune (or Hashimoto's) thyroiditis
	Postsurgical hypothyroidism
	Post-ablative (^{131}I) hypothyroidism
	Neck irradiation
	Central hypothyroidism due to hypothalamic or pituitary disorder
	Drug-induced hypothyroidism
	Lithium
	Amiodarone
	Sunitinib
	Excessive consumption of goitrogenic foods, such as raw Chinese white cabbage (bok choy)
	Information from Refs. [2–5]

Table 10.2 Common precipitating factors of myxedema coma

Infection, especially pneumonia or sepsis
Surgery
Cerebrovascular accident
Myocardial infarction
Congestive heart failure
Gastrointestinal hemorrhage
Acute trauma
Exposure to cold
Drugs
Sedatives (narcotics, tranquilizers, anesthetics)
Cardiac medications (amiodarone, beta-blockers)
Diuretics
Lithium
Phenytoin
Rifampin

Information from Refs. [2, 3, 6, 7]

be precipitated by an acute insult such as infection, surgery, myocardial infarction, or the use of sedative drugs (Table 10.2 [2, 3, 6, 7]).

The decrease in serum thyroxine (T4) results in lowering of serum and intracellular triiodothyronine (T3). This decrease in intracellular T3 can cause (a) decrease in thermogenesis resulting in hypothermia; (b) decrease sensitivity to adrenergic stimuli, with resulting decreased cardiac inotropism (decreased cardiac output), chronotropism (bradycardia), and vasoconstriction that may culminate in hypotension and shock [8]; (c) increase free water retention due to decrease in renal perfusion, excessive antidiuretic hormone secretion, and increase in vascular permeability, resulting in hyponatremia and effusions; (d) decrease in central nervous system sensitivity to hypercapnia and hypoxia and respiratory muscle weakness resulting in respiratory insufficiency [9]; and (e) slowing of central nervous system function leading to altered mental status. In myxedema coma, decreased mental status is multifactorial and related to the combination of the direct effect of low thyroid hormone action in the central nervous system, cerebral anoxia and hypercapnia from respiratory insufficiency, hemodynamic instability resulting in reduced brain perfusion, and electrolyte abnormalities [10].

Clinical Presentation

The classic presentation of myxedema coma is that of an elderly female with long-standing hypothyroidism who develops an intercurrent illness, is given sedatives or narcotics or exposed to cold weather, and develops lethargy and hypothermia. It is important to keep a high degree of clinical suspicion, as myxedema coma can occur in males and younger patients, and may be related due to some of the less common causal agents listed in Table 10.1. The features of severe hypothyroidism can be present, including dry skin, scaly elbows and knees, yellowness of the skin without scleral icterus, coarse hair, puffiness of the face and hands, thinning of the lateral aspects of the eyebrows, macroglossia, hoarseness, delayed relaxation phase of deep tendon reflexes, and bradycardia. Patients with severe hypothyroidism can develop effusions (pericardial and pleural) that do not cause organ compromise because of their slow rate of formation. Decreased mental status and hypothermia are characteristic of myxedema coma. The term myxedema coma, however, is a misnomer as most patients do not present with frank coma but only signs of cognitive deterioration, such as lethargy, confusion, or disorientation. Diastolic hypertension can be present, but hypotension that may progress to shock can occur due to sepsis or other causes of decreased cardiac output [8]. Hyponatremia is a common electrolyte abnormality in the severe hypothyroid state and results from decreased free water clearance due to increased release of antidiuretic hormone and decreased renal blood flow from hypotension or decreased cardiac output. Hypoglycemia results from decreased gluconeogenesis and reduced insulin clearance. Hypoglycemia also can be a sign of adrenal insufficiency which can be present in a small subset of patients with myxedema coma, especially those with hypopituitarism as the etiology of hypothyroidism or in patients with the polyglandular autoimmune failure syndrome. Hypoventilation with respiratory acidosis also can be encountered in myxedema coma. Late-onset epilepsy that resolves with thyroid hormone replacement is described in severe hypothyroidism [11], and myxedema coma presenting in status epilepticus is reported [12, 13]. Clinical features of myxedema

Table 10.3 Clinical finding in myxedema coma	
Hypothermia	
	Core body temperature (<35 °C or 95 °F)
	Infection with the absence of fever
Decreased mental status	
	Confusion, lethargy, obtundation, or coma
Cardiovascular abnormalities	
	Bradycardia
	Decreased myocardial contractility
	Low cardiac output
	Hypotension or shock
Respiratory abnormalities	
	Central depression of ventilator drive
	Respiratory muscle weakness
	Mechanical obstruction by large tongue or edema of vocal cords
Laboratory abnormalities	
	Respiratory acidosis due to hypoventilation
	Hypoglycemia, directly due to hypothyroidism or due to associated adrenal insufficiency
	Hyponatremia, due to impaired free water excretion
	Anemia, typically normocytic normochromic from decreased erythropoiesis
Acquired von Willebrand syndrome type 1 [15]	
	Elevation in muscle-derived creatinine phosphokinase, due to increased muscle permeability

coma are listed in Table 10.3. A more active presentation of hypothyroidism that includes psychotic manifestations (delusions, visual hallucinations, auditory hallucinations, perseveration, loose associations, and paranoia) can occur—a condition known as "myxedema madness." There is no clear correlation between the degree of thyroid dysfunction and development of psychiatric symptoms [14]. The precipitating insult should be sought, if not already clinically evident (Table 10.2). Infections can present without fever in patients with myxedema coma.

Diagnosis

The diagnosis should be considered in patients with altered mental status who have hypothermia and other features of severe hypothyroidism. Other causes of decreased mental status could lead or contribute to a similar presentation and should be sought on history and through investigation, including drugs (ethanol, toxins), infections of the central nervous system, severe sepsis, metabolic disorders (diabetes, uremia), or traumatic brain injury. The history obtained from family members can reveal a diagnosis of hypothyroidism or past radioactive iodine treatment. Evidence of a thyroidectomy by a surgical scar on examination is an important clue.

Essential laboratory tests include TSH, free T4, and cortisol. If possible, the cortisol axis should be investigated in more detail with cosyntropin (Cortrosyn™ ACTH) stimulation test (serum cortisol before, and 30 min, and 60 min after cosyntropin 250 μg as an intravenous bolus). Therapy can be started empirically if clinically indicated pending laboratory results, although laboratories in large clinical centers currently can provide a TSH result in 1–2 h.

In most patients, the etiology of myxedema coma is primary hypothyroidism, and the laboratory results will show elevated TSH and low free T4. TSH may not be as elevated as expected for the low level of free T4. This is usually due to intercurrent illness or the use of dopamine and/or glucocorticoids. On the other hand, a normal-to-low or low TSH coupled with a low free T4 value indicates central hypothyroidism, especially if associated with adrenal insufficiency and other clues such as inappropriately normal gonadotropins in postmenopausal women or a history of pituitary surgery. It can be difficult to differentiate patients with myxedema coma due to central hypothyroidism from ill patients with the nonthyroidal illness ("euthyroid sick") syndrome associated with decreased mental status. Nonthyroidal illness can present with a low TSH and a low total T3 due to critical illness and the drugs used to treat the patient in the intensive care unit setting, free T4 measured by immunoassays can be low due to interference with abnormally high levels of thyroid hormone-binding globulin, but free T4 measured by the equilibrium dialysis method is normal.

Management

Myxedema coma is associated with a high mortality and should be treated aggressively. Several factors on presentation may serve as indicators of a worse prognosis. One prospective study from India evaluated prognostic factors in 23 patients treated for myxedema coma. They noted that hypotension and bradycardia at presentation, hypothermia unresponsive to treatment, sepsis, the need for mechanical ventilation, sedative drugs, and a poor score on models that estimate outcome (Glasgow Coma Scale; Acute Physiology and Chronic Health Evaluation II (APACHEII); and Sequential Organ Failure Assessment (SOFA) scores) all were associated with increased mortality [16]. A Spanish study prospectively evaluated 11 patients treated for myxedema coma and found that, in addition to lower Glasgow Coma Scale and APACHEII scores, the lower level of consciousness on presentation was significantly associated with mortality [17]. A review of 87 cases of myxedema coma (8 new and 79 reported in the medical literature) revealed that increasing age and increasing frequency of cardiac abnormalities correlate with fatal outcomes [18]. Advanced age and the use of catecholamines were also associated with increased mortality [19].

Treatment of myxedema coma is based on thyroid hormone replacement, glucocorticoids, supportive care, and management of coexisting illness such as infection. Addressing all these components of care in a prompt and intense manner led to a considerable decrease in mortality from myxedema coma. Mortality dropped from close to 100% to the current rates of 30–50% [15–17].

There is no consensus on the optimal mode of thyroid hormone replacement in patients with myxedema coma, largely because the condition is so rare that there are no clinical trials comparing different treatment regimens. Therefore, most recommendations are based on expert opinion [20]. The preferred route of administration of thyroid hormone is intravenous, as oral medications may be poorly absorbed due to gastric atony or ileus. Although oral absorption of levothyroxine (LT4) is variable, the clinical response occurs promptly [17], and in one small observational study, the route of administration (oral or intravenous) did not affect mortality [16], suggesting that if intravenous thyroid hormone is not readily available, oral LT4 is a reasonable alternative.

Data on mortality and outcome comparing LT4 or liothyronine (LT3) only with combined LT4/LT3 regimens are lacking, again due to the rarity of the condition.

Table 10.4 Proposed methods of replacement with thyroid hormone in patients with myxedema coma

Method	Thyroid hormone	Loading dose[a]	Daily maintenance dose
1	Levothyroxine	200–500 µg IV	70–100 µg IV or
			100–150 µg (1.6 µg/kg) PO/NGT
2	Liothyronine	10–20 µg IV	10 µg IV/PO/NGT every 4–6 h
3[b]	Levothyroxine	200–300 µg IV	100 µg IV 24 h after loading dose, followed by 50 µg IV/PO daily
	Liothyronine	10 µg IV	10 µg IV every 8–12 h, until patient can take PO and then switch to LT4 PO regimen only

IV intravenous, PO oral administration, NGT nasogastric tube administration
[a]Thyroid hormone loading dose should be titrated to the lower end of recommended dose in elderly and patients with ischemic heart disease
[b]Replacement method suggested in [24]

We have chosen to describe all three methods of replacement (Table 10.4). The first approach is to replace with LT4 only. The average size of the extrathyroidal T4 pool is 500 µg per 1.73 m² in a normal person and may be reduced to lower than 250 µg per 1.73 m² in hypothyroidism [21]. Therefore, to restore this pool, the initial LT4 dose should be 200–500 µg IV given intravenously. Given that T4 has a volume of distribution of about 10 L, this dose will raise total serum T4 by 2–5 µg/dL. Thyroxine levels should be within the reference range in the first 48 h after starting replacement. The normal turnover rate of thyroid hormone is 10% or about 50 µg per day [22]. In one study, the daily production of thyroxine was estimated to range between 80 and 100 µg [19]. This is thought to be a little high by most authorities. Therefore, after the loading dose, the maintenance replacement dose of LT4 should be about 70-100 µg IV daily or 100–150 µg (1.6 µg/kg) oral daily dose (oral LT4 has bioavailability of approximately 70% of intravenous LT4).

The second approach is to treat with LT3 only. In hypothyroid patients without major intercurrent illness, LT4 alone may suffice to increase serum T3 levels to normal in 2–3 days due to normal activity of the 5′-deiodinase enzyme that converts T4 into T3. However, critically ill patients with multiple organ dysfunction may have reduced 5′-deiodinase activity. The patients, therefore, may benefit from supplemental LT3 replacement. Moreover, T3 works more rapidly than T4 [23]. The proportion of T4:T3 produced by the normal thyroid gland is approximately 80:20, with the normal daily production of triiodothyronine between 30 and 40 µg [19]. A dose of LT3 of 10–20 µg intravenously can be given initially, followed by 10 µg intravenously or per nasogastric tube every 4–6 h, depending on the patient's age and coexistent cardiac risk factors. This is followed by oral LT3 or LT4 therapy once there is improvement.

Finally, some authorities prefer to treat with a combination of LT4 and LT3. Wartofsky and associates recommend intravenous LT4 at a dose of 4 µg/kg lean body weight (~200–300 µg) initially and then 100 µg 24 h later, followed by 50 µg daily. LT3 is given initially as 10 µg intravenously and repeated every 8–12 h until the patient is alert enough to take maintenance oral doses of LT4 [24].

Elderly patients and those with ischemic heart disease may need smaller doses of thyroid hormone, and all patients should have the heart rhythm continuously monitored during the early phases of replacement. High daily doses of thyroid hormone replacement (LT4 ≥ 500 µg or LT3 ≥ 75 µg daily) are associated with increased mortality, especially in the elderly [17, 18].

The incidence of decreased adrenal function in patients with myxedema coma is about 5–10%. Thus, intravenous cortisol is indicated before initiating thyroid hormone therapy and should be continued until adrenal function is known to be normal [20]. Patients with myxedema coma could have associated hypopituitarism and secondary adrenal insufficiency or primary adrenal insufficiency due to concomitant autoimmune gland dysfunction. Patients should be treated with stress dose steroids, i.e., hydrocortisone 50 mg IV every 6–8 h. In critically ill patients, if serum cortisol is greater than 20–30 µg/dL, then steroid support is probably unnecessary. If serum cortisol is lower than 20 µg/dL, stress dose steroid should be continued for the first 48 h, and then the dose may be tapered over the next few days in parallel with clinical improvement, unless a diagnosis of adrenal insufficiency is made of the adrenal axis (Cortrosyn stimulation testing). In this situation, plans should be made to convert the patient over to oral glucocorticoids for the ongoing treatment of adrenal insufficiency.

Supportive measures are an important component of care for patients with myxedema coma. Early intubation and mechanical ventilation are life-saving for patients with hypoventilation and profound decrease in mental status. Posterior pharyngeal edema complicating endotracheal intubation is described in myxedema coma [25]. Passive rewarming is indicated for hypothermia, but active rewarming should be avoided since it can promote vasodilation and hypotension. Vasopressor agents are indicated for hemodynamic instability. Free water restriction may be needed to help correct hyponatremia. Fluid overload should be avoided. If necessary, small amounts of hypertonic saline can be used to treat severe hyponatremia (serum sodium <120 mEq/L). Sedative medications should be restricted when possible as their blood levels may accumulate due to decreased metabolism.

References

1. The Clinical Society of London—Report of a Committee nominated December 14, 1883 to Investigate the subject of myxoedema. Canton, MA: Science History Publications, a division of Watson Publishing International; 1888 (facsimile edition 1991).
2. Mazonson PD, Williams ML, Cantley LK, Dalldorf FG, Utiger RD, Foster JR. Myxedema coma during long-term amiodarone therapy. Am J Med. 1984;77(4):751–4.
3. Waldman SA, Park D. Myxedema coma associated with lithium therapy. Am J Med. 1989;87(3):355–6.
4. Chen SY, Kao PC, Lin ZZ, Chiang WC, Fang CC. Sunitinib-induced myxedema coma. Am J Emerg Med. 2009;27(3):370.e371–3.
5. Chu M, Seltzer TF. Myxedema coma induced by ingestion of raw bok choy. N Engl J Med. 2010;362(20):1945–6.
6. Olsen CG. Myxedema coma in the elderly. J Am Board Fam Pract. 1995;8(5):376–83.
7. Yuan Y, Hu Y, Xie T, Zhao Y. Myxedema coma after esophagectomy. Ann Thorac Surg. 2010;90(1):295–7.
8. Klein I. Thyroid hormone and the cardiovascular system. Am J Med. 1990;88(6):631–7.
9. Zwillich CW, Pierson DJ, Hofeldt FD, Lufkin EG, Weil JV. Ventilatory control in myxedema and hypothyroidism. N Engl J Med. 1975;292(13):662–5.
10. Gardner DG. Myxedema coma. In: David G, Gardner DS, editors. Greenspan's basic and clinical endocrinology. 9th ed. New York: McGraw-Hill; 2007.
11. Evans EC. Neurologic complications of myxedema: convulsions. Ann Intern Med. 1960;52:434–44.
12. Jansen HJ, Doebe SR, Louwerse ES, van der Linden JC, Netten PM. Status epilepticus caused by a myxoedema coma. Neth J Med. 2006;64(6):202–5.
13. Woods KL, Holmes GK. Myxoedema coma presenting in status epilepticus. Postgrad Med J. 1977;53(615):46–8.
14. Heinrich TW, Grahm G. Hypothyroidism presenting as psychosis: myxedema madness revisited. Prim Care Companion J Clin Psychiatry. 2003;5(6):260–6.
15. Manfredi E, van Zaane B, Gerdes VE, Brandjes DP, Squizzato A. Hypothyroidism and acquired von Willebrand's syndrome: a systematic review. Haemophilia. 2008;14:423–33.

16. Dutta P, Bhansali A, Masoodi SR, Bhadada S, Sharma N, Rajput R. Predictors of outcome in myxoedema coma: a study from a tertiary care centre. Crit Care. 2008;12(1):R1.
17. Rodriguez I, Fluiters E, Perez-Mendez LF, Luna R, Paramo C, Garcia-Mayor RV. Factors associated with mortality of patients with myxoedema coma: prospective study in 11 cases treated in a single institution. J Endocrinol. 2004;180(2):347–50.
18. Yamamoto T, Fukuyama J, Fujiyoshi A. Factors associated with mortality of myxedema coma: report of eight cases and literature survey. Thyroid. 1999;9(12):1167–74.
19. Ono Y, Ono S, Yasunaga H, Matsui H, Fushimi K, Tanaka Y. Clinical characteristics and outcomes of myxedema coma: analysis of a national inpatient database in Japan. J Epidemiol. 2017;20:117–22.
20. Jonklaas J, Bianco AC, Bauer AJ, Burman KD, Cappola AR, Celi FS, Cooper DS, Kim BW, Peeters RP, Rosenthal MS, Sawka AM. Guidelines for the treatment of hypothyroidism. Prepared by the American Thyroid Association Task Force on Thyroid Hormone Replacement. Thyroid. 2014;24:1670–751.
21. Sterling K, Chodos RB. Radiothyroxine turnover studies in myxedema, thyrotoxicosis, and hypermetabolism without endocrine disease. J Clin Invest. 1956;35(7):806–13.
22. Ingbar SH, Freinkel N. Simultaneous estimation of rates of thyroxine degradation and thyroid hormone synthesis. J Clin Invest. 1955;34(6):808–19.
23. Brent GAKR. Thyroid and Anti-thyroid Drugs. In: Brunton LLCB, Knollmann BC, editors. Goodman & Gilman's the pharmacological basis of therapeutics. 12th ed. New York: McGraw-Hill; 2011.
24. Klubo-Gwiezdzinska J, Wartofsky L. Thyroid emergencies. Med Clin North Am. 2012;96:385–403.
25. Lee CH, Wira CR. Severe angioedema in myxedema coma: a difficult airway in a rare endocrine emergency. Am J Emerg Med. 2009;27(8):1021.e1021–2.

Chapter 11
Acute Suppurative Thyroiditis

J. Stone Doggett and Brian Wong

Précis

1. Clinical Setting: Fever, leukocytosis, and neck pain, often associated with asymmetrical thyroid enlargement.
2. Diagnosis:

    (a) History: Thyroid infection is rare, and an underlying alteration in host susceptibility is usually present. These include congenital fistula from the pyriform sinus to the thyroid gland, persistent thyroglossal duct, thyroid nodules, and immunocompromised state.
    (b) Physical examination: Pain on palpating the thyroid gland is the primary finding. Most patients are euthyroid. Most patients will have fever (92%), dysphagia (91%), dermal erythema (82%), and dysphoria (82%).
    (c) Laboratory values: Most patients have leukocytosis of greater than 10,000 cells/mm^3, with a left shift. Thyroid function tests are usually in the normal range.

    Imaging: CT scan is the preferred first modality. Usually, an abscess is revealed if present. When possible, an ultrasound-guided fine needle aspiration of the abscess should be done. White cells and microbes revealed by gram stains strongly suggest a suppurative thyroiditis. Giant cells and granulomas point toward a painful nonsuppurative acute thyroiditis.

    Treatment: The initial antibiotic therapy should cover gram-positive, gram-negative, and anaerobic organisms. If the patient is not allergic to penicillin, ampicillin-sulbactam plus vancomycin should be administered intravenously.

J. S. Doggett (✉) · B. Wong
Division of Infectious Disease, Oregon Health and Science University, Portland, OR, USA
e-mail: doggettj@ohsu.edu

© Springer Nature Switzerland AG 2021   103
L. Loriaux, C. Vanek (eds.), *Endocrine Emergencies*, Contemporary Endocrinology,
https://doi.org/10.1007/978-3-030-67455-7_11

Penicillin-allergic patients should be treated with ceftriaxone plus metronidazole plus vancomycin. If an attempt to aspirate for abscess contents is anticipated, it should precede the administration of antibiotics of any kind.

Acute Suppurative Thyroiditis

Of the multiple types of thyroiditis, acute and chronic suppurative thyroiditis are the two types in which there is an ongoing infection of the thyroid gland. Although there is a presumed relationship between viral infections and painful subacute thyroiditis, painful subacute thyroiditis is typically self-limited, and treatment is aimed at decreasing inflammation and addressing fluctuations in thyroid hormone [1]. Chronic and acute suppurative thyroiditis can be caused by bacteria, mycobacteria, fungi, or parasites. Acute suppurative thyroiditis is most often caused by bacteria, can progress rapidly, and can be fatal if not treated emergently. Clinical knowledge of acute suppurative thyroiditis is based primarily on retrospective case reports and case series. Despite the paucity of clinical studies, recent attempts have been made to construct a treatment algorithm for acute suppurative thyroiditis [2, 3].

Predisposing Factors

Thyroid infection is rare, and an underlying host susceptibility is present in most cases. Frequently, immunocompetent patients with acute suppurative thyroiditis have a congenital fistula from the pyriform sinus that extends to the thyroid capsule. This defect provides a tract for pathogens to establish infection in or around the thyroid gland and is the most common predisposing factor in children [4]. Otherwise, in an immunocompetent host, the thyroid gland can become infected through a persistent thyroglossal duct or by direct spread from an adjacent tissue infection or from trauma. In individuals who are immunocompromised or have preexisting thyroid disease, such as thyroid nodules or thyroid malignancy, infection can develop through hematogenous or lymphatic spread. Case reports describe a wide range of nonbacterial pathogens that cause suppurative thyroiditis in immunocompromised patients. Patients with AIDS, as an example, are reported to develop suppurative thyroiditis due to the opportunistic fungal pathogen *Pneumocystis jirovecii* [5]. Preexisting thyroid disease has been observed in 61% of reported patients with suppurative thyroiditis [6].

Suppurative thyroiditis can occur within the first year of life or in the elderly. The average age of patients with acute suppurative thyroiditis in a literature review of 153 cases reported from 1900 to 1980 was 30 years for men and 35 years for women [6]. Twenty-two of these cases occurred in children under 10 years of age.

Microbiology

The majority of acute suppurative thyroiditis cases are caused by *Staphylococcus aureus* and *Streptococcus* species [6]. However, a broad range of pathogens are reported, and infections may be due to gram-negative, anaerobic, or polymicrobial infection [3]. Drug-resistant pathogens, such as methicillin-resistant *Staphylococcus aureus* (MRSA), have been reported as well [7].

Clinical Presentation

An acute suppurative thyroiditis can be difficult to distinguish from painful subacute thyroiditis or from head and neck infections such as parapharyngeal abscesses. Acute suppurative thyroiditis differs from Hashimoto's thyroiditis and other painless forms of thyroiditis in that pain is typically a prominent aspect of the patient's presentation. The majority of patients with acute suppurative thyroiditis are euthyroid, but hyperthyroidism may result from inflammation, or hypothyroidism may occur due to tissue destruction. In contrast, thyroid hormone abnormalities are common in painful subacute thyroiditis [8]. When there is thyrotoxicosis, both painful subacute thyroiditis and suppurative thyroiditis have low radioactive iodine uptake. Moreover, patients with acute suppurative thyroiditis tend to be acutely ill, and infection can occur after a respiratory tract infection or with concurrent pharyngitis.

Based on case reports, the most common features are anterior cervical pain (100%), fever (92%), dysphagia (91%), dermal erythema (82%), and dysphonia (82%) [6]. Leukocytosis of greater than 10,000 cells/mm^3 is present in 73% of patients. The left lobe is the most frequently involved area of the thyroid. The above features may be present in subacute thyroiditis, but they are much less common and should raise suspicion for acute suppurative thyroiditis [9].

Diagnosis

Initial imaging can be performed with ultrasound or CT. When there is concern for extensive infection outside of the thyroid, CT with intravenous contrast may be needed to define the extent of thyroid infection and the involvement of adjacent tissue. However, it should be noted that intravenous iodinated contrast will interfere with radioactive iodine thyroid uptake scans for several weeks. Typically, thyroid imaging in acute suppurative thyroiditis shows an abscess, whereas in painful subacute thyroiditis, the thyroid appears diffusely heterogeneous. If suppurative thyroiditis is suspected, and the patient is stable, evaluation with ultrasound-guided fine needle aspiration should be pursued to identify the pathogen. Fine needle aspiration can also be used to distinguish painful subacute thyroiditis from acute suppurative thyroiditis by demonstrating giant cells and granulomas as opposed to abscess formation with microorganisms. If there is airway compromise, cultures should be obtained during aggressive drainage of infection with surgery or percutaneous drainage. The identification of a pyriform fistula is often not possible during the acute inflammatory period but can be seen on imaging studies or endoscopically once the inflammation is decreased. Radiographic evaluation for a pyriform fistula can be done with a barium swallow or a CT scan with trumpet maneuver in which the patient inflates a syringe during the scan [2].

Treatment

The management of acute suppurative thyroiditis has been debated recently [2, 3]. While there are differing approaches to abscess drainage and the duration of antibiotic therapy, there is agreement that initial therapy includes broad antibacterial coverage. Empiric therapy should include coverage for gram-positive, gram-negative, and anaerobic bacteria and should be based on local antibiotic susceptibility patterns. Coverage for drug-resistant bacteria, particularly MRSA, should be considered. Once culture results are available, antibiotics can be tailored to the pathogen. Drainage of infection is indicated when there is airway obstruction or an abscess. In cases of extensive infection, or when there is no improvement with drainage and antibiotics, thyroidectomy may be required. Infection in the setting of preexisting thyroid disease is often more difficult to treat [2].

A pyriform fistula is more easily detected once acute inflammation resolves [10]. Endoscopic obliteration of the fistula can be performed with chemical or electrical cauterization during the infected period. It is more often done with a surgical fistulectomy after infection has resolved. The total duration of antibiotics should be determined on a case-by-case basis and guided by clinical response. After initial clinical improvement, parenteral antibiotics may be changed to oral antibiotics and targeted toward cultured pathogens. The total duration of antibiotic therapy has not been formally studied; however, a minimum duration of 14 days has been recommended [3].

Summary

Acute suppurative thyroiditis is a medical emergency that usually presents with anterior neck pain, fever, and dysphagia and can lead to airway obstruction. Differentiating acute suppurative thyroiditis from painful subacute thyroiditis or invasive head and neck infections usually requires diagnostic imaging with CT or ultrasound. In certain instances, tissue histology obtained by fine needle aspiration may be required to definitively diagnose acute suppurative thyroiditis. Obtaining cultures by aspiration, surgery, or percutaneous drainage is required to guide antibiotic therapy. Acute suppurative thyroiditis should be treated urgently with antibiotics and abscess drainage. Consultation with a surgeon and an infectious diseases specialist should be done when possible. The majority of immunocompetent patients will have a pyriform sinus fistula that can be detected endoscopically, by a barium swallow study or by a CT scan with the trumpet maneuver. Anatomic defects, such as a pyriform sinus fistula, should be corrected, to prevent recurrent infection:

- Acute suppurative thyroiditis is typically a bacterial infection of the thyroid that occurs in patients who have a congenital pyriform fistula but may occur in patients that are immunocompromised or have underlying thyroid disease.
- CT or ultrasound is the preferred initial diagnostic test.
- Acute suppurative thyroiditis should be treated emergently with parenteral antibiotics and abscess drainage.

References

1. Desailloud R, Hober D. Viruses and thyroiditis: an update. Virol J. 2009;6:5.
2. Miyauchi A. Thyroid gland: a new management algorithm for acute suppurative thyroiditis? Nat Rev Endocrinol. 2010;6(8):424–6.
3. Paes JE, Burman KD, Cohen J, et al. Acute bacterial suppurative thyroiditis: a clinical review and expert opinion. Thyroid. 2010;20(3):247–55.
4. Smith SL, Pereira KD. Suppurative thyroiditis in children: a management algorithm. Pediatr Emerg Care. 2008;24(11):764–7.
5. Golshan MM, McHenry CR, de Vente J, Kalajyian RC, Hsu RM, Tomashefski JF. Acute suppurative thyroiditis and necrosis of the thyroid gland: a rare endocrine manifestation of acquired immunodeficiency syndrome. Surgery. 1997;121(5):593–6.
6. Berger SA, Zonszein J, Villamena P, Mittman N. Infectious diseases of the thyroid gland. Rev Infect Dis. 1983;5(1):108–22.
7. Lethert K, Bowerman J, Pont A, Earle K, Garcia-Kennedy R. Methicillin-resistant Staphylococcus aureus suppurative thyroiditis with thyrotoxicosis. Am J Med. 2006;119(11):e1–2.
8. Pearce EN, Farwell AP, Braverman LE. Thyroiditis. N Engl J Med. 2003;348(26):2646–55.
9. Al-Dajani N, Wootton SH. Cervical lymphadenitis, suppurative parotitis, thyroiditis, and infected cysts. Infect Dis Clin N Am. 2007;21(2):523–41, viii.
10. Masuoka H, Miyauchi A, Tomoda C, et al. Imaging studies in sixty patients with acute suppurative thyroiditis. Thyroid. 2011;21(10):1075–80.

Chapter 12
Hyponatremia: SIADH

Raghav Wusirika and David H. Ellison

Précis

1. Clinical setting: Hyponatremia in the ambulatory or hospital setting.
2. Diagnosis:

    (a) History: The presence of cancer, especially of the lung or brain; infections of the lung or central nervous system; use of drugs known to predispose to syndrome of inappropriate antidiuretic hormone secretion (SIADH); recent use of "ecstasy" drug (3,4-methylenedioxymethamphetamine, MDMA); and other systemic infectious or malignant processes. Nonspecific symptoms, especially weakness, unsteadiness, confusion, and fatigue. A sensation of thirst may be prominent.

    (b) Physical examination: Neurological impairment, typically non-focal, including confusion, somnolence, or lethargy; neurological dysfunction may progress to grand mal seizures, in severe cases, and to death from uncal herniation. Most of the physical exam is notable for what is not present. Signs of depletion or expansion of the extracellular fluid (ECF) volume make a diagnosis of SIADH less likely. Thus, peripheral edema, ascites, pulmonary crackles, and jugular venous distension suggest that hyponatremia is the consequence of depletion of the "effective" arterial blood volume. This typically results from heart failure or cirrhosis of the liver. Conversely, postural hypotension, tachycardia, dry axillae, or mucus membranes raise the possibility that arginine vasopressin (AVP) secretion is, in fact, an appropriate response to true ECF volume depletion.

R. Wusirika (✉)
Division of Nephrology, Oregon Health and Science University, Portland, OR, USA
e-mail: wusirika@ohsu.edu

D. H. Ellison
Nephrology and Hypertension, Oregon Health and Science University, Portland, OR, USA

© Springer Nature Switzerland AG 2021   109
L. Loriaux, C. Vanek (eds.), *Endocrine Emergencies*, Contemporary Endocrinology,
https://doi.org/10.1007/978-3-030-67455-7_12

(c) Laboratory values: Hyponatremia is required to make a diagnosis and is typically the most prominent feature. A low serum uric acid supports that diagnosis; conversely, hyperuricemia suggests that depletion of the ECF volume may be responsible. Blood urea nitrogen concentration usually is low. A urine Na concentration less than 30 mmol/L argues strongly that ECF volume depletion is present and typically compels a trial of volume replacement. Conversely, a urine Na concentration ≥40 mmol/L is consistent with SIADH. Notably, measurement of plasma AVP is usually not a part of the diagnostic evaluation.

(d) Imaging: An MR or CT scan of the brain can be useful in distinguishing acute symptomatic hyponatremia from chronic hyponatremia. This is an important distinction since the approach to treatment depends on the acuity.

3. Treatment: Treatment of SIADH depends on its acuity, the associated symptoms and signs, and the cause. The initial decisions with respect to treatment involve a decision about treatment urgency. If the hyponatremia is symptomatic and deemed to be acute (typically defined as less than 48 h in duration), then rapid correction is safe and effective in preventing or correcting neurological sequelae. In this case, treatment with hypertonic saline (3% NaCl) is recommended at rates designed to increase serum Na concentration by 1–2 mmol/h for a total correction of 4–8 mmol/L during the first day (rates and approaches remain controversial and are discussed in detail, below).

When hyponatremia is chronic and asymptomatic, then a more conservative approach is recommended. This typically includes restriction of water intake. It may also include the use of pharmaceuticals to block vasopressin receptors in the kidney. Traditionally, demeclocycline has been employed. More recently, oral tolvaptan and urea have become available as treatment options.

Syndrome of Inappropriate Antidiuretic Hormone

The inappropriate secretion of antidiuretic hormone (ADH) was characterized by Schwartz, Bartter, and colleagues in 1957, when they described two patients with renal sodium loss and hyponatremia, associated with lung cancers, without apparent ECF volume depletion:

> These two patients with mediastinal tumors presented a syndrome in which the cardinal feature was hyponatremia. Renal and adrenal cortical function was normal. As hyponatremia and hypotonicity of the ECF developed, the urine was persistently hypertonic compared to the plasma. Since hypertonicity of the urine, in the presence of a normal glomerular filtration rate, constitutes prima facie evidence for the presence of ADH, it was postulated that there was sustained, inappropriate secretion of ADH in these subjects, and that this was responsible for the disorder of sodium metabolism [1].

They were aware that exogenous administration of vasopressin (Pitressin™) to normal subjects who were allowed to drink water as they desired led to a similar syndrome of hyponatremia and salt wasting. Although measurement of serum arginine vasopressin was not possible at the time, the authors inferred correctly that the peptide hormone was being produced inappropriately. Later analysis indicated that tumors themselves were usually the source of the antidiuretic hormone [2]. Subsequently, many other causes of the syndrome have been reported (see Table 12.1). Many of these involved disease of the lungs or the brain and included both malignant and infectious processes. It became clear that certain commonly administered drugs could lead to a similar syndrome, which was reversible on their discontinuation. Finally, other situations in which excessive ADH secretion occurs, such as the perioperative period, and during pain, further expanded the list of causes.

Table 12.1 Causes of the syndrome of inappropriate antidiuretic hormone secretion

Malignancies	Pulmonary disorders	Central nervous system disorders	Drugs	Miscellaneous
Carcinomas	Infections	Infections	Drugs that stimulate AVP release or enhance its actions	Inherited (gain of function V2R mutations)
Pulmonary	Bacterial pneumonia	Encephalitis	Chlorpropamide	Idiopathic
Small cell	Viral pneumonia	Meningitis	SSRIs	Transient
Mesothelioma	Pulmonary abscess	Brain abscess	Tricyclic	Endurance exercise
Oropharynx	Tuberculosis	Rocky Mountain spotted fever	Antidepressants	Surgery anesthesia
GI tract	Aspergillosis	AIDS	Clofibrate	Nausea
Stomach	Asthma	Bleeds and masses	Carbamazepine	Pain
Duodenum	Cystic fibrosis	Subdural hematoma	Vincristine	Stress
Pancreas	Positive-pressure breathing	Subarachnoid hemorrhage	Nicotine	
GU tract		Cerebrovascular accident	Narcotics	
Ureter		Brain tumors	Antipsychotics	
Bladder		Head trauma	Ifosfamide	
Prostate		Hydrocephalus	Cyclophosphamide	
Endometrial		Cavernous sinus thrombosis	Nonsteroidal anti-inflammatory drugs	
Endocrine		Miscellaneous	MDMA (ecstasy)	
Thymoma		Multiple sclerosis	AVP analogs	
Lymphomas		Guillain-Barré syndrome	Desmopressin (dDAVP)	
Sarcomas		Shy-Drager syndrome	Oxytocin	
Ewing's sarcoma		Delirium tremens	Vasopressin	
		Acute intermittent porphyria		

Source: From Ref. [3], with permission
SSRI selective serotonin reuptake inhibitors, *MDMA* 3,4-methylenedioxymethamphetamine, *AVP* arginine vasopressin

Antidiuretic Hormone Secretion

The human antidiuretic hormone is arginine vasopressin (AVP). This nonapeptide hormone (Cys-Tyr-Phe-Gln-Asn-Cys-Pro-Arg-Gly-NH$_2$; see Fig. 12.1) is produced by the hypothalamus and trafficked to the posterior pituitary, where it is stored (Fig. 12.2). In response to small increases in plasma tonicity (Fig. 12.3), AVP is secreted into the bloodstream, where its half-life is short (15–20 min). Secretion is also stimulated by effective arterial blood volume (EABV) depletion, although this response only occurs when ECF volume depletion amounts to approximately 10%. Thus, day-to-day control of AVP secretion is regulated primarily by the serum sodium concentration.

AVP binds to two classes of receptor, vascular receptors (V1R), which lead to vasoconstriction, and renal tubular receptors (V2R) on the basolateral membrane of principal cells in the collecting duct. Engagement with V2R leads to insertion of preformed water channels (aquaporin-2) into the apical plasma membrane, which increases transcellular water permeability (see Fig. 12.4). As the interstitium of the kidney is hypertonic, owing to countercurrent exchange, water is reabsorbed from the collecting duct and urine becomes concentrated. Via the action of this system, the urine osmolality can rise to 1200 mOsm/kg H$_2$O, although any value greater than 100 mOsm/kg H$_2$O is believed to reflect some AVP action (as urinary osmolality in the absence of AVP is as low as 50 mOsm/kg H$_2$O).

The AVP system typically acts in concert with thirst to regulate the serum Na concentration and, therefore, the effective osmolality of ECF. In contrast, ECF

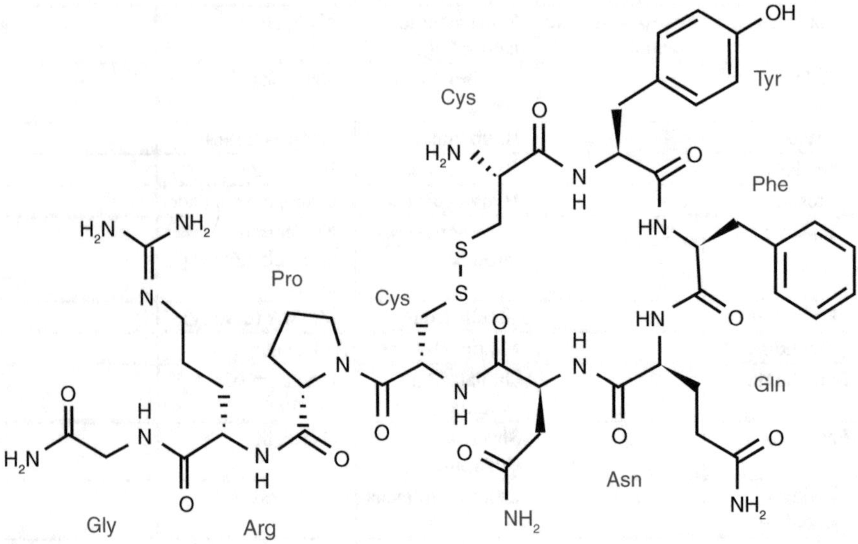

Fig. 12.1 Chemical structure of arginine vasopressin. Chemical structure of arginine vasopressin

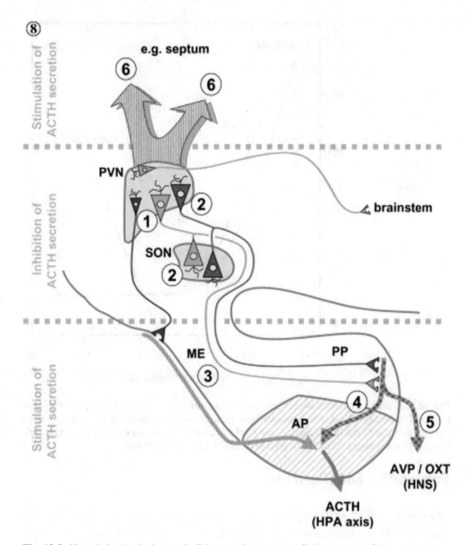

Fig. 12.2 Hypothalamic pituitary axis. Diagram shows parvocellular neurons of the paraventricular nucleus (PVN) mediate release of corticotropin-releasing hormone (*labeled 1*). Magnocellular neurons of the PVN (*labeled 2*) mediate AVP (*red*) and oxytocin (*green*) production. They not only traverse the median eminence (ME) to be stored in axonal terminals in the posterior pituitary (PP) but also innervate the supraoptic nucleus (SON). AVP is released from the PP upon signals discussed in the text (the hypothalamic neurohypophyseal system (HNS)) to have effects, both systemic (4) and local (5). Some work suggests that locally produced AVP may affect other central sites (6)). (From Ref. [4])

volume is regulated largely by the renin/angiotensin/aldosterone system, which modulates NaCl balance. Thus, *disorders of Na concentration* are analyzed as disorders of *water balance* (rather than salt balance) and typically result from disordered AVP secretion or action.

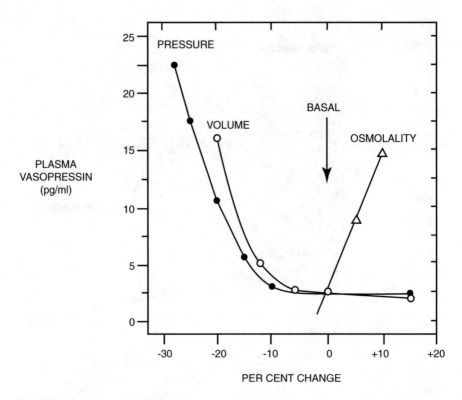

Fig. 12.3 Plasma vasopressin levels versus osmolality, volume, and pressure. Graph shows steep effects of percentage changes in plasma vasopressin with osmolality (*triangles*). Small percentage changes in extracellular fluid volume (*open circles*) and arterial pressure (*filled circles*) have little effect until the change exceeds 10%. (Graph from Ref. [5], with permission)

Presentation and Diagnosis

The patient with SIADH can be asymptomatic or suffer from severe neurological symptoms. The difference is determined largely by the acuity of the process. Severe hyponatremia ([Na]$_{serum}$ less than 125 mmol/L), especially when developing rapidly (duration less than 48 h), can lead to confusion, hallucinations, seizures, coma, decerebrate posturing, respiratory arrest, and death. Milder symptoms include headache, difficulty concentrating, impaired memory, muscle cramps, and weakness. Women are more prone to develop neurological symptoms and signs than are men.

Diagnostic criteria for SIADH are summarized in Table 12.2 [8]. It is important to measure serum osmolality to exclude pseudohyponatremia, a laboratory artifact that occurs when serum lipids or proteins are elevated and [Na]$_{serum}$ is measured using common indirect techniques [9]. Hypertonic hyponatremia occurs when osmotically active solutes (typically glucose or mannitol) draw water from cells. A correction factor (serum sodium concentration declines by 1.6–2.4 mmol/L for each 100 mg/dL increase in plasma glucose) can be used to determine whether the

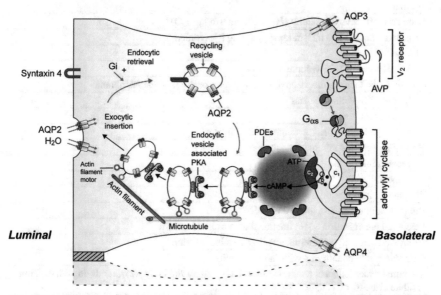

Outer and inner medullary collecting duct

Fig. 12.4 Mechanism of vasopressin effects on water. Cartoon shows a principal cell with G-protein-coupled V2 receptors on the basolateral cell surface. Agonist binding activates adenylyl cyclase, increases intracellular cyclic AMP, activates protein kinase A (PKA), and stimulates exocytic insertion of preformed aquaporin-2 (AQP2) molecules into the apical membrane. Other aquaporins (AQP3 and AQP4) permit constitutive water movement across the basolateral membrane. (From Ref. [6], with permission)

elevation of plasma glucose accounts for the decline in serum Na. Alternatively, the *effective* osmolality (sometimes called "tonicity") can be estimated as the *measured osmolality-blood urea nitrogen/2.8* (where BUN is measured in mg/dL). As the effective osmolality depends on properties of biological membranes, it cannot be measured in the laboratory [10]. To diagnose hypotonic hyponatremia, the *estimated* effective osmolality must be less than 275 mOsm/L (Table 12.2).

A second diagnostic criterion for SIADH is that the urine osmolality must exceed 100 mOsm/kg H_2O, when the plasma effective osmolality is low (Table 12.2). Although the urine may be highly concentrated, AVP secretion in SIADH is not necessarily continuous and at a high level (see Fig. 12.5). *Clinical euvolemia* is also considered essential, because EABV depletion also stimulates AVP secretion (Fig. 12.3). If AVP secretion is the result of an edematous disorder (such as heart failure or cirrhosis of the liver), then edema is typically easily detected, as hyponatremia only occurs in the setting of severe disease. In contrast, it can be difficult to discern ECF volume depletion as the cause of hyponatremia, because the sensitivity of clinical assessment is limited [12]. Laboratory tests can often provide additional guidance. A low serum uric acid or blood urea nitrogen or a urinary Na concentration greater than 40 mmol/L in hyponatremic patients suggest SIADH [13]; for

Table 12.2 Diagnosis of the syndrome of inappropriate antidiuresis

Essential
Decreased effective osmolality ($P_{eff} < 275$ mOsm/kg H_2O)
Urine osmolality >100 mOsm/kg H_2O during hypotonicity
Clinical euvolemia
No clinical signs of ECF volume depletion
No orthostasis, tachycardia, decreased skin turgor, or dry mucous membranes
No signs of ECF volume excess
No edema or ascites
Urine [Na] >40 mmol/L, on a normal NaCl intake
Normal thyroid and adrenal function
No recent diuretic use
Supplemental
Plasma uric acid less than 4 mg/dL
Blood urea nitrogen less than 10 mg/dL
Fractional Na excretion >1%; fractional urea excretion >55%
Failure to correct hyponatremia after 0.9% saline infusion
Correction of hyponatremia with fluid restriction
Abnormal water load test (excretion of <80% of 20 mL/kg body wt water during 4 h or failure to dilute urine to <100 mOsm/kg H_2O)[a]
Elevated plasma AVP levels, despite hypotonicity and clinical euvolemia[a]

Source: Adapted from Refs. [1, 7]. [a]Water load tests and AVP measurement are rarely recommended

example, a serum uric acid concentration lower than 4 mg/dL (when hyponatremia is present) has a positive predictive value for SIADH between 73% and 100%, whereas a urine [Na] <30 mmol/L has a predictive value of 71–100% that 0.9% saline infusion will effectively increase the serum [Na] [12, 14].

When diagnostic uncertainty remains and the patient's symptoms are mild, it is usually safe to infuse 2 L of 0.9% saline during 24 h. Even though 0.9% saline is not the preferred treatment for SIADH, correction of the hyponatremia suggests that ECF volume depletion was contributing to the hyponatremia. Although there is a concern that 0.9% saline may worsen hyponatremia in patients with severe SIADH, owing to the phenomenon of desalination [15], this maneuver is usually safe when baseline urinary osmolality is less than 500 mOsm/kg H_2O [14, 16, 17]. Measurement of the serum AVP level is not recommended routinely as part of the diagnostic evaluation.

Treatment of Symptomatic SIADH

The most important factors dictating the management of SIADH are its severity, duration, and the presence of symptoms [18–20]. Decisions about the best therapeutic approach always involve balancing competing risks; *undertreatment* may permit progressive neurological deterioration, possibly leading to death; whereas rapid

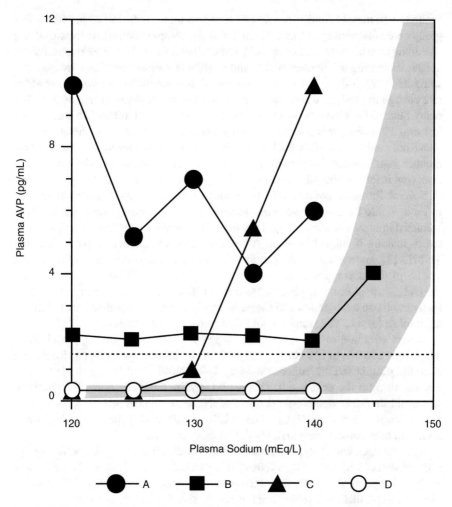

Fig. 12.5 Patterns of AVP secretion in SIADH. Patterns of plasma AVP (ADH) versus plasma sodium observed in patients with SIADH. Type A, unregulated secretion; Type B, elevated basal secretion, despite normal regulation by osmolality; Type C, reset osmostat; Type D, undetectable AVP. (From Ref. [11], with permission)

overtreatment may lead to osmotic demyelination, another dreaded and morbid complication.

For symptomatic patients with severe hyponatremia of less than 48 h duration, clinical experience suggests that treatment is safe and effective. The goal is to raise the [Na]$_{serum}$ enough to prevent neurological deterioration while avoiding complications. The target values for correction have changed during the past 20 years, and they remain highly controversial. Some experts advocate restricting the total correction to 6 mmol/L during the first 24 h of treatment and 12 mmol/L during 48 h, even when the hyponatremia is acute. An expert panel suggested that correction be limited to 10 mmol/L during the first 24 h and 18 mmol/L during 48 h, and yet this group noted that some patients are at high risk for complications from treatment and should be treated more cautiously [21]. Others, however, continue to emphasize the danger in treating too conservatively and suggest that more aggressive treatment is warranted [22]. Although it has been suggested that one should emphasize the absolute change in $[Na]_{serum}$ during the first 12 or 24 h, rather than the rate of rise [21], many authorities recommend increasing the $[Na]_{serum}$ by 1 mmol/L/h initially by infusing 3% saline; this approach is guided only by case series, in the absence of data from randomized trials, but it is widely accepted. Some authorities have recommended concomitant furosemide [23], but most recommend avoiding it [24] or reserving it for patients who become ECF volume expanded [7, 25].

Several formulas are available to estimate the rate at which saline should be infused. While the Adrogué-Madias formula [3] is commonly used and has been validated in some situations [26], it is a two-step procedure that is relatively complicated, making it subject to error. A simpler approach, advocated by Janicic and Verbalis [7], gives quite similar results [3]. Three percent saline is administered at a rate in mL/h that is equal to the body weight in kilograms. This is expected to raise the $[Na]_{serum}$ by 1 mmol/L per hour, as desired. Thus, if the goal is to raise $[Na]_{serum}$ by 6 mmol/L in a 6 h period and the patient weighs 70 kg, 3% saline can be infused at 70 mL/h for 6 h. The simplicity of this approach is advantageous.

Others continue to advocate more aggressive treatment. One approach is to administer 250 mL of 3% NaCl, giving 50 mL by intravenous push (which should raise the plasma sodium concentration by 1–2 mmol/L) and letting the remaining 200 mL drip for the next 4–6 h. This is said to raise the $[Na]_{serum}$ by 8–10 mmol/L and avoid the acute neurologic dangers of hyponatremia. In this case, the recommendation is to keep the $[Na]_{serum}$ below 120 mmol/L during the first 24 h of treatment and then correct the remaining deficit gradually [22].

The management of hyponatremia of unclear duration with nonspecific symptoms or signs (e.g., headache or lethargy) is particularly challenging. Some reports suggest that patients risk adverse outcomes if not treated aggressively [27], whereas others suggest that such patients are at higher risk from rapid correction [28] and that the reported morbidity results from the underlying disease [29]. It does seem clear that a longer duration of hyponatremia increases the risk of osmotic demyelination (OD) after sodium correction. This syndrome, which includes both central pontine and extrapontine myelinolysis, often begins following an initial symptomatic improvement and presents with lethargy and affective changes, followed by mutism or dysarthria, spastic quadriparesis, and pseudobulbar palsy [30]. Case series and experimental data indicate that this complication can result from rapid or too extreme correction of chronic hyponatremia [30]. Some authorities recommend initial evaluation with a CT scan or MRI of the brain to determine whether cerebral edema is present as a measure of the urgency of correction. It is not clear that this improves outcomes [31]. Many authorities recommend correcting such patients at 0.5–1 mmol/L/h using a lower rate of hypertonic saline infusion (half of that noted above). As above, many limit correction to 6–8 mmol/L in 24 h and 12–18 mmol/L in 48 h. Perhaps the one area in which all authorities agree is that close monitoring of $[Na]_{serum}$ (every 2–4 h) is imperative and can help prevent complications.

In patients who have exceeded recommended correction rates it is possible to re-lower $[Na]_{serum}$ by administering water and desmopressin (dDAVP, a synthetic analog of AVP that activates V2R selectively) [32]. Some patients, especially those with reversible causes of SIADH, will develop a spontaneous water diuresis upon admission to the hospital. This can lead to rapid and potentially harmful correction rates. When this has occurred, desmopressin, given as 1–2 µg doses intravenously or subcutaneously, can be administered to slow the water losses, and dextrose in water can be administered as needed to achieve the $[Na]_{serum}$ target level [33]. An even more aggressive approach is to start both desmopressin and 3% saline simultaneously, to prevent sudden water diuresis and excessive correction [34]. While this approach may be considered in selected individuals, it should be used cautiously, since experience with it is very limited.

A more recent option for treating SIADH is VR antagonists. For acute use, conivaptan is available. In a double-blind, randomized trial, $[Na]_{serum}$ increased by 6 mmol/L more in groups assigned to conivaptan than placebo for 4 days. Other studies have suggested that the drug effectively raises $[Na]_{serum}$. Yet, there are concerns about its use. In a single-center trial, conivaptan led to correction more rapidly than desired in approximately 50% of treatments, and hypotension (presumably because conivaptan blocks both types of VR) and phlebitis were noted. Thus, the appropriate role for conivaptan in the treatment of symptomatic hyponatremia remains to be determined.

Another more recent treatment for SIADH is oral urea. Similar to hypertonic saline, oral urea provides an osmolar load which must be excreted with free water. In comparison to hypertonic saline, a single 15 gm dose of urea contains 250 mOsms as compared to 92 mOsms in a 100 ml of hypertonic saline. Oral urea has been studied in long-term care but has been shown to be effective short term [35].

Chronic treatment of SIADH is beyond the scope of this chapter but, in addition to eradication of the underlying disorder, it involves restricting fluid intake, demeclocycline, and perhaps oral vaptans or urea. The interested reader is referred to reviews, for more information [3].

References

1. Schwartz WB, Bennett W, Curelop S, Bartter FC. A syndrome of renal sodium loss and hyponatremia probably resulting from inappropriate secretion of antidiuretic hormone. Am J Med. 1957;23:529–42.
2. Vorherr H, Massry SG, Utiger RD, Kleeman CR. Antidiuretic principle in malignant tumor extracts from patients with inappropriate ADH syndrome. J Clin Endocrinol Metab. 1968;28:162–8.
3. Ellison DH, Berl T. Clinical practice. The syndrome of inappropriate antidiuresis. N Engl J Med. 2007;356:2064–72.

4. Engelmann M, Landgraf R, Wotjak CT. The hypothalamic-neurohypophysial system regulates the hypothalamic-pituitary-adrenal axis under stress: an old concept revisited. Front Neuroendocrinol. 2004;25:132–49.
5. Robertson GL. Diseases of the posterior pituitary. In: Felig P, Broadus A, editors. Endocrinology and metabolism. 2nd ed. New York: McGraw-Hill; 1987. p. 338–85.
6. Bichet DG. Lithium, cyclic AMP signaling, A-kinase anchoring proteins, and aquaporin-2. J Am Soc Nephrol. 2006;17:920–2.
7. Janicic N, Verbalis JG. Evaluation and management of hypo-osmolality in hospitalized patients. Endocrinol Metab Clin N Am. 2003;32:459–81, vii.
8. Saeed BO, Beaumont D, Handley GH, Weaver JU. Severe hyponatraemia: investigation and management in a district general hospital. J Clin Pathol. 2002;55:893–6.
9. Turchin A, Seifter JL, Seely EW. Clinical problem-solving. Mind the gap. N Engl J Med. 2003;349:1465–9.
10. Bhave G, Neilson EG. Body fluid dynamics: back to the future. J Am Soc Nephrol. 2011;22:2166–81.
11. Robertson GL. Regulation of arginine vasopressin in the syndrome of inappropriate antidiuresis. Am J Med. 2006;119:S36–42.
12. Chung H-M, Kluge R, Schrier RW, Anderson RJ. Clinical assessment of extracellular fluid volume in hyponatremia. Am J Med. 1987;83:905–8.
13. Berghmans T, Paesmans M, Body JJ. A prospective study on hyponatraemia in medical cancer patients: epidemiology, aetiology and differential diagnosis. Support Care Cancer. 2000;8:192–7.
14. Musch W, Thimpont J, Vandervelde D, Verhaeverbeke I, Berghmans T, Decaux G. Combined fractional excretion of sodium and urea better predicts response to saline in hyponatremia than do usual clinical and biochemical parameters. Am J Med. 1995;99:348–55.
15. Steele A, Gowrishankar M, Abrahamson S, Mazer CD, Feldman RD, Halperin ML. Postoperative hyponatremia despite near-isotonic saline infusion: a phenomenon of desalination. Ann Intern Med. 1997;126:20–5.
16. Musch W, Decaux G. Treating the syndrome of inappropriate ADH secretion with isotonic saline. QJM. 1998;91:749–53.
17. Milionis HJ, Liamis GL, Elisaf MS. The hyponatremic patient: a systematic approach to laboratory diagnosis. CMAJ. 2002;166:1056–62.
18. Berl T. Treating hyponatremia: what is all the controversy about? Ann Intern Med. 1990;113:417–9.
19. Chonchol M, Berl M. Hyponatremia. In: Dubose T, Hamm LL, editors. Acid-base and electrolyte disorders. Philadelphia: Saunders; 2002. p. 229–39.
20. Decaux G, Soupart A. Treatment of symptomatic hyponatremia. Am J Med Sci. 2003;326:25–30.
21. Verbalis JG, Goldsmith SR, Greenberg A, Schrier RW, Sterns RH. Hyponatremia treatment guidelines 2007: expert panel recommendations. Am J Med. 2007;120:S1–21.
22. Kokko JP. Symptomatic hyponatremia with hypoxia is a medical emergency. Kidney Int. 2006;69:1291–3.
23. Adrogue HJ, Madias NE. Hyponatremia. N Engl J Med. 2000;342:1581–9.
24. Smith DM, McKenna K, Thompson CJ. Hyponatraemia. Clin Endocrinol. 2000;52:667–78.
25. Palmer BF, Gates JR, Lader M. Causes and management of hyponatremia. Ann Pharmacother. 2003;37:1694–702.
26. Liamis G, Kalogirou M, Saugos V, Elisaf M. Therapeutic approach in patients with dysnatraemias. Nephrol Dial Transplant. 2006;21:1564–9.
27. Ayus JC, Arieff AI. Chronic hyponatremic encephalopathy in postmenopausal women: association of therapies with morbidity and mortality. JAMA. 1999;281:2299–304.
28. Sterns RH. The treatment of hyponatremia: first, do no harm. Am J Med. 1990;88:557–60.
29. Chawla A, Sterns RH, Nigwekar SU, Cappuccio JD. Mortality and serum sodium: do patients die from or with hyponatremia? Clin J Am Soc Nephrol. 2011;6:960–5.
30. Laureno R, Karp BI. Myelinolysis after correction of hyponatremia. Ann Intern Med. 1997;126:57–62.

31. Gross P, Reimann D, Henschkowski J, Damian M. Treatment of severe hyponatremia: conventional and novel aspects. J Am Soc Nephrol. 2001;12(Suppl 17):S10–4.
32. Soupart A, Ngassa M, Decaux G. Therapeutic relowering of the serum sodium in a patient after excessive correction of hyponatremia. Clin Nephrol. 1999;51:383–6.
33. Perianayagam A, Sterns RH, Silver SM, Grieff M, Mayo R, Hix J, Kouides R. DDAVP is effective in preventing and reversing inadvertent overcorrection of hyponatremia. Clin J Am Soc Nephrol. 2008;3:331–6.
34. Sterns RH, Hix JK, Silver S. Treating profound hyponatremia: a strategy for controlled correction. Am J Kidney Dis. 2010;56:774–9.
35. Decaux G, Andres C, Gankam Kengne F, Soupart A. Treatment of euvolemic hyponatremia in the intensive care unit by urea. Crit Care. 2010;14(5):R184.

Chapter 13
Diabetes Insipidus

Raghav Wusirika and David H. Ellison

Précis

1. Clinical setting: Urine output greater than 3 L daily.
2. Diagnosis: Exclude primary polydipsia, and then determine whether the process reflects (a) central diabetes insipidus (CDI, owing to a lack of antidiuretic hormone (ADH), also known as *arginine vasopressin*, AVP) production or (b) nephrogenic diabetes insipidus (NDI, owing to the failure of the kidney to respond to AVP):

   (a) History: The most prominent symptom or sign is polyuria, typically including nocturia. In most affected individuals, this is accompanied by polydipsia, which is a secondary phenomenon. There may be a history of a central nervous system event (with CDI), the ingestion of a drug known to damage the urinary concentrating capacity (such as lithium, for NDI), or a family history (for inherited disease). When thirst is impaired or when fluid intake is impossible (such as during acute hospitalization or anesthesia), hypernatremia will develop unless water losses are replaced. In this case, lethargy, confusion, weakness, and irritability, sometimes progressing to twitching, seizures, and coma, can occur.

   (b) Physical examination: Often, the physical exam is relatively normal. Signs of depletion or expansion of the extracellular fluid (ECF) volume are typically absent. Thus, peripheral edema, ascites, pulmonary crackles, or jugular venous distension suggest that other processes have supervened. Neurological

R. Wusirika (✉)
Division of Nephrology, Oregon Health and Science University, Portland, OR, USA
e-mail: wusirika@ohsu.edu

D. H. Ellison
Nephrology and Hypertension, Oregon Health and Science University, Portland, OR, USA

© Springer Nature Switzerland AG 2021   123
L. Loriaux, C. Vanek (eds.), *Endocrine Emergencies*, Contemporary Endocrinology,
https://doi.org/10.1007/978-3-030-67455-7_13

impairment, which occurs during frank hypernatremia, is typically non-focal unless the result of a specific neurological insult (such as a stroke).

(c) Laboratory values: Most laboratory tests are normal, including serum Na concentration and osmolality. Hypernatremia is only observed when there is a defect in thirst or in the ability to drink; thus hypernatremia is typically observed only in the very young (who cannot access fluids by themselves), the very old (who tend to experience a mild to moderate loss of thirst as they age), or the very ill (who are unable to gain access to, or indicate the need for, fluids). The urine is typically dilute, with an osmolality <250 mOsm/kg water. A low serum [Na] concentration suggests primary polydipsia. Further testing, classically a water deprivation test or levels of stimulated copeptin which is a stable peptide precursor of AVP (see below), may be necessary to distinguish between polydipsia and DI, but this is not necessary if the basal serum [Na] concentration exceeds 145 mmol/L. Measurement of a random copeptin level can also be used to distinguish CDI (low levels) from NDI in most cases.

(d) Imaging: Imaging is not typically employed to make a diagnosis of diabetes insipidus; it is, however, important to determine whether processes within the central nervous system are contributing to any observed defects in urinary concentration.

3. Treatment: The two goals of therapy are to replace the free water deficit and to stop the ongoing inappropriate loss of free water. The free water deficit can be calculated by the formula:

$$\text{Water deficit} = \frac{\left(\text{Plasma } Na^+ - 140\right)}{140} \times \text{Total body water.}$$

Total body water is about 60% of body weight in men and 50% of body weight in women. That deficit, typically between 2.5 and 5 L, should be corrected slowly over 48–72 h. The serum sodium should be lowered no faster than 0.5 mmol/L/h or 12 mmol/L/day. Half-normal saline, 0.45% NS, is the usual choice for rehydration. 5% dextrose, D5W, is used for acute, symptomatic hypernatremia.

Ongoing water loss will be corrected by dDAVP (desmopressin) in most cases of CDI. The usual adult dose is 50 μg by mouth twice a day or 1–2 μg IV twice a day.

NDI will not respond to dDAVP, but can often be helped by a low-sodium diet and a thiazide diuretic.

Diabetes Insipidus

Diabetes insipidus means the excessive production of dilute urine; the term *diabetes* indicates excessive urine production (Greek: διαβετεσ = siphon), and the term *insipidus* implies "tasteless," in contrast to the taste of urine from patients with diabetes mellitus. A syndrome in which copious amounts of dilute urine are produced has been recognized since at least the mid-eighteenth century, when William Cullen stressed that the urine in "diabetes" might be sweet or not. He stated, "I myself, indeed, think I have met with one instance of diabetes in which the urine was perfectly insipid; and it would seem that a like observation had occurred to Dr. Martin Lister. I am persuaded, however, that such instances are very rare; and that the other is much more common and perhaps the almost universal occurrence. I judge therefore, that the presence of such a saccharine matter may be considered as the principal circumstance in idiopathic diabetes" [1].

Over the ensuing years, it gradually became clear that there is a circulating factor (endocrine hormone) responsible for concentrating the urine and that the circulating factor is produced by hypothalamic neurons and secreted from the posterior lobe of the pituitary. The chemical structure of this factor, AVP, was finally determined by du Vigneaud, which led, together with his work on oxytocin, to the Nobel Prize in 1955. The kidney receptor for vasopressin (the type 2 vasopressin receptor, V2R) was cloned in 1992 by Birnbaumer, Rosenthal, and colleagues [2]. Water channels were identified first in 1992 by Peter Agre [3], a discovery also leading to the Nobel Prize. In the collecting duct apical membrane, aquaporin 2 (AQP2) mediates vasopressin-sensitive water reabsorption.

Although primary polydipsia (psychogenic polydipsia) also leads to copious amounts of dilute urine, this disorder, which affects individuals with serious psychiatric disease, with anxiety disorders, and occasionally with infiltrative diseases of the brain, is not typically considered to be a cause of diabetes insipidus. Instead, the diagnosis of diabetes insipidus is given only to individuals in whom the elaboration of copious amounts of highly dilute urine results from defective urinary concentrating *ability* (the dilute urine is, therefore, inappropriate).

Antidiuretic Hormone Secretion

The human ADH is AVP. This nonapeptide hormone (Cys-Tyr-Phe-Gln-Asn-Cys-Pro-Arg-Gly-NH_2; see Fig. 12.1) is produced by the hypothalamus and trafficked to the posterior pituitary, where it is stored (see Fig. 12.2). In response to small increases in plasma tonicity (see Fig. 12.3), AVP is secreted into the bloodstream, where its half-life is short (15–20 min). Secretion is also stimulated by depletion of the effective arterial blood volume (EABV), although this response only occurs when ECF volume depletion amounts to approximately 10% (see Fig. 12.3); thus day-to-day control of AVP secretion is regulated primarily by plasma osmolality. AVP is released as a larger prohormone that is cleaved. A nonfunctional portion of that prohormone, copeptin, is a 39 amino acid peptide that is stable in circulation and released in equimolar amounts to AVP. Much like C-peptide measurement is used as a surrogate of insulin secretion, copeptin can be used as a surrogate for circulating AVP levels.

AVP binds to two classes of receptor, vascular receptors (V1R), which lead to vasoconstriction, and renal tubular receptors (V2R) on the basolateral membrane of principal cells in the collecting duct. Engagement with V2R leads to insertion of preformed water channels (AQP2) into the apical plasma membrane, which increases transcellular water permeability (see Fig. 12.4). As the interstitium of the kidney is hypertonic, owing to countercurrent exchange, water is reabsorbed from the collecting duct, and urine becomes concentrated. Via the action of this system, the urine osmolality can rise to 1200 mOsm/kg H_2O; conversely, in the presence of copious water intake, the urinary osmolality can be as low as 50 mOsm/kg H_2O.

The AVP system typically acts in concert with thirst to regulate the serum osmolality (usually reflected by the serum Na^+ concentration). In contrast, ECF volume is regulated largely by the renin/angiotensin/aldosterone system, which modulates NaCl balance. Thus, *disorders of Na concentration* are typically analyzed as disorders of *water balance* (rather than salt balance) and result from disordered AVP secretion or action or water intake or excretion.

Causes and Classification of Diabetes Insipidus

Diabetes insipidus is classified as *central* (CDI), resulting from deficient AVP secretion, and *nephrogenic* (NDI), resulting from renal resistance to AVP (see Table 13.1). Although some patients are completely unable to concentrate their urine, others can increase urine osmolality moderately, in response to increases in plasma osmolality (see Fig. 13.1). Such individuals have been labeled as suffering from "partial" DI, to reflect this. It is believed that their disease can become complete in some cases.

Although there are hereditary causes of both CDI and NDI, most cases are acquired, especially in adults. A urinary concentrating defect can be observed during pregnancy when the placenta elaborates vasopressinase, resulting in a deficiency of circulating AVP, but not from inadequate secretion (thus, this is neither CDI nor NDI). Finally, a distinct disorder results when hypothalamic lesions impair both AVP secretion and thirst simultaneously. Here, the natural compensatory process of increased fluid intake is absent, and affected individuals invariably present with the symptoms of hypernatremia. This syndrome has been called *essential hypernatremia* because of this presentation.

There are hereditary causes of both CDI and NDI (see Table 13.1) [4]. These are rare, accounting for less than 10% of cases. Individuals with *autosomal dominant neurohypophyseal diabetes insipidus* typically retain some capacity for AVP secretion, so that symptoms usually appear after the first year. In contrast, individuals with *X-linked NDI* as a result of AVPR2 mutations present with severe failure to thrive after birth that can lead to physical and mental retardation because of the recurrent episodes of dehydration. A similar presentation can be seen with mutations of AQP2, but this variant is observed in both boys and girls, as it is autosomal.

Table 13.1 Causes of polydipsia and hypertonic polyuria

Central DI
Congenital
Inherited neurohypophyseal DI (autosomal dominant, OMIM 125700)
Acquired
Trauma (neurosurgery, deceleration injury)
Vascular incident (cerebral hemorrhage or infarction)
Infectious (meningitis, encephalitis)
Inflammatory (lymphocytic infundibuloneurohypophysitis)
Drug-/toxin-induced
Ethanol
Phenytoin
Snake venom
Nephrogenic DI
Congenital
X-Linked recessive (AVPR$_2$ mutations, OMIM 304800)
Autosomal recessive (AQP2 mutations, OMIM 2222000)
Dominant (AQP2 mutations, OMIM 125800)
Acquired
Infiltrating lesions (sarcoidosis, amyloidosis)
Vascular (sickle cell)
Drug-/toxin-induced
Lithium, cisplatin, methoxyflurane, demeclocycline, vaptans
Metabolic
Hypercalcemia
Hypokalemia
AVP metabolism
Pregnancy (vasopressinase)
Primary polydipsia
Psychogenic (schizophrenia) - can present with hyponatremia
Dipsogenic (resetting of the thirst threshold, same causes as central DI)
Osmoreceptor dysfunction (essential hypernatremia, both thirst and concentration defects)
Granulomatous
Neoplastic
Vascular
Others

Acquired processes are much more common causes of polyuric syndromes, especially in adults. These include multiple central processes, such as traumatic, neoplastic, infectious, or surgical events (Table 13.1). NDI can be caused by kidney disease, but the most common cause is therapeutic drugs. Lithium treatment of bipolar disease is the most frequent cause of drug-induced NDI. Between 20% and 50% of patients taking lithium develop this complication [5].

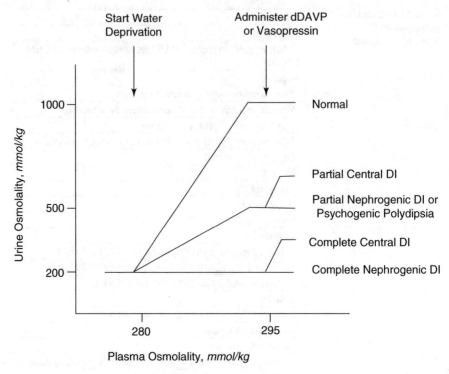

Fig. 13.1 Effect of plasma osmolality on urine osmolality in complete and partial diabetes insipidus. Typical response to water deprivation in healthy individuals and patients with complete or partial DI. The 200 mOsm/kg H$_2$O line is for schematic representation, because patients with the full phenotypes have urine osmolalities less than 100 mOsm/kg H$_2$O. (From Ref. [6], with permission)

Presentation and Diagnosis

The patient typically presents with polyuria. A sudden increase in urine output suggests CDI, whereas a more gradual onset suggests NDI. Presentation during infancy clearly suggests an inherited cause. Historical features are crucial in distinguishing CDI from NDI. The history of a neurological event points toward CDI, whereas the use of offending drugs points toward NDI. Conversely, a history of psychiatric disease suggests that the disorder may be primary polydipsia, rather than DI. Oftentimes, progressive nocturia in the absence of prostatic hypertrophy can be a clue to the development of a concentrating defect. A family history of polyuria suggests the possibility of an inherited defect.

Although hypernatremia and hyperosmolality are not the most common presenting features (owing to compensatory fluid intake), they are the most common emergent complications. This is most often observed, as noted, in situations where fluid intake is difficult. In adults, it is most common in the elderly or in those who require intensive care. Signs and symptoms of hypertonic dehydration include prerenal azotemia, hypotension, and, sometimes, shock. In a person with a urinary concentrating defect, rapidly developing hypernatremia can occur when the underlying process is not recognized. When this occurs, symptoms resulting from neurological dysfunction are common. These include lethargy, confusion, weakness, irritability, twitching, seizures, and coma. The severity of symptoms resulting from a given rise in serum [Na] concentration is dependent upon the time period over which the change occurs. A rapid rise will cause confusion, weakness, or extreme thirst. In contrast, chronic hypernatremia is often asymptomatic because of the adaptive processes of neurons which accumulate electrolyte and nonelectrolyte ("idiogenic") osmoles to balance the hypertonicity of the plasma (see below).

To make the diagnosis of DI in the setting of polyuria (or hypernatremia), the urine concentration must be less than 250 mOsm/kg H_2O, despite a stimulus for AVP secretion (typically, plasma hypertonicity). Although these criteria appear straightforward, their application is not always so easy. Although low serum [Na] concentration in the presence of polyuria suggests the presence of primary polydipsia, a formal water deprivation test (see Table 13.2) is often recommended to

Table 13.2 Water deprivation test

Before the test
Ask the patient to cease fluid consumption 2 h before coming to the office or clinic
On arrival
Measure the body weight and serum [Na] and osmolality at the baseline
Ask the patient to void
Record each urine void, record its volume, and determine the specific gravity and osmolality
Obtain weight and vital signs every 2 h for the first 4 h and then hourly
Measure serum [Na] and osmolality at 4 h and then every other hour
A testing threshold is reached when the:
1. Urine specific gravity ≥1.020
2. Serum Na >145 mmol/L
3. Plasma osmolality ≥300 mOsm/kg H_2O
4. Urine osmolality reaches a plateau (<10% change over three periods)
For safety reasons, stop the test when any of the following occur:
1. There is a weight loss ≥3% or patient exhibits signs of volume depletion
2. A preselected time point is reached: this may be 6 h if <6 months old, 8 h is <2 years, and 12 h for children older than 2
At the end of the test, measure weight, vital signs, plasma sodium, and plasma and urine osmolality and urine-specific gravity
Measure plasma AVP
Then administer 1 µg desmopressin subcutaneously, and follow the urine osmolality for 2 h more
Interpretation
CDI is diagnosed if the urine osmolality rises by >50% following desmopressin
NDI is diagnosed if the urine osmolality rises <10%
Intermediate cases (urine osmolality rise 10–50%) can be assessed by examining the plasma AVP

differentiate primary polydipsia from DI. In contrast, if the serum [Na] concentration exceeds 145 mmol/L *at baseline*, and the urine osmolality is less than the plasma osmolality, *the diagnosis of DI has been established*; the diagnostic workup only involves determining whether the DI is central or nephrogenic (see below).

Although water deprivation can sometimes be necessary to confirm a diagnosis, it does present risk and is not always recommended. Caution is required when evaluating newborns and young children and individuals at risk for a thirst defect. Patients with a history of lithium ingestion and dilute urine also may not need a formal water deprivation test. Some authorities do not recommend overnight fluid restriction for patients with substantial polyuria, as this can prove hazardous [6]. Others suggest that overnight deprivation can be tried in routine cases [7]. A protocol for water deprivation is presented in Table 13.2, along with guidelines to interpret the test. In general, to make a diagnosis of CDI, the urine osmolality should rise by at least 50% following AVP or desmopressin administration. On the other hand, a less robust response can be observed in patients with partial DI. Both AVP and desmopressin can be used to assess diabetes insipidus. Some authorities prefer desmopressin because it is selective for the V2 receptor and does not have the vasoconstrictive properties of AVP (Pitressin™).

Although the water deprivation test is physiologically sound and has been done for decades, given the safety limitations above, there has been an interest in a safer test for diagnosis. A random copeptin level of >21.4 pmol/L has been shown to be 100% sensitive and specific for the diagnosis of NDI [8]. Furthermore, the stimulated copeptin level by water deprivation or hypertonic saline infusion to raise the serum sodium level to 150 mmol/L has also been shown to be effective at differentiating CDI and primary polydipsia since there is some instances in which diagnosing partial CDI versus primary polydipsia is difficult. A stimulated copeptin level of <4.9 pmol/L suggested CDI as a cause for polyuria. Hypertonic saline infusion does also have risks including significant risk of CNS symptoms such as headache, vertigo, and nausea but can be done over the course of a few hours rather than an overnight water deprivation and was preferred by most patients [9]. To improve on the safety of the infusion strategy, arginine infusion has been used as an alternative to hypertonic saline as a non-osmolar stimulate for AVP which was better tolerated than hypertonic saline infusions but as it is a non-osmotic stimulus does decrease diagnostic accuracy of the test [10].

Treatment of Hypernatremia

Hypernatremia is the most dreaded complication of diabetes insipidus. In diabetes insipidus, the hypernatremia is generally driven by the loss of water only, meaning that repletion with water (as opposed to hypotonic saline) is generally recommended. A key determinant of the rate at which hypernatremia should be corrected is its duration. When hypernatremia has been present for a short period of time (<12 h), then correcting it promptly is important to prevent neurological consequences. In contrast, when the hypernatremia is chronic, rapid correction is hazardous owing to the appearance of organic osmolytes (previously called idiogenic osmoles) within cells of the central nervous system. These organic osmolytes help maintain the intracellular osmolality in the face of high extracellular osmolality, permitting the brain to re-expand (see Fig. 13.2). If overly rapid correction is begun once these adaptations have occurred, cerebral edema can result. When hypernatremia is demonstrably acute (<12 h), the serum [Na] concentration can be corrected at a rate of 1 mmol/h to reduce the risk of neurological complications [11]. In contrast, when the hypernatremia is of unknown or longer duration, such rapid correction can lead to cerebral edema. In this case, a slower rate of correction is typically recommended, often 0.5 mmol/h [11]. In either case, it is recommended to restrict the total correction to 10 mmol during the first 24 h.

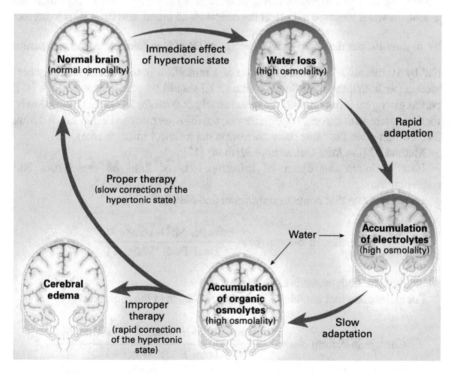

Fig. 13.2 Effects of hypernatremia on brain water. During acute hypertonicity, the brain loses water. Volume regulatory processes rapidly lead to some accumulation of electrolytes within brain cells, attenuating the shrinkage that would otherwise occur. Over time, these electrolytes are replaced by organic osmolytes, which help equalize the intracellular osmolality without cellular toxicity, leading to brain re-expansion. If aggressive sodium lowering occurs at this time, brain edema can result. (Used, with permission, from Ref. [11])

Correcting the Water Deficit

It is important to assess the magnitude of the existing water deficit to guide the rate at which free water should be administered. Two approaches are commonly recommended. The first involves estimating the water deficit.

Method #1 (the *Water Deficit Method*) [12]:

$$\text{Water Deficit} = \text{Total Body Water} \times \left(\frac{[Na]}{[140]} - 1 \right),$$

where *total body water* is estimated as the current weight × 0.6 (for men) or 0.5 (for women). [Na] is the current serum Na^+ concentration [13].

For example, in a 70-kg man with a [Na] concentration of 165 mmol/L, the TBW = 42 L. The water deficit is estimated as 42 × 0.179 = 7.5 L. As this is the amount of water required to correct the deficit by 25 mmol, and the goal is to correct

by 10 mmol/L per day, then $7.5 \times \frac{10}{25} = 3L$ of D5W is required to reduce the serum

Na^+ by 10 mmol/L. To correct at a rate of 1 mmol/L/h (one-tenth of the daily correction per hour), the total fluid volume (3 L) should be administered over a 10-h period giving an infusion rate of approximately 300 mL/h. To correct more slowly, for the patient with chronic hypernatremia, the infusion rate can be 125 mL/h during 24 h (which gives the same daily correction but a slower infusion rate).

Method #2 (the *Rate Calculation Method*) [11]:

First, estimate the effect of infusing 1 L of fluid on the serum Na^+ concentration.

For an infusate that contains only water and Na^+, the

$$\text{Change in Serum } Na = \frac{\text{infusate } Na^+ - \text{serum } Na^+}{\text{Total Body Water} + 1},$$

where the total body water is estimated as above.

For an infusate that contains K^+, as well as Na^+, then the formula is

$$\text{Change in Serum } Na = \frac{\left(\text{infusate } Na^+ + \text{infusate } K^+ \right) - \text{serum } Na^+}{\text{Total Body Water} + 1}.$$

For the same example as above, where D5W is infused (infusate Na^+ is 0), 1 L will reduce Na^+ by −165/43 = 3.8 mmol/L. To reduce Na^+ by 10 mmol/L, the second formula recommends infusing 2.63 L (= 10 mmol/3.8 mmol/L) [8].

Thus, the two formulas give similar, but not identical, recommended infusion rates. *The first approach has the benefit of greater simplicity.* The second approach can be used when the infusion rate for fluids contains both Na^+ and K^+.

Ongoing Losses

The predicted infusion rates for hypotonic fluid often underestimate water needs. This is most common because insensible losses (typically 0.5 L per day) and ongoing urinary losses have not been fully accounted for. To estimate urinary losses, especially in the setting of NDI, where urinary water losses may be relatively fixed, it is generally recommended to calculate the electrolyte-free water excretion [14]:

$$CH_2O^e = V \times \left(1 - \frac{\left(U_{Na} + U_k \right)}{P_{Na}} \right).$$

Thus, if the individual above is making 4 L per day of urine, with a urine $[Na^+] = 41$ and a $[K^+] = 41$, then the electrolyte-free water clearance will be approximately 2 L per day. This amount should be added to the infusion rate, calculated from the deficit, using the formulas above.

The greatest importance of these formulas and approaches is to provide an initial estimate of water infusion rates. These are only estimates, and rates of ongoing water loss can increase or decrease unexpectedly. As the goal of treatment is to achieve a measured reduction in serum [Na], the physician must remain vigilant during treatment, monitoring the serum electrolytes frequently (every 4 h initially) and adjusting infusion rates appropriately. If dextrose-containing infusion solutions are employed, the patient should also be monitored for the possible development of hyperglycemia.

Treating the Underlying Disorder

Once a plan for correction of any water deficit has been devised, attention turns to the underlying disorder and to the major symptoms associated with DI, namely, polyuria. In the case of CDI with an urgent need to treat (such as a patient going to surgery), parenteral desmopressin is typically preferred. This drug has the advantage of high specificity for V2R, over V1R, therefore avoiding the side effects associated with AVP. For the urgent situation, desmopressin should be administered parenterally, intravenously, intramuscularly, or subcutaneously, in doses of 1–2 µg every 8–12 h.

For longer-term treatment of CDI, especially when complete, desmopressin represents the best approach. In the absence of thirst defects, the treatment of CDI is directed toward amelioration of bothersome symptoms, especially nocturia. Complete correction of the water excretory defect runs a risk of water retention and is not generally recommended. Dose finding is empiric. One approach is to start 0.05–0.2 mg orally or 5–10 µg intranasally at bedtime [9]. If this dose controls nocturia, and polyuria does not return until afternoon, then it may be sufficient. The patient should be instructed to detect inadvertent hyponatremia and report these symptoms immediately. Once a stable dose is reached, twice yearly monitoring may be sufficient. Patients should be monitored for a potential return of concentrating capacity during the annual visits.

The efficacy of endogenous AVP in partial CDI can be enhanced using pharmacological agents, including chlorpropamide (250–500 mg/day), clofibrate (500 mg 3–4 times daily), or carbamazepine (400–600 mg daily) [12]. Alone, these agents are typically only marginally effective, but when combined with endogenous AVP and oral solute restriction, they may be useful. Unfortunately, as all are used primarily for other conditions, such as diabetes or seizures, side effects are common.

The treatment of NDI is more difficult, as no specific agents are available. For patients with acquired disease, it is always best to eradicate the underlying cause. Factors such as hypokalemia, hypercalcemia, or the use of drugs such as demeclocycline, glyburide, or colchicine should be removed, if possible. Many times, however, lithium is found to be essential for control of bipolar disease. Amiloride (5 mg/day), which apparently competes for lithium for uptake into distal cells [15], can improve polyuria in such patients [16]. For other patients with NDI, thiazides are well-known to reduce urine flow, probably by inducing mild volume depletion and by increasing water reabsorption along the collecting duct [17, 18].

Finally, for gestational diabetes insipidus resulting from the placental secretion of vasopressinase, desmopressin is recommended. The secreted vasopressinase does not metabolize the synthetic drug, and the drug has a good safety record in pregnant individuals [19].

References

1. Lindholm J. Diabetes insipidus: historical aspects. Pituitary. 2004;7:33–8.
2. Birnbaumer M, Seibold A, Gilbert S, Ishido M, Barberis C, Antaramian A, Brabet P, Rosenthal W. Molecular cloning for the receptor for human antidiuretic hormone. Nature. 1992;357:333–5.
3. Preston GM, Carroll TP, Guggino WB, Agre P. Appearance of water channels in Xenopus Oocytes expressing red cell CHIP28 protein. Science. 1992;256:385–7.
4. Fujiwara TM, Bichet DG. Molecular biology of hereditary diabetes insipidus. J Am Soc Nephrol. 2005;16:2836–46.
5. Grunfeld JP, Rossier BC. Lithium nephrotoxicity revisited. Nat Rev Nephrol. 2009;5:270–6.
6. Sands JM, Bichet DG. Nephrogenic diabetes insipidus. Ann Intern Med. 2006;144:186–94.
7. Verbalis JG. Diabetes insipidus. Rev Endocr Metab Disord. 2003;4:177–85.
8. Timper K, et al. Diagnostic accuracy of copeptin in the differential diagnosis of the polyuria-polydipsia syndrome: prospective multicenter study. J Clin Endocrinol Metab. 2015;100(6):2268–74.
9. Fenske W, et al. A copeptin-based approach in the diagnosis of diabetes insipidus. N Engl J Med. 2018;379(5):428–39.
10. Winzeler B, et al. Arginine-stimulated copeptin measurements in the differential diagnosis of diabetes insipidus: a prospective diagnostic study. Lancet. 2019;394(10198):587–95. https://doi.org/10.1016/S0140-6736(19)31255-3.
11. Adrogue HJ, Madias NE. Hypernatremia. N Engl J Med. 2000;342:1493–9.

12. Thurman JM, Haltermman TJ, Berl T. Therapy of dysnatremic disorders. In: Brady HR, Wilcox CS, editors. Therapy in nephrology and hypertension. 2nd ed. London: Saunders; 2003. p. 335–48.
13. Bichet DG, Mallié J-P. Hypernatremia and the polyuric disorders. In: Dubose Jr TD, Hamm LL, editors. Acid–base and electrolyte disorders. Philadelphia: Saunders; 2002. p. 241–70.
14. Rose BD. New approach to disturbances in the plasma sodium concentration. Am J Med. 1986;81:1033–40.
15. Kortenoeven ML, Li Y, Shaw S, Gaeggeler HP, Rossier BC, Wetzels JF, Deen PM. Amiloride blocks lithium entry through the sodium channel thereby attenuating the resultant nephrogenic diabetes insipidus. Kidney Int. 2009;76:44–53.
16. Wells BG. Amiloride in lithium-induced polyuria. Ann Pharmacother. 1994;28:888–9.
17. Kim GH, Lee JW, Oh YK, Chang HR, Joo KW, Na KY, Earm JH, Knepper MA, Han JS. Antidiuretic effect of hydrochlorothiazide in lithium-induced nephrogenic diabetes insipidus is associated with upregulation of aquaporin-2, Na-Cl co-transporter, and epithelial sodium channel. J Am Soc Nephrol. 2004;15:2836–43.
18. Loffing J. Paradoxical antidiuretic effect of thiazides in diabetes insipidus: another piece in the puzzle. J Am Soc Nephrol. 2004;15:2948–50.
19. Durr JA, Hoggard JG, Hunt JM, Schrier RW. Diabetes insipidus in pregnancy associated with abnormally high circulating vasopressinase activity. N Engl J Med. 1987;316:1070–4.

Chapter 14
Pheochromocytoma Hypertensive Crisis

Vitaly Kantorovich and Karel Pacak

Précis

1. Clinical setting: Severe, often episodic, arterial hypertension resistant to the usual therapeutic interventions or any acute hypertensive event in an otherwise non-hypertensive person. There can be an associated family history of pheochromocytoma, von Hippel-Lindau syndrome, multiple endocrine neoplasia type 2, neurofibromatosis type 1, or one of the hereditary paraganglioma (extra-adrenal pheochromocytoma) syndromes, or the incidentally discovered adrenal mass.
2. Diagnosis:

    (a) History: The classic "paroxysmal attack" begins abruptly and can last for minutes to hours. The frequency of attacks varies between several attacks per day and a single attack every few months. Patients usually complain of palpitations, diaphoresis, and headache. Some patients complain of light-headedness on rising from a lying or sitting position. Other symptoms include anxiety, tremulousness, chest and abdominal pain, weakness, and weight loss.

    (b) Physical examination: Sustained or episodic hypertension with or without orthostatic hypotension is usually the initial finding. Tachycardia and pallor are often present. Physical findings suggesting a hereditary pheochromocytoma syndrome include renal tumor, retinal angioma, thyroid nodule, mucosal neuroma, and neurofibroma.

V. Kantorovich
Division of Endocrinology and Metabolism, University of CT Health Center,
Farmington, CT, USA

K. Pacak (✉)
Eunice Kennedy Shriver National Institute of Child Health and Human Development,
National Institutes of Health, Bethesda, MD, USA
e-mail: karel@mail.nih.gov

© Springer Nature Switzerland AG 2021
L. Loriaux, C. Vanek (eds.), *Endocrine Emergencies*, Contemporary Endocrinology,
https://doi.org/10.1007/978-3-030-67455-7_14

(c) Laboratory evaluation: Plasma or urinary metanephrines should be measured. If the plasma or urinary metanephrine values are equivocal (usually less than four times above the upper reference limit) and no interfering medication effect can be shown, a clonidine suppression test is confirmatory.

(d) Imaging studies: CT of the adrenal glands is the preferred imaging modality. MRI is also useful, especially in where radiation exposure must be minimized. "Brightening" of the tumor with T_2-weighted images on MRI is highly suggestive of pheochromocytoma. Functional imaging— ^{123}I-MIBG scintigraphy and Octreoscan—can improve diagnostic accuracy. Most tumors are intra-adrenal (80%), unilateral (90%), and benign (80%).

3. Initial treatment: Treatment of the hypertensive crisis should be carried out in an intensive care unit when possible. Nitroprusside is the first line of therapy with an initial intravenous dose of 0.3 µg/kg/min. This dose can be increased by increments of 0.1–0.3 µg/kg/min at 3–5 min intervals until the hypertension is controlled, likely within 10 min. The maximum recommended dose is 10 µg/kg/min.

Phentolamine, a nonselective α-adrenoceptor antagonist, can be used outside the ICU. The usual dose for adults is 5 mg intravenously which can be repeated every several minutes until the blood pressure is controlled.

Patients who present with tachyarrhythmia should receive a β-adrenoceptor antagonist. Labetalol is recommended at an initial dose of 20 mg administered intravenously over a 2-min period. Additional doses of 40 mg, up to 80 mg, can be administered at 10-min intervals until the tachycardia is controlled. The total dose should not exceed 300 mg in a 24-h period. Metoprolol can be given IV at an initial dose of 2.5–5.0 mg every 6–12 h and titrated as needed up to 15 mg every 3 h. Alternatively, atenolol is very effective, especially outside the ICU.

Once satisfactory control of the hypertensive crisis is achieved, treatment is transitioned to oral phenoxybenzamine, an α-adrenoceptor antagonist, 10 mg twice daily, adjusted upward in 10 mg increments every 2 or 3 days, to a maximum of 50–100 mg three times daily. Intravenous β-adrenoceptor blockade can be transitioned to oral atenolol 25–50 mg every 8–12 h. β-Adrenoceptor blockade should never be introduced before α-adrenoceptor blockade is at a satisfactory therapeutic level.

Pheochromocytoma

Fränkel and colleagues reported the first case of pheochromocytoma in 1886. The patient was a previously healthy 18-year-old woman from Wittenweier, Germany, who presented to the University Hospital of Freiburg in 1884 and died 10 days after admission. Her medical history included recurrent attacks of sudden-onset palpitations, anxiety, dizziness, headache, vomiting, and constipation. Weakness appeared and progressed during the year before her death. She was found to be malnourished and pale with an "agitated heart action and strong pulse." She had hypertension, retinopathy, proteinuria, and microhematuria. She had paroxysmal tachycardia (up to 180 beats per minute), sweating attacks, headaches, vomiting, visual deterioration, epistaxis, anxiety, and, in the end, severe chest pain [1]. Her autopsy showed all the signs of acute and chronic hypertension. She had two adrenal tumors. A retrospective family history points to the diagnosis of MEN-2 with bilateral adrenal pheochromocytomas [1].

Pheochromocytoma is a rare disease. It is hard to estimate the exact prevalence because of its variable clinical features. It is estimated that the overall prevalence of pheochromocytoma is between 1:1,700 and 1:4,500, with an annual incidence of 3–8 cases per one million per year [2]. It occurs at any age, most often in the fourth and fifth decades. It has an equal gender distribution. Most of the tumors (80%) are in the adrenal gland. The rest are extra-adrenal paragangliomas. Paragangliomas can be found anywhere from the head and neck to the urinary bladder and pelvis where they are usually in and around the Organ of Zuckerkandl. About 10–20% of pheochromocytomas are malignant [3], but there are "patient subgroups" in which a much higher prevalence of malignancy is reported [4]. Recently, there has been a significant shift in the patient population undergoing the "workup" for pheochromocytoma—most of the patients are now referred because of an incidentally discovered adrenal mass and less often because of poorly controlled hypertension.

Clinical signs and symptoms of pheochromocytoma relate to catecholamine action through adrenergic and dopaminergic receptors. The net effect of α-adrenergic stimulation is an increase in systemic vasoconstriction, peripheral pressure, and a decrease in target organ (myocardial, cerebral, renal, GI) perfusion. Activation of β-adrenoceptors induces pronounced myocardial inotropic and chronotropic effects, as well as the release of renin (Table 14.1). The "classic" symptoms and signs of a pheochromocytoma are headache, palpitations, and sweating. Hypertension, often the only sign of the disease, occurs in 90% of patients. Other symptoms and signs include tachycardia, anxiety, pallor, and orthostatic hypotension [5]. Sustained hypertension occurs in 50% of patients. Episodic or paroxysmal hypertension occurs in 45%. Five percent of patients are normotensive [3]. Sustained hypertension strongly correlates with high levels of plasma norepinephrine. Paroxysmal hypertension is seen more frequently with epinephrine-secreting tumors and is typical of MEN-2-related pheochromocytoma [6]. The frequency of hypertensive spells can vary from "rare" to daily, but most occur at 7- to 10-day intervals. The length of each attack varies from minutes to an hour. The longer-lasting ones often evolve into a hypertensive crisis [7, 8]. A hypertensive crisis refers to markedly increased arterial blood pressure that is resistant to the usual antihypertensive indications. Because of potentially devastating consequences that include acute myocardial infarction, congestive heart failure, renal failure, acute cerebrovascular accident, retinal detachment, and aortic dissection, crises are usually treated in the ICU. These spells are related to a sudden release of catecholamines from the tumor induced by factors such as physical activity, smoking, abdominal pressure, postural changes, and anxiety [6, 9]. Foods or beverages with a high tyramine content (aged cheese,

Table 14.1 Pathogenesis and organ-specific clinical features of pheochromocytoma

Organ	Syndrome	Mechanism	Receptor	Receptor action
Heart	Angina	Coronary spasm	Coronary α_1, β_2	Constriction
	Heart attack	Positive inotropy	Conducting system β_1, β_2	Increased conduction, automaticity, and contractility
	Cardiomyopathies	Positive chronotropy	Conducting system β_1, β_2	
	Myocarditis	Unmatched O_2 demand	Cardiomyocyte β_1, β_2	
	Acute failure	Hypoperfusion		
	Arrhythmias			
Brain	Stroke	Vasoconstriction	Cerebral arterioles α_1	Mild constriction
	Encephalopathy	Unmatched O_2 demand		Most of the effect related to systemic hypertension
		Hypoperfusion		
Vascular	Shock	Vasoconstriction	Skeletal muscle α_1, α_2, β_2	Arteriolar constriction
	Postural hypotension	Unmatched O_2 demand		Venous dilation
	Aortic dissection	Hypoperfusion		
	Organ ischemia			
	Limb ischemia			
Kidneys	ARF	Vasoconstriction	Vascular α_1, α_2, β_1, β_2	Dilation > constriction
	Hematuria	Unmatched O_2 demand		
		Hypoperfusion		
Lungs	Pulmonary edema	Cardiac decompensation	Vascular α_1, β_2	Dilation > constriction bronchodilation
	ARDS	Increased permeability	Smooth muscle β_2	
	Fibrosis			
	Pulmonary HTN			
GI	Intestinal ischemia (necrosis, peritonitis)	Vasoconstriction	Visceral arterioles α_1, β_2	Constriction
		Unmatched O_2 demand		
		Hypoperfusion		
Ocular	Acute blindness	Vasoconstriction		
	Retinopathy			
Death	All of the above			Acute multiorgan failure

beer, and wine) and certain medications (histamine, phenothiazine, and tricyclic antidepressants) can precipitate a hypertensive paroxysm in patients with pheochromocytoma [10]. Metoclopramide, used to treat nausea, when given to a patient who has pheochromocytoma, can precipitate a severe life-threatening hypertensive crisis [11]. Glucocorticoids used to treat many inflammatory diseases also can cause a pheochromocytoma crisis [12]. Pheochromocytomas that secrete predominantly dopamine usually present with normotension. These tumors are often extra-adrenal and are diagnosed biochemically by increased plasma levels of free methoxy-tyramine, a metabolite of dopamine [13].

The complications associated with catecholamines excess are shown in Table 14.1. Catecholamines, mainly norepinephrine, induce peripheral vasocon-striction and elevated blood pressure, leading to increased arterial stiffness [14]. Hypercatecholaminemia can lead to hypoxic myocardial damage, aseptic myocar-ditis, and cardiomyopathy [8]. In most of these events, the coronary arteries are patent. The pathophysiology of asymmetric myocardial ballooning in takotsubo cardiomyopathy is poorly understood, but we suggest that it is related to the differ-ential expression of adrenergic receptors in endocardium and myocardium, with an increased concentration in the region of the pacemaker. Increased myocardial oxy-gen demand shortens diastolic relaxation, resulting in worsening of myocardial damage. Peripheral vascular disease can be the result of intense vasoconstriction and result in limb ischemia, necrosis, gangrene, and aortic dissection. Pheochromocytoma can cause neurologic complications, including hypertensive encephalopathy with headache, papilledema, altered mental status, and stroke. Paroxysmal hypertension usually causes hemorrhagic stroke, while postural hypo-tension is associated with ischemic stroke. The renal effects of pheochromocytoma include hypertensive nephropathy, renovascular hypertension, renal artery stenosis, and, eventually, renal failure. Rarely, severe peripheral vasoconstriction can cause rhabdomyolysis due to muscular ischemia and acute tubular necrosis caused by myoglobinuria. Renal artery stenosis can coexist with extra-adrenal pheochromocy-toma, making both diagnosis and treatment more complicated [15]. Acute intestinal ischemia is one of the most feared complications of pheochromocytoma. It presents with severe abdominal pain due to a spasm of the visceral arteries [16]. Paralytic ileus with pseudo-obstruction can be associated with pheochromocytoma and may respond to high-dose phentolamine and metyrosine (see below) [17]. Eye disease associated with pheochromocytoma includes hypertensive retinopathy, secondary retinal arteriosclerosis, retinal microaneurysms, hemorrhages, cotton wool spots, and venous hemorrhage. Pheochromocytoma in pregnancy is associated with increased maternal and fetal morbidity and mortality [18]. Pheochromocytoma should be suspected with resistant hypertension and hypertensive crisis.

Diagnosis: The diagnostic approach is based on the assessment of either plasma or urine metanephrines [19]. Plasma catecholamines should not be used in the bio-chemical diagnosis of pheochromocytoma since they often are secreted episodically, and elevated levels can be missed with a single plasma sample (Fig. 14.1). Metanephrines are produced continuously and independently of catecholamine release. Therefore, metanephrines are more reliable than catecholamines in the detection of patients with pheochromocytoma (Figs. 14.2 and 14.3). Metanephrine levels correlate with tumor size. Failure to suppress plasma normetanephrine levels with clonidine is supportive of the diagnosis of pheochromocytoma (97% sensitivity, 100% specificity). CT and MRI provide high-resolution images that allow for the assessment of size, consistency, contrast washout rate, and lipid content (Fig. 14.4). Functional imaging that detects specific transporters/receptors associated with pheo-chromocytoma are ^{123}I-MIBG scintigraphy and Ga-68 DOTATATE PET.

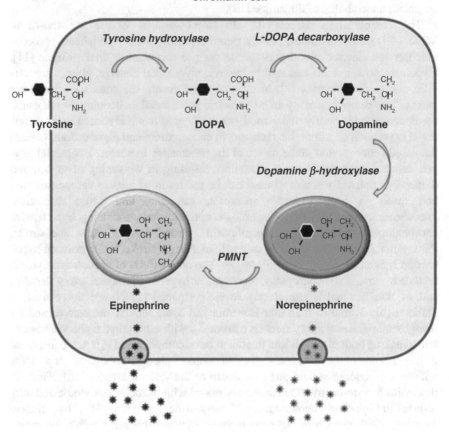

Fig. 14.1 Catecholamine synthesis

Treatment rests on two main principles: (a) medical treatment in preparation for surgery and (b) surgery for the definitive treatment of pheochromocytoma. The mainstay of medical therapy is the use of a noncompetitive α1- or α2-adrenoceptor antagonist. Phenoxybenzamine is the drug of choice. The usual dose is 10–30 mg twice a day. Postoperative hypotension is sometimes a complication of phenoxybenzamine treatment. Selective α1-adrenoceptor blockade with doxazosin, prazosin, or terazosin are suitable alternatives and more readily available than phenoxybenzamine. When treatment with α-adrenoceptor antagonists leads to tachycardia, β-adrenoceptor blockade can be very helpful. An alpha-methyl-L-tyrosine (metyrosine, Demser™) is the only medication that causes an actual decrease in catecholamine production. It blocks tyrosine hydroxylase and is effective in preoperative preparation and in the treatment of patients with metastatic disease [20]. Medical treatment to control hypertension should ideally be in place for at least 7 days prior to surgery.

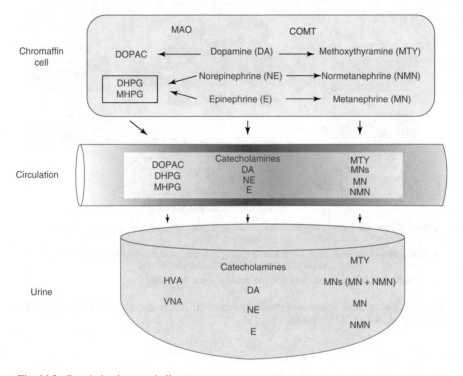

Fig. 14.2 Catecholamine metabolism

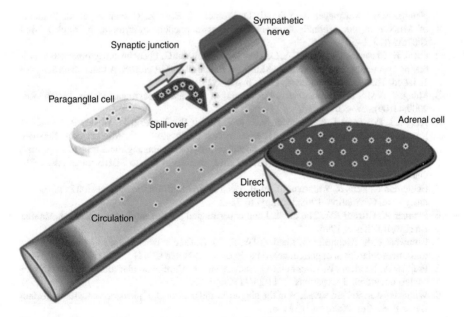

Fig. 14.3 Catecholamine secretion from the adrenal medulla and paraganglia

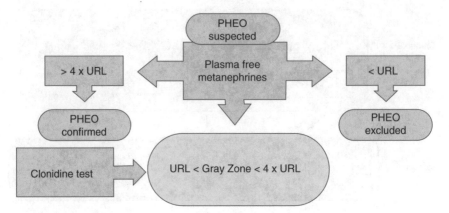

- Use clonidine test coupled with the measurement of plasma <u>normetanephrine</u> (NMN; sensitivity 97%, specificity 100%)
- Distinguishes increased sympathetic activity (false-positives) (NMN decrease more than 40% or below URL) from PHEO/PGL (true-positives)
- Glucagon test: sensitivity less than 50%; not recommended to be used

Fig. 14.4 Biochemical diagnosis of pheochromocytoma. (Eisenhofer et al. *JCEM*. 2003;88:2656; Lenders et al. *JCEM*. 2010;95:238)

References

1. Neumann HP, Vortmeyer A, Schmidt D, Werner M, Erlic Z, Cascon A, et al. Evidence of MEN-2 in the original description of classic pheochromocytoma. N Engl J Med. 2007;357:1311–5.
2. Pacak K, Chrousos GP, Koch CA, Lenders JW, Eisenhofer G. Pheochromocytoma: progress in diagnosis, therapy, and genetics. In: Margioris A, Chrousos GP, editors. Adrenal disorders, vol. 1. 1st ed. Totowa: Humana Press; 2001. p. 479–523.
3. Manger WM. The protean manifestations of pheochromocytoma. Horm Metab Res. 2009;41(09):658–63.
4. King KS, Prodanov T, Kantorovich V, Fojo T, Hewitt JK, Zacharin M, Wesley R, Lodish M, Raygada M, Gimenez-Roqueplo AP, McCormack S, Eisenhofer G, Milosevic D, Kebebew E, Stratakis CA, Pacak K. Metastatic pheochromocytoma/paraganglioma related to primary tumor development in childhood or adolescence: significant link to SDHB mutations. J Clin Oncol. 2011;29(31):4137–42.
5. Engleman K, Zelis R, Waldmann T, et al. Mechanism of orthostatic hypotension in pheochromocytoma. Circulation. 1968;38(Suppl 6):71–2.
6. Manger W, Gifford RW. The clinical and experimental pheochromocytoma. 2nd ed. Malden: Blackwell Science; 1996.
7. Brouwers FM, Eisenhofer G, Lenders JW, Pacak K. Emergencies caused by pheochromocytoma, neuroblastoma, or ganglioneuroma. Endocrinol Metab Clin N Am. 2006;35(4):699–724.
8. Prejbisz A, Lenders JW, Eisenhofer G, Januszewicz A. Cardiovascular manifestations of phaeochromocytoma. J Hypertens. 2011;29(11):2049–60.
9. Widimský J Jr. Recent advances in the diagnosis and treatment of pheochromocytoma. Kidney Blood Press Res. 2006;29(5):321–6.

10. Manger WM. An overview of pheochromocytoma: history, current concepts, vagaries, and diagnostic challenges. Ann N Y Acad Sci. 2006;1073:1–20.
11. Eisenhofer G, Rivers G, Rosas AL, Quezado Z, Manger WM, Pacak K. Adverse drug reactions in patients with phaeochromocytoma: incidence, prevention and management. Drug Saf. 2007;30(11):1031–62.
12. Rosas AL, Kasperlik-Zaluska AA, Papierska L, Bass BL, Pacak K, Eisenhofer G. Pheochromocytoma crisis induced by glucocorticoids: a report of four cases and review of the literature. Eur J Endocrinol. 2008;158(3):423–9.
13. Eisenhofer G, Goldstein DS, Sullivan P, et al. Biochemical and clinical manifestations of dopamine-producing paragangliomas: utility of plasma methoxytyramine. J Clin Endocrinol Metab. 2005;90(4):2068–75.
14. Petrak O, Strauch B, Zelinka T, et al. Factors influencing arterial stiffness in pheochromocytoma and effect of adrenalectomy. Hypertens Res. 2010;33(5):454–9.
15. Hill FS, Jander HP, Murad T, et al. The coexistence of renal artery stenosis and pheochromocytoma. Ann Surg. 1983;197(4):484–90.
16. Salehi A, Legome EL, Eichhorn K, et al. Pheochromocytoma and bowel ischemia. J Emerg Med. 1996;15(1):35–8.
17. Sawaki D, Otani Y, Sekita G, Kobayakawa N, Fukushima K, Takeuchi H, Aoyagi T. Pheochromocytoma complicated with refractory paralytic ileus dramatically improved with intravenous administration of alpha-adrenergic receptor antagonist, phentolamine. J Clin Gastroenterol. 2003;37(2):194.
18. Schenker JG, Chowers I. Pheochromocytoma and pregnancy. Review of 89 cases. Obstet Gynecol Surv. 1971;26(11):739–47.
19. Lenders JW, Pacak K, Walther MM, Linehan WM, Mannelli M, Friberg P, Keiser HR, Goldstein DS, Eisenhofer G. Biochemical diagnosis of pheochromocytoma: which test is best? JAMA. 2002;287(11):1427–34.
20. Pacak K. Preoperative management of the pheochromocytoma patient. J Clin Endocrinol Metab. 2007;92(11):4069–79.

Chapter 15
Hypocalcemia

Robert Klein and Chaim Vanek

Précis

1. Clinical setting: Hypocalcemia, defined as an ionized calcium level of less than 1.1 mmol/L, is a common electrolyte disturbance complicating nearly one-quarter of hospital admissions. It is found in the majority of patients admitted to an intensive care unit (ICU) [10].
2. Diagnosis: The potential causes of hypocalcemia are diverse and numerous. In general terms, hypocalcemia can result from inadequate parathyroid hormone (PTH) or vitamin D production, resistance to the actions of PTH or vitamin D, and the consequence of an underlying medical condition in which multiple factors (e.g., sepsis, critical illness) are contributing. Correct management depends on an accurate diagnosis. If the patient has severe symptoms, therapy should be initiated immediately, and the diagnosis pursued after the patient's condition is stabilized.

    (a) The initial evaluation of a patient with hypocalcemia should include a detailed family history (searching for a genetic cause) and a relevant medical history (e.g., inadequate nutrition, prior neck surgery, infiltrative disorders, autoimmune disease, intestinal or renal dysfunction, and medications that interfere with calcium homeostasis).
    (b) Physical examination: The clinical presentation of hypocalcemia depends on the chronicity and severity of the disturbance and ranges from few if any symptoms with long-standing minor hypocalcemia to severe life-threatening symptoms if an acute and dramatic decline has taken place. Circumoral anesthesia, cataracts, papilledema, and laryngeal stridor can be observed in

R. Klein · C. Vanek (✉)
Division of Endocrinology, Diabetes and Clinical Nutrition, Oregon Health and Science University, Portland, OR, USA
e-mail: vanekc@ohsu.edu

© Springer Nature Switzerland AG 2021
L. Loriaux, C. Vanek (eds.), *Endocrine Emergencies*, Contemporary Endocrinology, https://doi.org/10.1007/978-3-030-67455-7_15

hypocalcemic patients. The bedside Trousseau's sign (indicative of latent tetany) is a sensitive and specific indicator for hypocalcemia.

(c) Laboratory evaluation: It is important to verify results with a repeat measurement of ionized calcium or total serum calcium corrected for albumin to confirm a true decrease in the serum calcium concentration. Additional laboratory testing should include measurements of phosphorus, magnesium, vitamin D metabolites, alkaline phosphatase, and intact PTH levels. An electrocardiogram can reveal a prolonged QT interval and alert the treating physician to the increased likelihood of ventricular arrhythmias.

3. Treatment: Hypocalcemia with neurological, muscular, or cardiac dysfunction is associated with significant morbidity and mortality and should be handled as a medical emergency. Parenteral infusions of calcium are indicated when a rapid correction of the serum calcium level is required. Emergency treatment should be initiated with 2 g calcium gluconate (1 g calcium gluconate contains 93 mg of elemental calcium) in 100 mL of normal saline given intravenously over a 10-min period. This should be followed by an infusion of 6 g calcium gluconate in 500 mL normal saline over 4–6 h. Serum calcium should be measured at 4-h intervals, and the infusion rate adjusted to maintain the serum calcium between 8 and 9 mg/mL.

Introduction

Calcium is the single most abundant mineral in the human body, and it serves as a critical ion for many physiological processes including blood coagulation, platelet adhesion, neuromuscular activity, endocrine and exocrine secretory functions, and bone metabolism. The adult human body contains approximately 1000 g of calcium [1]. Most of this calcium (99%) is stably incorporated into bone as hydroxyapatite, with less than 1% in the serum [1]. Plasma normally contains 8.9–10.1 mg/dL of calcium. Approximately 40–50% of calcium in the blood is bound to plasma proteins, primarily albumin. An equivalent amount is ionized or "free," and the remainder is complexed to phosphate, citrate, bicarbonate, and other ions. Only the free calcium is physiologically active. Ionized serum calcium is closely regulated by the endocrine system and, as such, is a better indicator of the functional status of calcium metabolism than total calcium levels [2]. The normal range for ionized serum calcium concentration is 1.20–1.30 mmol/L.

The regulation of ionized calcium concentration is primarily accomplished by the coordinated actions of PTH and calcitriol (the activated form of vitamin D or 1,25-dihydroxyvitamin D) at the three main sites of calcium transport (intestine, bone, kidney) [3]. Calcium-sensing receptors on the surface of parathyroid cells constantly sense the extracellular ionized calcium concentration and, when the concentration falls, direct the synthesis and release of PTH [4]. PTH exerts effects in several target organs, including the skeleton, where it increases osteoclast-mediated bone resorption, leading to the release of calcium and phosphorus, and the kidney, where PTH increases reabsorption of calcium into the extracellular space from the distal convoluted tubules and decreases the reabsorption of phosphorus from the proximal convoluted tubules. Additionally, PTH increases renal 1α(alpha)-hydroxylase activity, which increases the conversion of 25-hydroxyvitamin D to its hormonally active form 1,25-dihydroxyvitamin D (calcitriol). Calcitriol, in turn, binds to nuclear receptors in the intestine where it directs the expression of calcium transport proteins to enhance calcium uptake, augments the actions of PTH on distal convoluted tubules in the kidney, and stimulates the mobilization of calcium and phosphorus from the skeleton into the circulation.

In the short-term serum proteins, chiefly albumin, can serve to stabilize the ionized calcium concentration by acting as a calcium buffer. A transient drop in the ionized calcium concentration is compensated for by a concomitant release of calcium from some of the 30 calcium-binding sites on an albumin molecule. The albumin-calcium buffer is highly sensitive to pH. Changes in pH alter the fraction of charged amino acid residues in albumin, and, thus, the number of calcium ions bound. This results in a change in the fraction of total calcium that is free. Increases in pH, such as respiratory alkalosis caused by hyperventilation, will cause the ionized calcium to fall, while decreases in pH will cause ionized calcium to rise [2].

Although an ionized calcium determination is the most physiologically relevant measure of calcium homeostasis, it is neither the easiest nor the cheapest to measure. In comparison, the laboratory costs for total serum calcium and albumin assays (part of the most large automated chemistry analyzers) are much lower than those associated with an ionized calcium analysis. The total serum calcium concentration is a reliable indicator of the serum ionized calcium concentration under most, but not all, circumstances. One important situation in which total serum calcium poorly reflects the ionized calcium concentration is when serum albumin levels are abnormal. As the primary calcium-binding site in serum is albumin, and because albumin molecules bind a relatively predictable quantity of calcium at a given pH, it is possible to estimate ionized calcium levels from protein and total calcium measurements [5]. The adjustment is accomplished by adding 0.8 mg/dL to the measured total serum calcium for every 1 g/dL of albumin: below 4 g/dL albumin: ((4-measured albumin)*0.8). The "albumin-adjusted" total calcium value is then compared to a standard (non-adjusted) total calcium reference range. Total calcium- or albumin-corrected calcium measures, however, can still misclassify a significant proportion of patients due to alterations in blood pH, drugs, fatty acids bound to albumin, the presence of calcium-binding immunoglobulins, gadolinium-containing agents that interfere with the colorimetric detection of total calcium, etc. [6–9]. Consequently, in critically ill patients, the direct measurement of ionized calcium concentration is strongly recommended [2].

Etiology

A low circulating ionized calcium level can be the consequence of the decreased entry of calcium into the vascular space, accelerated removal of calcium from the vascular space, or by sequestration of ionized calcium. Clinical disorders associated with hypocalcemia are listed in Table 15.1. The most common cause of acute hypo-calcemia is postoperative hypoparathyroidism in the context of neck surgery during which damage or unintentional removal of most or all functioning parathyroid tissue has taken place [11, 12]. Damage to the parathyroid glands may also be caused by immune-mediated destruction of the parathyroid glands [13], iron (hemochromatosis), or copper (Wilson's disease) accumulation in the parathyroid glands [14–16] or, in rare cases, by iodine-131 therapy for thyroid diseases [17] or metastatic infiltration of the parathyroid glands by tumor [18]. Hypoparathyroidism causes hypocalcemia because PTH secretion is inadequate to mobilize calcium from bone, reabsorb calcium from the urine, or stimulate renal 1α(alpha)-hydroxylase activity. As a result, insufficient 1,25-dihydroxyvitamin D is produced for optimal intestinal absorption of calcium [12]. Parathyroid secretory reserve is sizable, so considerable damage must take place for hypocalcemia to develop. It is estimated that one normal gland is sufficient for maintaining PTH and calcium homeostasis [12]. A number of genetic disorders have been identified in patients with inherited hypoparathyroidism (e.g., DiGeorge, or velocardiofacial, syndrome, activating mutations in the extracellular calcium-sensing receptor, pseudohypoparathyroidism) and should be considered a possible cause of hypocalcemia in the appropriate clinical setting [19, 20].

Magnesium is essential for PTH secretion and receptor activation [21]. Thus, magnesium depletion can cause hypocalcemia by inducing a functional hypoparathyroid state. Hypomagnesemia as the underlying cause for hypocalcemia should be considered in a variety of clinical situations (malnutrition, pancreatitis, chronic

Table 15.1 Causes of hypocalcemia

Reduced PTH action	Reduced vitamin D action	Calcium deposition/ complexation
Hypoparathyroidism	*Vitamin D deficiency*	*Hyperphosphatemia*
Surgical	Dietary lack or limited sunlight exposure	Rhabdomyolysis
Idiopathic	Malabsorption	Renal insufficiency
Autoimmune		Tumor lysis syndrome
Infiltrative (Fe, Cu, tumor)	*Abnormal vitamin D metabolism*	Phosphate administration
Postradiation	Liver or kidney disease	
Genetic (DiGeorge, activating CaSR mutation, etc.)	Abnormal enterohepatic circulation	*Acute pancreatitis*
Hypomagnesemia (functional)	Anticonvulsants	
	Nephrotic syndrome	*Blood transfusions*
PTH resistance	*Vitamin D resistance*	*Excessive skeletal mineralization*
Pseudohypoparathyroidism	Vitamin D-dependent rickets	Hungry bone syndrome
Renal insufficiency		Osteoblastic metastases

alcohol abuse, diarrhea) or as a consequence of certain therapies (diuretics, antibiotics, and chemotherapeutic agents such as cisplatin derivatives).

Vitamin D deficiency (resulting from dietary insufficiency, sunlight deprivation, or hepatic or renal impairment) or reduced vitamin D-mediated signaling can be a primary cause of hypocalcemia or aggravate the hypocalcemia initiated by other processes [22, 23]. Excessive remineralization of bone can occur after successful parathyroid surgery for hyperparathyroidism ("hungry bone" syndrome) [24] and in the setting of osteoblastic bone metastases (e.g., breast or prostate cancer) [25, 26]. Hyperphosphatemia, commonly seen in renal impairment, tumor lysis syndrome, and rhabdomyolysis, causes hypocalcemia by complexing with circulating free calcium ions. Acute pancreatitis is associated with the formation of calcium complexes within the abdominal cavity. Calcium chelation can occur iatrogenically with citrate-containing blood transfusions but is rare if renal and hepatic functions are normal. Acute and critical illness, often in the ICU setting, is frequently accompanied by low ionized calcium values. This entity is typically multifactorial with poor nutrition, vitamin D insufficiency, renal dysfunction, acid-base disturbances, release of inflammatory cytokines, magnesium abnormalities, frequent transfusions, and other factors all likely contributing to some degree. Finally, a number of medications are associated with symptomatic hypocalcemia (e.g., foscarnet, calcitonin, bisphosphonates, denosumab, phenobarbital, and phenytoin) especially in the setting of unrecognized calcium and/or vitamin D deficiency [27].

Clinical Signs and Features

The clinical manifestations of hypocalcemia depend on the degree of hypocalcemia (ionized calcium level) and the rate of its development. An acute decrease in the blood calcium level enhances neuron excitability, but chronic hypocalcemia can be asymptomatic even at quite low levels of serum calcium. Conversely, severe or acute hypocalcemia is usually associated with predictable signs (Table 15.2). Patients with acute hypocalcemia will present with neurologic complaints ranging from circumoral tingling and distal paresthesias to severe central nervous system symptoms such as confusion, delirium, and/or seizure. Laryngospasm and bronchospasm, which could lead to respiratory compromise, also can indicate hypocalcemia. Cardiovascular manifestations of hypocalcemia can include decreased myocardial contractility, congestive heart failure, and arrhythmias due to prolonged QT intervals. Tetany is typically seen when the ionized calcium drops below 1.0 mmol/L, but chronic hypocalcemia can be asymptomatic even with these low serum calcium levels. In this situation, the clinician can attempt to draw out latent tetany due to hypocalcemia by demonstrating Trousseau's sign. A sphygmomanometer cuff is inflated 20 mmHg above systolic pressure for 3 min to occlude the brachial artery. Flexion of the wrist and metacarpophalangeal joints, hyperextension of the fingers, and flexion of the thumb result. This response to anoxia is known as the "main d'accoucheur" (*French* for "hand of the obstetrician") (Fig. 15.1). Chvostek's

Table 15.2 Clinical manifestations of hypocalcemia

Acute neuromuscular features
Paresthesias
Perioral numbness
Muscle cramps and weakness
Confusion, delirium
Carpopedal spasm
Tetany
Seizure
Laryngospasm and bronchospasm
Congestive heart failure
Arrhythmia, prolonged QT interval
Other features more common with chronic hypocalcemia
Subcapsular cataracts
Dry skin and hair
Papilledema
Pseudotumor cerebri
Basal ganglia calcification
Depression
Dementia

sign, an abnormal contraction of the ipsilateral facial muscles in response to tapping the facial nerve 2 cm in front of the tragus of the ear, is also indicative of hypocalcemic neural irritability. However, perioral twitching occurs in up to 25% of normal individuals, and the Chvostek's sign is negative in approximately 30% of those with hypocalcemia [28]. By contrast, the Trousseau's sign is considerably more sensitive (94%) and specific for hypocalcemia [28]. Other manifestations of chronic hypocalcemia include premature cataracts, alopecia, depression, dementia, pseudotumor cerebri, calcification of the basal ganglia, and seizures.

The etiology of hypocalcemia may be obvious from the clinical history. A family history of hypocalcemia suggests a genetic cause (e.g., activating mutation of the calcium-sensing receptor, pseudohypoparathyroidism). In contrast, acquired hypoparathyroidism is most often the result of postsurgical or autoimmune damage to the parathyroid glands. A history of head and neck surgery or the presence of a neck scar suggests postsurgical hypoparathyroidism, while the presence of chronic mucocutaneous candidiasis, diabetes mellitus type 1, and adrenal insufficiency suggests a polyglandular autoimmune syndrome. Other causes of hypocalcemia include acute or chronic kidney disease, acute pancreatitis, metastatic disease, and malnutrition.

Laboratory Evaluation

Based upon the patient's history and physical examination, there are several laboratory measurements that can confirm the underlying etiology of the hypocalcemia.

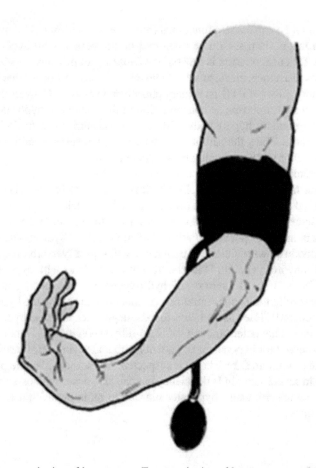

Fig. 15.1 Trousseau's sign of latent tetany. Trousseau's sign of latent tetany can be observed in patients with low calcium. To elicit the sign, a blood pressure cuff is placed around the upper arm and inflated to a pressure greater than the systolic blood pressure and held in place for 3 min. In the absence of brachial artery blood flow, the patient's hypocalcemia and resultant neuromuscular irritability will induce spasm of the muscles of the hand and forearm. The wrist and metacarpophalangeal joints flex, the DIP and PIP joints extend, and the fingers adduct. The sign is also known as main d'accoucheur (*French* for "hand of the obstetrician") because of its resemblance to the position of an obstetrician's hand in delivering a baby. Importantly, this sign may become positive before other gross manifestations of hypocalcemia such as hyperreflexia and tetany are manifest. (Reproduced from TheFreeDictionary.com)

Serum intact PTH is the most important. It only can be interpreted correctly when serum calcium is measured simultaneously. The most potent stimulus of PTH secretion is a reduced ionized calcium level. A low or normal serum PTH concentration in a patient with hypocalcemia is a strong proof of hypoparathyroidism. In contrast, patients with hypocalcemia as a result of vitamin D deficiency or pseudohypoparathyroidism (PTH resistance) will have elevated levels of PTH (secondary hyperparathyroidism). Hypomagnesemia (serum magnesium concentration below 1 mg/

dL or 0.4 mmol/L) can cause a functional (but reversible) form of hypoparathyroidism. Serum magnesium should be measured in any patient with hypocalcemia in whom the PTH concentration is low but the cause is not obvious. In states of PTH deficiency or resistance, elevated serum phosphate levels will occur due to a loss of the stimulatory effect of PTH on urinary phosphate excretion. Conversely, the presence of a low serum phosphate concentration in the context of hypocalcemia indicates either secondary hyperparathyroidism or poor nutrition with limited dietary phosphate intake. Thus, the serum phosphate level can serve as an important discriminating factor when evaluating hypocalcemic patients.

When vitamin D deficiency is suspected, serum 25-hydroxyvitamin D should be assessed first rather than serum 1,25-dihydroxyvitamin D (calcitriol). The diminished intestinal calcium absorption seen in vitamin D deficiency results in a state of secondary hyperparathyroidism. As increased circulating PTH levels and hypophosphatemia are both potent stimulators of renal 1,25-dihydroxyvitamin D production, individuals with vitamin D deficiency will typically exhibit normal or high serum 1,25-dihydroxyvitamin D levels. In contrast, patients with hypoparathyroidism can have normal serum 25-hydroxyvitamin D but generally low 1,25-dihydroxyvitamin D concentrations (in that clinical setting the hyperphosphatemia and reduced PTH levels attenuate, to some degree, renal 1,25-dihydroxyvitamin D production). The determination of 1,25-dihydroxyvitamin D concentrations should be reserved for hypocalcemic patients with underlying renal insufficiency or when a state of vitamin D resistance is suspected. An elevated alkaline phosphatase is common in severe vitamin D deficiency but can also occur with osteoblastic bone metastases, which can cause hypocalcemia due to rapid deposition of calcium in bone metastases.

Treatment

The treatment of hypocalcemia should vary with its severity and the underlying cause (Table 15.3). For example, asymptomatic hypocalcemia due to hypoalbuminemia requires no therapy, while severe hypocalcemia (total serum calcium concentration of less than 7.5 mg/dL or ionized calcium concentration below 0.9 mmol/L) or acute symptomatic hypocalcemia requires urgent medical attention. It is important for the treating physician to recognize that patients with acute hypocalcemia can be quite symptomatic (e.g., tetany, seizures, laryngospasm, or cardiac dysfunction) at serum calcium values that would not usually cause symptoms in patients with chronic hypocalcemia. Clinical manifestations can also vary with other factors such as acid-base status and underlying illness.

Parenteral infusions of either calcium gluconate or calcium chloride are indicated when rapid correction of serum calcium levels is required. Although calcium chloride provides nearly four times more elemental calcium than an equivalent

Table 15.3 Therapeutic options for hypocalcemia

Agent	Dosing information	Notes
Acute management		
Parenteral calcium infusion		
Calcium chloride	10 mL ampule (272 mg elemental calcium) diluted in 200 mL of 5% dextrose in water given intravenously over 30–90 min	$CaCl_2$ solutions can be irritating to surrounding tissues if extravasated, so this agent should be administered by a central venous catheter, if possible
Calcium gluconate	10 mL ampules (93 mg elemental calcium); 1–3 ampules diluted in 200 mL of 5% dextrose or normal saline given intravenously over 30–90 min	Therapy should be individualized and guided by frequent serum ionized calcium determinations
Calcium gluconate infusion	10 ampules (930 mg elemental calcium) diluted in 1 L 5% dextrose in water	Infusion rate should be 1–3 mg/kg/h to maintain serum calcium levels within the targeted range
Long-term management		
Calcium supplements		
Calcium carbonate	40% elemental calcium by weight	Best absorbed in small, multiple doses with meals and with acid present in the stomach
Calcium citrate	21% elemental calcium by weight	Preferred option for patients with achlorhydria
Vitamin D preparations		
D_2 (ergocalciferol) D_3 (cholecalciferol)	2000–100,000 IU once daily; onset of action 10–14 days; offset of action 14–75 days	Wide dose range reflects the various disorders these agents are used. Careful attention to serum levels of calcium, phosphorus, and creatinine is necessary for safe use
25-Hydroxyvitamin D_3 (calcifediol)	20–200 µg daily; onset of action 5–10 days; offset of action 14–75 days	Used in hepatic failure when renal function is intact to insure 1-alpha hydroxylation available to activate this metabolite
Dihydrotachysterol	0.2–1 mg once daily; onset of action 4–7 days; offset of action 7–21 days	Active D metabolite that does not require renal conversion
1α(Alpha)-hydroxyvitamin D_3 (alfacalcidol)	0.5–3 µg daily; onset of action 1–2 days; offset of action 5–7 days	Rapidly converted to active 1,25-dihdroxyvitamin D_3 in vivo
1,25-Dihydroxyvitamin D_3 (calcitriol)	0.25–1 µg once or twice daily; onset of action 1–2 days; offset of action 2–3 days	Active D metabolite that does not require renal conversion – *preferred agent*
Thiazide diuretic		
Hydrochlorothiazide Chlorthalidone	25–100 mg daily	Used in concert with a low-sodium diet (80–100 mmol per day) to promote renal calcium retention; hypokalemia and hyponatremia are adverse events

Table adapted from Table 3 in Shoback [12]

amount of calcium gluconate, calcium gluconate is the preferred salt for peripheral venous administration as calcium chloride can cause tissue necrosis in the event of local extravasation. Initially, 1 g of calcium chloride (272 mg of calcium) or up to 3 g of calcium gluconate (279 mg of calcium) can be delivered over 30–90 min to control symptoms (Table 15.3). However, a single intravenous injection of calcium is usually only effective for a few hours [29]. A continuous infusion of calcium gluconate will be required to fully control symptoms and achieve a safe and stable ionized calcium level, usually above 1.0 mmol/L. In patients receiving parenteral calcium replacement, the serum ionized calcium level should be measured every 1–2 h until the patient's condition has stabilized and then every 4–6 h in order to monitor therapy. The recurrence of hypocalcemic symptoms can necessitate an increase in the infusion rate but should always be correlated with a simultaneous ionized calcium value. The infusion rate should not exceed 1–2 mg/min because of the potential risk for cardiac arrhythmias associated with rapid calcium infusion. Oral calcium and vitamin D therapy should be started as soon as possible and the intravenous calcium infusion tapered slowly (over a period of 24–48 h or longer), while oral therapy is adjusted.

When magnesium depletion is present, hypocalcemia is frequently difficult to correct without first normalizing the serum magnesium concentration. If the serum magnesium concentration is low, 2 g of magnesium sulfate in 20 mL of D5W should be infused over 10–20 min, followed by 1 g in 100 mL D5W per hour as long as the serum magnesium concentration remains less than 1 mg/dL. As intracellular magnesium deficits are generally large and inadequately mirrored by the serum magnesium level, continued supplementation with oral magnesium salts over an extended period of time may be necessary. Careful monitoring is required in patients with impaired renal function who are at greater risk of developing hypermagnesemia.

The chronic management of hypocalcemia should be tailored to the underlying etiology and will almost always rely on oral calcium supplements, vitamin D metabolites, and, sometimes, thiazide diuretics (Table 15.3). Synthetic parathyroid hormone, Natpara™, a daily subcutaneous injection, is FDA approved for hypocalcemia due to hypoparathyroidism but is on manufacturer recall at the time of this writing. It is not used for acute hypocalcemia. Although calcium supplements of all types can be used for hypocalcemia, the most efficient means of supplementation is in the form of either carbonate or citrate salts. The former contains 40% calcium by weight and the latter 21%. A reasonable starting dose is 0.5–1 g of elemental calcium two or three times each day. Subsequent dosing can then be adjusted based on patient compliance, side effects, and clinical objectives.

In addition to calcium, patients with vitamin D deficiency will require vitamin D supplementation [22]. For vitamin D-deficient subjects with intact renal function, either ergocalciferol (vitamin D_2) or cholecalciferol (vitamin D_3) can be used. Patients who choose to avoid the ingestion of animal products should be aware that cholecalciferol is of animal origin. Although the recommended regimen to reach a 25-hydroxyvitamin D concentration of 25–30 ng/mL is 50,000 international units (IU) of vitamin D weekly for 8–12 weeks, a daily 50,000 IU dose of ergocalciferol can be safely administered for 5 days at the beginning of therapy in patients with severe vitamin D deficiency. Because of their long-term storage in fat, these forms of vitamin D have an extended tissue half-life (up to months), and toxicity may be difficult to anticipate and/or correct quickly. Hypercalcemia, should it occur, can persist for weeks after the vitamin D supplement is stopped. For this reason calcitriol, despite its increased expense compared to vitamin D, is preferred by many clinicians because of its rapid onset and offset of action. Calcitriol is most useful in diseases in which the activity of renal 1α(alpha)-hydroxylase is impaired, such as renal failure or hypoparathyroidism. Although hypercalcemic events are more common with calcitriol than with vitamin D, halting treatment is followed by resolution of hypercalcemia in a few days rather than a few weeks. Calcifediol (25-hydroxyvitamin D) does not require hepatic 25-hydroxylation and therefore can be useful in patients with liver disease. The pharmacokinetics of calcifediol are intermediary—more rapid and not as prolonged as that of vitamin D, but slower in onset and more prolonged than that of calcitriol.

Serum calcium, phosphorus, and creatinine along with a measure of urinary calcium excretion should be monitored regularly to avoid toxicity from calcium and vitamin D therapy. In patients who develop hypercalciuria (urinary calcium excretion greater than 300 mg/day), thiazide diuretics (along with a low-salt diet) can be employed to promote urinary calcium retention [30]. Effective doses of hydrochlorothiazide are generally between 50 and 100 mg/d. Patients should be monitored for alterations in serum potassium, sodium, and magnesium. Soft tissue calcification and nephrocalcinosis can be prevented by keeping the serum calcium × phosphate product below 55 mg^2 / dl^2 [31]. Hyperphosphatemia can be managed by reducing the patient's dietary intake of phosphate-rich foodstuffs (e.g., meats, eggs, and dairy products) and, if necessary, with oral phosphate binders.

References

1. Committee to Review Dietary Reference Intakes for Vitamin D and Calcium FaNB, Institute of Medicine. Dietary reference intakes for calcium and vitamin D. Washington, DC: The National Academies Press; 2011. http://www.iom.edu/Reports/2010/Dietary-Reference-Intakes-for-Calcium-and-Vitamin-D/Report-Brief.aspx.
2. Baird GS. Ionized calcium. Clin Chim Acta. 2011;412(9–10):696–701.
3. Bushinsky DA, Krieger NS. Integration of calcium metabolism in the adult. In: Coe FL, Favus MJ, editors. Disorders of bone and mineral metabolism. New York: Raven; 1992. p. 417–32.
4. Tfelt-Hansen J, Brown EM. The calcium-sensing receptor in normal physiology and pathophysiology: a review. Crit Rev Clin Lab Sci. 2005;42(1):35–70.
5. McLean FC, Hastings AB. Clinical estimation and significance of calcium-ion concentrations in the blood. Am J Med Sci. 1935;189:601–13.
6. Koch SM, Warters RD, Mehlhorn U. The simultaneous measurement of ionized and total calcium and ionized and total magnesium in intensive care unit patients. J Crit Care. 2002;17(3):203–5.
7. Lin J, Idee JM, Port M, Diai A, Berthommier C, Robert M, Raynal I, Devoldere L, Corot C. Interference of magnetic resonance imaging contrast agents with the serum calcium measurement technique using colorimetric reagents. J Pharm Biomed Anal. 1999;21(5):931–43.

8. Prince MR, Erel HE, Lent RW, Blumenfeld J, Kent KC, Bush HL, Wang Y. Gadodiamide administration causes spurious hypocalcemia. Radiology. 2003;227(3):639–46.
9. Zaloga GP, Willey S, Tomasic P, Chernow B. Free fatty acids alter calcium binding: a cause for misinterpretation of serum calcium values and hypocalcemia in critical illness. J Clin Endocrinol Metab. 1987;64(5):1010–4.
10. Zivin JR, Gooley T, Zager RA, Ryan MJ. Hypocalcemia: a pervasive metabolic abnormality in the critically ill. Am J Kidney Dis. 2001;37(4):689–98.
11. Bilezikian JP, Khan A, Potts JT Jr, Brandi ML, Clarke BL, Shoback D, Juppner H, D'Amour P, Fox J, Rejnmark L, Mosekilde L, Rubin MR, Dempster D, Gafni R, Collins MT, Sliney J, Sanders J. Hypoparathyroidism in the adult: epidemiology, diagnosis, pathophysiology, target-organ involvement, treatment, and challenges for future research. J Bone Miner Res. 2011;26(10):2317–37.
12. Shoback D. Clinical practice. Hypoparathyroidism. N Engl J Med. 2008;359(4):391–403.
13. Eisenbarth GS, Gottlieb PA. Autoimmune polyendocrine syndromes. N Engl J Med. 2004;350(20):2068–79.
14. Angelopoulos NG, Goula A, Rombopoulos G, Kaltzidou V, Katounda E, Kaltsas D, Tolis G. Hypoparathyroidism in transfusion-dependent patients with beta-thalassemia. J Bone Miner Metab. 2006;24(2):138–45.
15. Carpenter TO, Carnes DL Jr, Anast CS. Hypoparathyroidism in Wilson's disease. N Engl J Med. 1983;309(15):873–7.
16. de Seze S, Solnica J, Mitrovic D, Miravet L, Dorfmann H. Joint and bone disorders and hypoparathyroidism in hemochromatosis. Semin Arthritis Rheum. 1972;2(1):71–94.
17. Winslow CP, Meyers AD. Hypocalcemia as a complication of radioiodine therapy. Am J Otolaryngol. 1998;19(6):401–3.
18. Goddard CJ, Mbewu A, Evanson JM. Symptomatic hypocalcaemia associated with metastatic invasion of the parathyroid glands. Br J Hosp Med. 1990;43(1):72.
19. Brown EM. Clinical lessons from the calcium-sensing receptor. Nat Clin Pract Endocrinol Metab. 2007;3(2):122–33.
20. Kobrynski LJ, Sullivan KE. Velocardiofacial syndrome, DiGeorge syndrome: the chromosome 22q11, 2 deletion syndromes. Lancet. 2007;370(9596):1443–52.
21. Tong GM, Rude RK. Magnesium deficiency in critical illness. J Intensive Care Med. 2005;20(1):3–17.
22. Holick MF. Vitamin D deficiency. N Engl J Med. 2007;357:266–81.
23. Pearce SH, Cheetham TD. Diagnosis and management of vitamin D deficiency. BMJ. 2010;340:b5664.
24. Brasier AR, Nussbaum SR. Hungry bone syndrome: clinical and biochemical predictors of its occurrence after parathyroid surgery. Am J Med. 1988;84(4):654–60.
25. Riancho JA, Arjona R, Valle R, Sanz J, Gonzalez-Macias J. The clinical spectrum of hypocalcaemia associated with bone metastases. J Intern Med. 1989;226(6):449–52.
26. Sackner MA, Spivack AP, Balian LJ. Hypocalcemia in the presence of osteoblastic metastases. N Engl J Med. 1960;262:173–6.
27. Liamis G, Milionis HJ, Elisaf M. A review of drug-induced hypocalcemia. J Bone Miner Metab. 2009;27(6):635–42.
28. Fonseca OA, Calverley JR. Neurological manifestations of hypoparathyroidism. Arch Intern Med. 1967;120(2):202–6.
29. Kraft MD, Btaiche IF, Sacks GS, Kudsk KA. Treatment of electrolyte disorders in adult patients in the intensive care unit. Am J Health Syst Pharm. 2005;62(16):1663–82.
30. Martinez-Maldonado M, Eknoyan G, Suki WN. Diuretics in nonedematous states. Physiological basis for the clinical use. Arch Intern Med. 1973;131(6):797–808.
31. Cozzolino M, Dusso AS, Slatopolsky E. Role of calcium-phosphate product and bone-associated proteins on vascular calcification in renal failure. J Am Soc Nephrol. 2001;12(11):2511–6.

Chapter 16
Hypercalcemia

Robert Klein and Chaim Vanek

Précis

1. Clinical setting: Hypercalcemia (serum calcium >10.5 mg/dL or ionized calcium level >1.3 mmol/L) is a disorder commonly encountered by primary care physicians and is usually well tolerated if calcium levels remain below 12 mg/dL (ionized calcium level of 1.5 mmol/L). Calcium levels above this threshold are associated with increasingly severe volume contraction, neurological, cardiac, and gastrointestinal dysfunction and require urgent treatment to prevent life-threatening consequences.

2. Diagnosis: The differential of hypercalcemia is broad and can be categorized based on parathyroid hormone (PTH) levels. The principal challenges in the management of hypercalcemia are distinguishing primary hyperparathyroidism (PHPT) from conditions that will not respond to parathyroidectomy (e.g., cancer, granulomatous disorders, vitamin D intoxications). Correct management depends on an accurate diagnosis. However, in the setting of hypercalcemic crisis, therapy should be initiated immediately, and the diagnosis pursued after the patient's condition has been stabilized.

   (a) History: Important complaints include polyuria and altered mental status which together can contribute to volume contraction and worsening hypercalcemia. Calcium levels elevated to the extent that overt symptoms are present nearly always indicate PHPT or malignancy. The most frequent presentation of PHPT is that of relatively "asymptomatic" disease. Constitutional symptoms (fevers, night sweats, weight loss) raise concern for a malignant or infectious etiology. A careful family history should provide clues as to

R. Klein · C. Vanek (✉)
Division of Endocrinology, Diabetes and Clinical Nutrition, Oregon Health and Science University, Portland, OR, USA
e-mail: vanekc@ohsu.edu

© Springer Nature Switzerland AG 2021
L. Loriaux, C. Vanek (eds.), *Endocrine Emergencies*, Contemporary Endocrinology, https://doi.org/10.1007/978-3-030-67455-7_16

whether the patient has a familial form of hyperparathyroidism or familial hypocalciuric hypercalcemia (FHH). Calcium and vitamin D supplement use or ongoing treatment with a thiazide or lithium represents other obvious causes.

(b) Physical examination: Just as with hypocalcemia, the clinical presentation of hypercalcemia depends on the chronicity and severity of the disturbance—ranging from few if any symptoms with longstanding mild hypercalcemia to severe life-threatening symptoms if an acute and dramatic change has taken place. The term hypercalcemic crisis describes a severely debilitated patient with profound volume depletion, cardiac decompensation, and altered neurocognitive function. This can present as obtundation and even coma.

(c) Laboratory evaluation: Hypercalcemia is defined as a serum calcium >10.5 mg/dL or ionized calcium level >1.3 mmol/L. Once the diagnosis is considered, a repeat measurement (ionized calcium or total serum calcium corrected for albumin) should be obtained to confirm a true increase in the serum calcium concentration. The first step in evaluating hypercalcemia is to establish whether the process is PTH-dependent. Additional laboratory testing should include measurements of serum creatinine, phosphorus, vitamin D metabolites, thyroid function, serum electrophoresis, and renal calcium excretion. The QT interval on the electrocardiogram can be shortened by hypercalcemia due to the increased rate of cardiac repolarization.

3. Treatment: Severe hypercalcemia is an endocrine emergency that requires prompt action to prevent severe neurological, cardiac, and renal consequences. The diagnosis should be considered in any patient with known parathyroid disease or malignancy who presents with acute clinical decline, especially in the event of neurological deterioration. The emergent treatment of hypercalcemia must focus on restoring intravascular volume and increasing renal calcium excretion. In most situations, 500–1000 mL 0.9% saline should be infused over the first hour and an additional 2–5 L over the next 24 h. The goal is to achieve a urine output of 200 mL/h. This can be continued for several days and will usually lower serum calcium by 1–3 mg/dL. If this degree of hydration leads to pulmonary edema or pitting edema, loop diuretics should be added. In this case, potassium and magnesium levels must be closely monitored. If hypophosphatemia occurs, it should be replaced with enteral phosphate to achieve a plasma level of phosphate of 2.5–3.0 mg/dL. For patients with congestive heart failure and end-stage renal disease, hemodialysis or peritoneal dialysis, with a low-calcium dialysate, can be very helpful.

The most important element of treatment is swift volume resuscitation, followed by the administration of specific therapies tailored to the underlying pathophysiologic process (e.g., calcitonin and bisphosphonates to slow bone resorption; glucocorticoids to limit 1,25-dihyroxyvitamin D synthesis). It is essential that physicians know how to evaluate and optimally manage patients with hypercalcemia, because treatment and prognosis vary according to the underlying disorder. Surgery remains the only effective therapy for PHPT, and all patients whose course has been complicated by severe hypercalcemia should be referred for parathyroidectomy. Despite encouraging developments in pharmacologic management, the prognostic implications related to malignancy-associated hypercalcemia (MAH) remain relatively bleak. Only patients for whom effective antineoplastic therapy is available can be expected to experience a longer survival.

Etiology

Hypercalcemia is defined as a serum calcium more than two standard deviations above the laboratory's population mean, commonly 10.5 mg/dL for total serum calcium and 1.30 mmol/L for ionized serum calcium. Under normal conditions, the flux of ionized calcium between the vascular space and the skeleton, the intestine, and the kidney is very tightly regulated [1]. Consequently, for hypercalcemia to develop, one or more of the following disturbances must be in play: (a) increased intestinal calcium absorption, (b) increased bone resorption, or (c) decreased renal calcium excretion. Approaching hypercalcemia from this physiological perspective can serve as a very practical means to establish the correct diagnosis and devise an effective treatment strategy.

The main function of PTH is to maintain the serum calcium concentration by promoting the release of calcium from bone, stimulating renal calcium conservation by the kidney, and augmenting intestinal calcium absorption by increasing renal 1,25-dihydroxyvitamin D synthesis. Accordingly, in the event of hypocalcemia, PTH release into the bloodstream should be enhanced, while hypercalcemia should prompt a decrease in circulating PTH concentrations. It is for this reason that the underlying causes of hypercalcemia can be conveniently divided into those associated with an elevated or inappropriately normal PTH level and those where PTH levels are appropriately suppressed (Table 16.1).

PHPT is a relatively common endocrine disease, with an incidence as high as 1 in 500 to 1 in 1000 [2]. As such, PHPT accounts for the vast majority of hypercalcemia (>90%) detected in the outpatient clinic setting [3]. PHPT occurs at all ages but is most frequent in those over the age of 50 with women affected nearly three times more often than men [2]. Most cases of the disease (~80%) are caused by a benign, solitary adenoma. Parathyroid adenomas are most commonly sporadic but can be part of an endocrine neoplastic syndrome such as multiple endocrine neoplasia (MEN-1 or MEN-2a), especially if discovered in the young patient [2]. Less commonly (~15–20% of cases), the disease is caused by hyperplasia of all four parathyroid glands. Rarely, hyperparathyroidism can result from a parathyroid carcinoma. In adenomas, the parathyroid cell loses its normal sensitivity to calcium (altered "set point"), whereas in hyperplasia of the parathyroid glands, the overall increase in the number of parathyroid cells is responsible for the hypercalcemia.

Other causes of hypercalcemia in the setting of parathyroid hyperplasia and inappropriately normal or high PTH secretion are tertiary hyperparathyroidism, familial hypocalciuric hypercalcemia (FHH), and lithium therapy [4]. Physiologically

Table 16.1 Causes of hypercalcemia

Parathyroid hormone-dependent etiologies
Primary hyperparathyroidism
Adenoma
Hyperplasia
Sporadic
Familial
Multiple endocrine neoplasia, type 1 and type 2a
Carcinoma
Familial hypocalciuric hypercalcemia (does not cause calcium levels greater 12.0 mg/dl)
Lithium therapy/toxicity
Tertiary (severe secondary) hyperparathyroidism
Parathyroid hormone-independent etiologies
Malignancy
Humoral hypercalcemia of malignancy (PTHrP)
Local osteolytic hypercalcemia
1,25-Dihyroxyvitamin D-mediated
Vitamin D-related
Vitamin D intoxication
Granulomatous disorder (excessive 1,25-dihyroxyvitamin D production)
Milk-alkali syndrome
Immobilization
Hyperthyroidism
Pheochromocytoma
VIP-oma syndrome
Vitamin A intoxication

appropriate (or secondary) hyperparathyroidism that accompanies long-standing calcium insufficiency or renal insufficiency can sometimes lead to parathyroid autonomy that persists even after resolution of the stimulus (calcium and vitamin D repletion; renal transplant). When hypercalcemia develops under these circumstances, the condition is referred to as tertiary hyperparathyroidism, and four-gland hyperplasia is the rule. FHH is an autosomal-dominant genetic disorder resulting from an inactivating mutation in the calcium-sensing receptor (CaSR) [5]. The diminished ability of renal tissue to detect calcium results in enhanced renal tubular reabsorption of calcium and mild hypercalcemia. Similarly, parathyroid tissue in FHH inadequately senses circulating calcium so that parathyroid hyperplasia occurs and inappropriately normal PTH levels are maintained despite the chronic mild hypercalcemia. Lithium therapy produces a physiologic picture that mimics FHH as the calcium "set point" for suppression of PTH release is raised above normal [6].

In contrast to PHPT, MAH accounts for up to 90% of the hypercalcemia encountered among hospitalized patients, and hypercalcemia complicates 10–30% of malignancies [7–10]. The most common form of MAH is humoral hypercalcemia of malignancy (HHM), which derives from tumor-associated PTH-related protein

(PTHrP), a peptide with significant homology to PTH [11] but not detected on a PTH assay. Based on its structural similarity to PTH, PTHrP can activate skeletal and renal PTH receptors. As a result, enormous amounts of calcium (up to 1 g/d) are delivered into the circulation and, combined with the anticalciuric effects of PTHrP to restrict renal calcium clearance, marked hypercalcemia ensues. In contrast to PHPT, HHM is associated with suppressed PTH levels and normal or low calcitriol levels. Many solid tumors are associated with HHM and include squamous cell carcinomas of the lung, skin, cervix, head, neck, and esophagus, renal cell carcinoma, and breast carcinoma. Humoral-mediated bone resorption accounts for the majority of hypercalcemia in these malignancies even when osteolytic metastases are present.

A second form of MAH is local osteolytic hypercalcemia (LOH) that occurs in cancer subjects with widespread skeletal involvement [12]. The tumors most commonly associated with LOH are breast cancer and hematological neoplasms such as leukemia, lymphoma, and myeloma. Locally produced, tumor-derived osteoclast-activating cytokines (including interleukins-1 and -6, PTHrP, and macrophage inflammatory protein-1α(alpha)) are thought to be responsible for most instances of LOH. As such, LOH is primarily a resorptive (skeletally derived) form of hypercalcemia in which massive removal of skeletal calcium overwhelms the ability of the kidney to eliminate calcium.

In the third form of MAH, certain lymphomas and ovarian dysgerminomas can cause 1,25-dihydroxyvitamin D-mediated hypercalcemia. Malignant cells (or perhaps adjacent normal cells) overexpress 1α(alpha)-hydroxylase that converts normal levels of circulating 25-dihydroxyvitamin D into elevated concentrations of 1,25-dihydroxyvitamin D [13]. Because 1,25-dihydroxyvitamin D activates intestinal calcium absorption, this syndrome is principally considered an absorptive form of hypercalcemia. Finally, extremely rare cases in which ectopic production of authentic PTH, and not PTHrP, by tumors has been shown to cause MAH [14–16].

Together, PHPT and malignancy account for the vast majority (>90%) of hypercalcemia cases. Among the remaining miscellaneous etiologies are granulomatous disorders, a few endocrine disorders, immobilization, and a number of medications. Just as is the case with certain lymphomas and dysgerminomas, granulomas possess 1α(alpha)-hydroxylase activity that can result in absorptive hypercalcemia due to increased circulating levels of 1,25-dihydroxyvitamin D [17]. Hypercalcemia has been described in virtually every disease associated with granuloma formation, and the mineral disturbance resolves with elimination of the granulomas. The accelerated bone resorption that accompanies hyperthyroidism can cause mild hypercalcemia [18]. Hypercalcemia has been associated with pheochromocytoma, and the VIP-oma (vasoactive intestinal polypeptide) syndrome though the mechanisms are not well understood [19, 20]. Immobilization can also cause hypercalcemia through accelerated osteoclastic bone resorption [21]. A number of medications may result in hypercalcemia [22]. Thiazide diuretics are well-recognized for the ability to cause mild hypercalcemia due to stimulation of renal calcium reabsorption [23]. Consumption of large amounts of calcium carbonate (daily doses in excess of 4000 mg/d taken for esophageal reflux of peptic ulcer symptoms) can lead to a disorder termed milk-alkali syndrome that is characterized by hypercalcemia, alkalosis, and renal insufficiency [24]. Similarly, vitamin D intoxication from over-the-counter supplements or prescribed forms of ergocalciferol and calcitriol may also cause hypercalcemia due to a combination of increased intestinal calcium absorption and reduced renal calcium clearance. Vitamin A intoxication has also been associated with hypercalcemia, and the effect appears to be mediated through increased bone resorption [25].

Clinical Signs and Features

Just as is the case with hypocalcemia, the clinical manifestations of hypercalcemia depend on the degree of hypercalcemia (ionized calcium level) and the rapidity of its onset (Table 16.2). In general, however, overt symptoms are rare in patients with serum calcium concentrations below 12 mg/dL (ionized calcium below 1.5 mmol/L), but at concentrations above 14 mg/dL (ionized calcium of 1.75 mmol/L), most patients are symptomatic [26]. Neuromuscular function depends upon a normal extracellular calcium concentration. So it is not surprising that, as with hypocalcemia, a spectrum of neurologic symptoms can accompany hypercalcemia, ranging from slight cognitive difficulties, mild fatigue, lethargy, and depression to confusion, agitation, obtundation, and even coma. The effect of hypercalcemia to raise the depolarization threshold of skeletal and smooth muscle cells results in skeletal myopathy and diffuse gastrointestinal complaints (e.g., constipation, abdominal pain, nausea, vomiting, and anorexia). In a similar fashion, bradyarrhythmias, cardiac conduction defects, and digitalis sensitivity are associated with increased ionized calcium levels. Beyond its neuromuscular impact, hypercalcemia also exerts clinically important renal effects. The increased delivery of calcium to the nephron impairs normal renal tubular reabsorption of water, leading to polyuria and increased thirst. Aquaporin-2 water channels are decreased by hypercalcemia, and tubulointerstitial injury can result from direct calcium deposition [27]. When fluid intake fails to match the obligatory renal fluid losses, volume contraction and prerenal azotemia develop, which in turn limit renal clearance of calcium and further worsen the hypercalcemia. Long-standing hypercalcemia can cause precipitation of calcium salts in the renal interstitium (nephrocalcinosis), urinary tract (nephrolithiasis), cornea ("band keratopathy"), vasculature, myocardium, and cardiac valves as well as accelerated bone loss and a predisposition to fragility fractures.

As the clinical presentation of hypercalcemia is, for the most part, the same regardless of the underlying etiology, the history and physical examination of the hypercalcemic patient should focus on signs and symptoms relevant to the causal disorder. In the acute setting, hypercalcemia is most commonly seen in the context of parathyroid dysfunction and malignancy. MAH is generally a late development in the course of disease, and thus tumors causing hypercalcemia are rarely occult. Palpable neck masses are extremely unusual in PHPT unless the patient has a parathyroid carcinoma. Osteoporosis of cortical bone is frequently observed in PHPT

Table 16.2 Clinical manifestations of hypercalcemia

Neuromuscular
Muscle weakness
Lethargy, fatigue
Poor recent memory
Impaired cognition
Confusion, stupor, coma
Renal
Polyuria
Dehydration
Nephrolithiasis
Nephrocalcinosis
Gastrointestinal
Nausea, vomiting
Anorexia
Abdominal pain
Constipation
Skeleton
Bone pain, fracture
Cardiovascular
Arrhythmia
Cardiovascular calcification
Band keratopathy

[28]. A careful family history should provide clues as to whether the patient has FHH or another variant of familial hyperparathyroidism. Hyperthyroidism should be suspected from physical examination findings, as should a history of recent ingestion of any medication known to cause hypercalcemia.

Laboratory Evaluation

After taking a careful history and physical examination, laboratory testing should be designed to assess the extent of the alteration in calcium homeostasis and to ascertain the underlying etiology. A single raised serum calcium value should be repeated (along with an ionized calcium, if available) to confirm that the disorder is clinically genuine and not the consequence of a lab artifact. Hypercalcemia without a concomitant elevation in ionized calcium can occur in the setting of hyperalbuminemia, severe dehydration, thrombocythemia, or in multiple myeloma with a calcium-binding M-paraprotein [29]. If accessible, previous values for serum calcium should also be reviewed. Evidence of long-standing asymptomatic hypercalcemia would suggest PHPT or FHH as likely explanations. The degree of hypercalcemia also can be useful. Serum calcium concentrations above 13 mg/dL (1.6 mmol/L) are infrequent in PHPT and, in the absence of another apparent cause, are more commonly the result of malignancy.

Fig. 16.1
Immunoradiometric assay
for intact parathyroid
hormone. Intact PTH
measured by two-site
immunoradiometric assay
in sera from 72 normal
individuals, 37 patients
with surgically proven
primary
hyperparathyroidism, and
24 patients with
malignancy-associated
hypercalcemia. The normal
reference range is
12–65 pg/
mL. (Reproduced from
Nussbaum et al. [30])

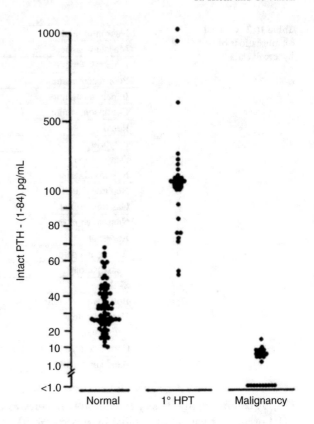

Once confirmed the next step in the laboratory evaluation of hypercalcemia is to establish whether or not the process is PTH-dependent (Fig. 16.1). Two-site immunoradiometric assays for the intact PTH molecule are now performed routinely and have eliminated most of the problems related to circulating biologically inactive fragments (present in patients with impaired renal function) [30]. The finding of an elevated or at least incompletely suppressed PTH level in the setting of hypercalcemia is virtually diagnostic of PHPT. Cancer patients appear to have a higher incidence of PHPT than the general population [31]. Thus, the intact PTH assay is an important component of the routine evaluation for all hypercalcemic patients, even those with a known malignancy.

A low or low-normal serum PTH level (below 20 pg/mL) points to the presence of a PTH-independent cause of hypercalcemia. In this clinical situation, malignancy should be regarded as the most likely cause, especially if the hypercalcemia is of relatively recent onset. An elevated serum concentration of PTHrP, the primary mediator of HHM, would confirm the diagnosis [32]. However, this assay is often superfluous. In most such patients, the malignancy is readily apparent. In the rare situation where the circulating PTHrP value indicates the presence of an occult malignancy, further evaluation should focus on localizing the primary site and determining the extent of spread of the neoplasm. MAH generally develops in patients with advanced disease, and its appearance has grave prognostic signifi-cance. Consequently, if the patient has a low serum PTH but long-standing hyper-calcemia, a PTH-independent disorder, apart from malignancy, should be pursued.

A disturbance in the serum levels of vitamin D metabolites should be considered if there is no obvious malignancy and neither PTH nor PTHrP levels are elevated. An elevated serum concentration of 25-hydroxyvitamin D is indicative of vitamin D intoxication due to the ingestion of over-the-counter supplements or prescribed forms of vitamin D (D_2, ergocalciferol or D_3, cholecalciferol). Assessment of 1,25-dihydroxyvitamin D is only required if the patient is taking calcitriol or has a confirmed or suspected diagnosis of a granulomatous disease or lymphoprolifera-tive disorder. Additional testing for specific clinical disorders based on findings from the history and physical examination could include a TSH determination if signs of thyrotoxicosis are present, a serum retinol level if hypervitaminosis A is possible, serum and urine protein electrophoresis if multiple myeloma is suspected, or a 24-h urine collection for calcium if the family history suggests FHH.

Treatment

Optimal management of hypercalcemia requires aggressively dealing with the underlying pathophysiologic process. Although there are dozens of clinical entities that can cause hypercalcemia, PHPT and malignancy account for 80–90% of cases. Hypercalcemia is generally a late feature of malignancy, and thus it is rare for an underlying malignancy not to be clinically evident when hypercalcemia is first noted. Consequently, hypercalcemia in otherwise healthy outpatients is usually the result of PHPT, while malignancy is more often responsible for hypercalcemia in hospitalized patients. If the patient's serum calcium concentration is less than 12 mg/dL (1.5 mmol/L), treatment should primarily be directed toward the underly-ing disorder, for example, discontinuing or reducing the dose of an offending medi-cation such as vitamin D or lithium, removal of a parathyroid adenoma, or elimination of a tumor responsible for HHM with chemotherapy or surgery if pos-sible. When the patient has symptoms and signs of acute hypercalcemic crisis (azo-temia, somnolence, and/or coma) and the serum calcium is greater than 12 mg/dL (1.5 mmol/L), a series of urgent calcium-specific measures should be instituted (Table 16.3).

The emergent treatment of hypercalcemia must first focus on correcting dehydra-tion, restoring intravascular volume, and enhancing renal calcium excretion. As delineated above, hypercalcemia induces a severe extracellular fluid deficit due to nausea, vomiting, and polyuria. Within the kidney, calcium is actively reabsorbed via PTH action in the distal tubule and passively reabsorbed because of the favor-able electrochemical gradient created by reabsorption of sodium and chloride ions in the proximal tubule and in the thick ascending limb of the loop of Henle. Restoration of intravascular volume will thus enhance urinary calcium excretion by increasing glomerular filtration of calcium and decreasing proximal tubular and

Table 16.3 Therapeutic options for hypercalcemia

Agent	Dosing information	Mechanism of action	Notes
Normal saline	2–5 L daily	Corrects volume depletion and enhances calciuria	May be poorly tolerated by patients with cardiac or renal failure
Loop diuretic (furosemide, ethacrynic acid)	Furosemide 10–20 mg. Ethacrynic acid 50 mg	Inhibits distal tubular calcium reabsorption	Can worsen hypercalcemia by reducing intravascular volume
Calcitonin	4–8 IU/kg intramuscularly or subcutaneously every 6 h	Inhibits osteoclastic bone resorption	Efficacy declines after 6–8 doses
Bisphosphonate	Pamidronate 60–90 mg intravenously over 4 h. Zoledronic acid 4 mg intravenously over 15 min	Inhibits osteoclastic bone resorption	Potent inhibition of bone resorption can result in hypophosphatemia. Effects can last weeks
Glucocorticoids	Hydrocortisone 100–200 mg intravenously daily. Prednisone 60 mg orally daily	Inhibits vitamin D conversion to active calcitriol	Side effects include hyperglycemia, immune suppression, and myopathy
Denosumab [38]	120 mg subcutaneously weekly x 3 weeks	Inhibits osteoclast bone resorption	Effective for bisphosphonate refractory hypercalcemia of malignancy

loop sodium reabsorption. Although a necessity in the management of a hypercalcemic crisis, parenteral fluid resuscitation must be administered cautiously in patients with compromised cardiovascular or renal function. Appropriate fluid administration depends on the patient's volume status, but in most situations of 500–1000 mL of 0.9%, saline should be infused over the first hour and then an additional 2–5 L over the first 24 h. The goal is to achieve a urine output of 200 mL per hour. This regimen can be continued for several days and usually succeeds in lowering calcium levels by 1–3 mg/dL. The addition of loop diuretics (e.g., furosemide, ethacrynic acid) to ongoing saline infusion has been advocated to enhance calciuria, but if administered before adequate hydration has taken place, the diuretic-induced volume contraction can instead worsen the hypercalcemia [33]. Therefore, loop diuretics are best reserved for those patients where vigorous fluid resuscitation may provoke cardiogenic fluid overload. Central venous access with hemodynamic monitoring should be considered in patients who do not tolerate initial attempts at fluid administration. With aggressive hydration and diuretic-induced diuresis, potassium and magnesium levels should be carefully monitored and appropriately replaced, as required. Hypophosphatemia also can occur and should be repleted enterally to a level of 2.5–3 mg/dL. Parenteral administration of phosphate is contraindicated as it can cause severe hypocalcemia and renal failure [34]. For patients with renal insufficiency or congestive heart failure in whom isotonic saline infusion is not feasible, hemodialysis or peritoneal dialysis with low calcium levels in the dialysate can be an effective strategy for removing calcium from the circulation [35].

In severe hypercalcemia, increased mobilization of skeletal calcium is often an important contributor. A parenteral bisphosphonate is the treatment of choice for inhibition of bone resorption in this situation [36]. Bisphosphonates (e.g., pamidronate, zoledronic acid) target and adhere to actively remodeling bone surfaces where they interfere with the ability of osteoclasts to resorb bone. Pamidronate 60–90 mg is administered intravenously in 500 mL of 0.9% saline over 4 h, and zoledronic acid 4 mg is administered intravenously in 5 mL of 0.9% saline over 15–30 min. These agents can cause transient fever, flu-like symptoms or myalgias for a day or two. The effect of a parenteral bisphosphonate to lower serum calcium is apparent within 3–4 days, with a maximal effect within 7–10 days after commencing treatment. The effect can persist for 7–30 days. Transient hypophosphatemia can occur, especially in malnourished patients. Due to the prolonged period of activity of bisphosphonates, it is crucial to first ascertain the etiology of the underlying disorder and correct reversible causes of hypercalcemia before administering one of these agents. Bisphosphonates are contraindicated if parathyroid surgery is imminent as their use can lead to profound postoperative hypocalcemia. Calcitonin is another therapeutic option to inhibit osteoclastic resorption. It has a rapid onset of action, causing serum calcium levels to fall by as much as 2 mg/dL within 2–6 h of administration. Consequently it may be used in conjunction with a bisphosphonate to more rapidly reduce the serum calcium level [37]. It is usually given intramuscularly or subcutaneously at a dose of 4–8 IU/kg. However, the efficacy of parenteral calcitonin is transient (lasting 24–48 h) due to rapidly acquired resistance. Denosumab, a RANKL inhibitor, which inhibits osteoclast-mediated bone resorption has shown efficacy in treating hypercalcemia of malignancy previously refractory to bisphosphonate therapy [38].

To optimally address severe hypercalcemia, multiple therapies should be started as soon as possible. For example, aggressive parenteral rehydration and calcitonin along with a potent bisphosphonate can all be used in the first few days. Any drugs that inhibit urinary calcium excretion, decrease renal blood flow, or augment PTH action as well as supplements that contain calcium, vitamin D, vitamin A, or other retinoids should be discontinued as soon as possible. Immobilization promotes osteoclastic bone resorption; hence early ambulation should be encouraged. Though the gut has an important role in normal calcium homeostasis, intestinal absorption is usually diminished in the setting of hypercalcemia, making dietary calcium restriction unnecessary.

Once the acute episode of hypercalcemia has been successfully addressed and the patient is stable, clinical efforts should then be directed toward the underlying hypercalcemic disorder per se. Ultimately, definitive therapy directed at the underlying disorder is necessary to prevent the redevelopment of hypercalcemia. Parathyroidectomy should be considered at the earliest safe opportunity in all patients with hypercalcemic crises as a result of underlying parathyroid disease (e.g., parathyroid adenoma, hyperplasia, or carcinoma). Definitive cytoreductive therapies (surgery, radiation, or chemotherapy) for cancer patients with HHM can prevent further hypercalcemic events, while, for other patients with LOH, improvement may come with radiation therapy directed at the lesion(s). Treatment of granulomatous disorders with standard regimens including glucocorticoids and/or immunosuppressants can usually succeed in reducing circulating 1,25-dihydroxyvitamin D levels. Substituting an alternative psychotropic agent effective in bipolar disease can be an effective approach in those patients with lithium-induced hypercalcemia.

References

1. Bushinsky DA, Krieger NS. Integration of calcium metabolism in the adult. In: Coe FL, Favus MJ, editors. Disorders of bone and mineral metabolism. New York: Raven; 1992. p. 417–32.
2. Wermers RA, Khosla S, Atkinson EJ, Achenbach SJ, Oberg AL, Grant CS, Melton LJ III. Incidence of primary hyperparathyroidism in Rochester, Minnesota, 1993–2001: an update on the changing epidemiology of the disease. J Bone Miner Res. 2006;21(1):171–7.
3. Silverberg SJ, Lewiecki EM, Mosekilde L, Peacock M, Rubin MR. Presentation of asymptomatic primary hyperparathyroidism: proceedings of the third international workshop. J Clin Endocrinol Metab. 2009;94(2):351–65.
4. Broome JT, Solorzano CC. Lithium use and primary hyperparathyroidism. Endocr Pract. 2011;17(Suppl 1):31–5.
5. Brown EM. Clinical lessons from the calcium-sensing receptor. Nat Clin Pract Endocrinol Metab. 2007;3(2):122–33.
6. Mallette LE, Eichhorn E. Effects of lithium carbonate on human calcium metabolism. Arch Intern Med. 1986;146(4):770–6.
7. Adami S, Rossini M. Hypercalcemia of malignancy: pathophysiology and treatment. Bone. 1992;13(Suppl 1):S51–5.
8. Clines GA. Mechanisms and treatment of hypercalcemia of malignancy. Curr Opin Endocrinol Diabetes Obes. 2011;18(6):339–46.
9. Mundy GR, Guise TA. Hypercalcemia of malignancy. Am J Med. 1997;103(2):134–45.
10. Ralston SH. Pathogenesis and management of cancer associated hypercalcaemia. Cancer Surv. 1994;21:179–96.
11. Strewler GJ. The physiology of parathyroid hormone-related protein. N Engl J Med. 2000;342(3):177–85.
12. Clines GA, Guise TA. Hypercalcaemia of malignancy and basic research on mechanisms responsible for osteolytic and osteoblastic metastasis to bone. Endocr Relat Cancer. 2005;12(3):549–83.
13. Hewison M, Kantorovich V, Liker HR, Van Herle AJ, Cohan P, Zehnder D, Adams JS. Vitamin D-mediated hypercalcemia in lymphoma: evidence for hormone production by tumor-adjacent macrophages. J Bone Miner Res. 2003;18(3):579–82.
14. Iguchi H, Miyagi C, Tomita K, Kawauchi S, Nozuka Y, Tsuneyoshi M, Wakasugi H. Hypercalcemia caused by ectopic production of parathyroid hormone in a patient with papillary adenocarcinoma of the thyroid gland. J Clin Endocrinol Metab. 1998;83(8):2653–7.
15. Mahoney EJ, Monchik JM, Donatini G, De Lellis R. Life-threatening hypercalcemia from a hepatocellular carcinoma secreting intact parathyroid hormone: localization by sestamibi single-photon emission computed tomographic imaging. Endocr Pract. 2006;12(3):302–6.

16. Nielsen PK, Rasmussen AK, Feldt-Rasmussen U, Brandt M, Christensen L, Olgaard K. Ectopic production of intact parathyroid hormone by a squamous cell lung carcinoma in vivo and in vitro. J Clin Endocrinol Metab. 1996;81(10):3793–6.

17. Sharma OP. Hypercalcemia in granulomatous disorders: a clinical review. Curr Opin Pulm Med. 2000;6(5):442–7.

18. Alikhan Z, Singh A. Hyperthyroidism manifested as hypercalcemia. South Med J. 1996;89(10):997–8.

19. Ghaferi AA, Chojnacki KA, Long WD, Cameron JL, Yeo CJ. Pancreatic VIPomas: subject review and one institutional experience. J Gastrointest Surg. 2008;12(2):382–93.

20. Stewart AF, Hoecker JL, Mallette LE, Segre GV, Amatruda TT Jr, Vignery A. Hypercalcemia in pheochromocytoma. Evidence for a novel mechanism. Ann Intern Med. 1985;102(6):776–9.

21. Stewart AF, Adler M, Byers CM, Segre GV, Broadus AE. Calcium homeostasis in immobilization: an example of resorptive hypercalciuria. N Engl J Med. 1982;306(19):1136–40.

22. Buckley MS, Leblanc JM, Cawley MJ. Electrolyte disturbances associated with commonly prescribed medications in the intensive care unit. Crit Care Med. 2010;38(6 Suppl):S253–64.

23. Desai HV, Gandhi K, Sharma M, Jennine M, Singh P, Brogan M. Thiazide-induced severe hypercalcemia: a case report and review of literature. Am J Ther. 2010;17(6):e234–6.

24. Orwoll ES. The milk-alkali syndrome: current concepts. Ann Intern Med. 1982;97(2):242–8.

25. Bhalla K, Ennis DM, Ennis ED. Hypercalcemia caused by iatrogenic hypervitaminosis a. J Am Diet Assoc. 2005;105(1):119–21.

26. Bilezikian JP. Clinical review 51: management of hypercalcemia. J Clin Endocrinol Metab. 1993;77(6):1445–9.

27. Nielsen S, Frokiaer J, Marples D, Kwon TH, Agre P, Knepper MA. Aquaporins in the kidney: from molecules to medicine. Physiol Rev. 2002;82(1):205–44.

28. Rubin MR, Bilezikian JP, McMahon DJ, Jacobs T, Shane E, Siris E, Udesky J, Silverberg SJ. The natural history of primary hyperparathyroidism with or without parathyroid surgery after 15 years. J Clin Endocrinol Metab. 2008;93(9):3462–70.

29. Jacobs TP, Bilezikian JP. Clinical review: rare causes of hypercalcemia. J Clin Endocrinol Metab. 2005;90(11):6316–22.

30. Nussbaum SR, Zahradnik RJ, Lavigne JR, Brennan GL, Nozawa-Ung K, Kim LY, Keutmann HT, Wang CA, Potts JT Jr, Segre GV. Highly sensitive two-site immunoradiometric assay of parathyrin, and its clinical utility in evaluating patients with hypercalcemia. Clin Chem. 1987;33(8):1364–7.

31. Nilsson IL, Zedenius J, Yin L, Ekbom A. The association between primary hyperparathyroidism and malignancy: nationwide cohort analysis on cancer incidence after parathyroidectomy. Endocr Relat Cancer. 2007;14(1):135–40.

32. Casez J, Pfammatter R, Nguyen Q, Lippuner K, Jaeger P. Diagnostic approach to hypercalcemia: relevance of parathyroid hormone and parathyroid hormone-related protein measurements. Eur J Intern Med. 2001;12(4):344–9.

33. LeGrand SB, Leskuski D, Zama I. Narrative review: furosemide for hypercalcemia: an unproven yet common practice. Ann Intern Med. 2008;149(4):259–63.

34. Stewart AF. Clinical practice. Hypercalcemia associated with cancer. N Engl J Med. 2005;352(4):373–9.

35. Wang CC, Chen YC, Shiang JC, Lin SH, Chu P, Wu CC. Hypercalcemic crisis successfully treated with prompt calcium-free hemodialysis. Am J Emerg Med. 2009;27(9):1174.e1–3.

36. Drake MT, Clarke BL, Khosla S. Bisphosphonates: mechanism of action and role in clinical practice. Mayo Clin Proc. 2008;83(9):1032–45.

37. Ljunghall S. Use of clodronate and calcitonin in hypercalcemia due to malignancy. Recent Results Cancer Res. 1989;116:40–5.

38. Hu MI, Glezerman IG, Leboulleux S. Denosumab for treatment of hypercalcemia of malignancy. J Clin Endocrinol Metab. 2014;99(9):3144–52.

Chapter 17
Pituitary Apoplexy

Pouyan Famini and Shlomo Melmed

Précis

1. Clinical setting—acute development of neurological symptoms and signs often accompanied by resistant shock and other symptoms of hypopituitarism.
2. Diagnosis

    (a) History: Most common presenting symptoms include sudden severe headache, double vision, visual loss including field deficits, nausea, and vomiting. Altered mental status may be present. Complaints of hypopituitarism, such as loss of libido and sexual function, may precede or accompany the development of neurological complaints. History of a pituitary adenoma and precipitating factors that may result in pituitary apoplexy include acute hypotension, hypertension, diabetes mellitus, coagulopathy, pregnancy, head trauma, and major surgical procedures. Medications that increase bleeding risk including anticoagulants, antiplatelets, and thrombolytics as well as medications that act directly on pituitary function such as dopamine agonists may all increase risk.

    (b) Physical examination: Fever, orthostatic hypotension, ophthalmoplegia, decrease or loss of visual acuity, visual field loss, and meningismus are commonly seen. Rarely encountered physical findings include hemiplegia, trigeminal neuralgia, photophobia, proptosis, eyelid edema, rhinorrhea, and epistaxis.

P. Famini · S. Melmed (✉)

Division of Endocrinology, Diabetes, and Metabolism, Cedars-Sinai Medical Center, Los Angeles, CA, USA

e-mail: melmed@cshs.org

© Springer Nature Switzerland AG 2021

L. Loriaux, C. Vanek (eds.), *Endocrine Emergencies*, Contemporary Endocrinology, https://doi.org/10.1007/978-3-030-67455-7_17

(c) Laboratory values: Hyponatremia, hypoglycemia, and elevated leukocyte count are often observed. Most patients also present with partial or complete hypopituitarism including hypocortisolism. Prolactin may be elevated or below normal.

(d) Imaging: Computerized tomography (CT) and magnetic resonance imaging (MRI) findings are consistent with intrasellar hemorrhage and/or necrosis of a pituitary and or adenoma.

3. Treatment—High-dose corticosteroids (200 mg IV Hydrocortisone bolus) in addition to intravenous fluids and vasopressors are the mainstay of treatment in the acute period. Surgical decompression can restore neuro-ophthalmic and pituitary function. Patients with altered mental status, severe reduced visual acuity, and/or severe or deteriorating visual field deficits should be managed with timely surgery. A conservative approach may be undertaken in patients with milder symptoms such as ophthalmoplegia or headache. Assessment of normal adrenal function, defined as elicited cortisol levels >20 μg/dL, should be urgently determined upon presentation. High-dose corticosteroid therapy should be titrated with improvement of clinical status and serial adrenal evaluations to prevent side effects of over-therapy. Assessments of other hypothalamic–pituitary function may be determined weeks after initial presentation with replacement of hormone therapy initiated at that time. Long-term endocrine reassessments are essential as anterior pituitary function may fully or partially recover from initial presentation. Follow-up radiological imaging is also essential as recurrent apoplexy may occur.

Introduction

Pituitary apoplexy is a life-threatening, acute clinical syndrome of pituitary infarction, hemorrhage, and/or necrosis presenting as abrupt onset headache, nausea and vomiting, fever, meningismus, visual disturbances, and altered sensorium [1]. Varying degrees of transient or persistent hypopituitarism accompany the syndrome [2–5]. Bailey first described hemorrhage into a pituitary adenoma in 1898 in a male with acromegaly presenting with sudden onset headache, nausea, vomiting, fever, visual loss, and oculomotor palsies [6]. Autopsy demonstrated hemorrhage in an intrasellar adenoma with endarteritis of the adenohypophyseal vasculature [6]. It can be imagined that David felled Goliath with a simple stone by inducing apoplexy in the acromegalic giant. However, the clinical syndrome [7–11] was not fully recognized until 1950 when Brougham et al. coined the phrase "pituitary apoplexy" [1].

Apoplexy describes hemorrhagic and necrotic changes, usually of vascular origin. Derived from the Greek word *apoplēssein*, which means to strike down and incapacitate, the ancient Greeks believed that those suffering from cerebrovascular accidents had been struck down by the gods. Historically, failure to diagnose this condition until autopsy resulted in significant neurological morbidity and death, sometimes hours within presentation [1, 9, 12]. In contrast, diagnosis and surgical removal of hemorrhagic and necrotic tumor resulted in prompt neurological recovery as early as the 1920s [13, 14]. Physicians also became aware of the valuable effects of hormone replacement by the early 1950s, although corticosteroids could not yet be synthesized and administered. Early attempts included implantation of adrenal cortex extract [15] and fresh calf pituitaries [16]. By the end of the 1950s, preoperative cortisone administration was advocated [17]. Following such improvements in therapy, mortality cases reviewed in the literature became exceedingly rare [12].

Significant advances have been made in both diagnostics and surgical techniques. MRI is now the radiological modality of choice due to its ability to demonstrate hemorrhage and infarction, as well as disease impact on neighboring parasellar structures [18–20]. Transsphenoidal decompression and immediate institution of high-dose intravenous corticosteroid replacement therapy are generally considered the standard of care [2, 21–24]. However, there is also considerable literature advocating conservative management in a carefully selected group of patients [25–27]. Yet, pituitary apoplexy remains a frequently misdiagnosed and poorly understood condition with often vision-threatening and sometimes life-threatening consequences [4, 22].

Pathogenesis of Pituitary Apoplexy and Clinical Manifestations

Pituitary apoplexy results from hemorrhage, infarction, or combination hemorrhagic infarction of a pituitary adenoma and normal pituitary gland [28]. However, the exact pathogenesis is not completely understood nor well delineated. The unusual pituitary blood supply likely contributes to this process (Fig. 17.1). Presentation of pituitary apoplexy varies from relatively benign events to clinical catastrophes involving severe neurological deficits, endocrine dysfunction, and even death [2, 21, 24, 29]. The clinical spectrum may be explained by three mechanisms (see Table 17.1) [30]: (1) destruction or compression of the pituitary gland causing hypopituitarism; (2) sudden development of pressure and compression of neighboring parasellar neurovascular structures due to upward or lateral enlargement of hemorrhagic and/or necrotic pituitary gland; (3) subarachnoid leakage of blood or necrotic tissue within the basal cisterns leading to inflammatory responses similar to subarachnoid hemorrhage or aseptic meningitis.

Pituitary Anatomy

The pituitary gland lies within the sella turcica (see Fig. 17.2), surrounded by the anterior and posterior clinoid processes, and is composed of three sections. The tuberculum sella is an olive-shaped swelling on the anterior slope between the

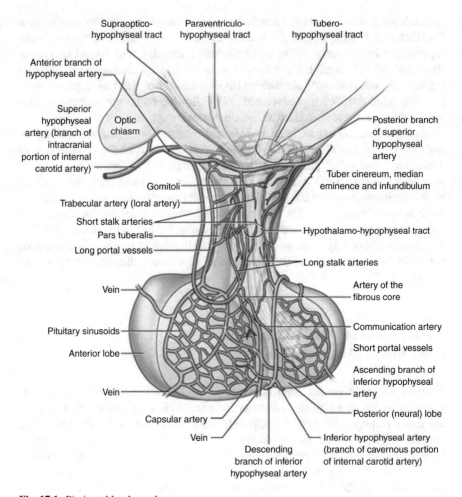

Fig. 17.1 Pituitary blood supply

chiasmal sulcus and the sella turcica. The hypophyseal fossa, which contains the pituitary gland, lies immediately posterior to the tuberculum sellae. The dorsum sella forms the posterior aspect of the sella turcica and terminates at the posterior clinoid process.

The anterior and posterior pituitary lobes are separated by a section of avascular tissue called the pars intermedia. The pituitary gland is connected via the pituitary stalk to the hypothalamus at the median eminence, a thin plate of tissue making up the floor of the anterior part of the third ventricle. The optic chiasm is located superiorly in a cerebrospinal fluid-filled space, and the lateral walls of the pituitary fossa are formed by the cavernous sinuses, which contain the internal carotid arteries, branches of sympathetic chain, and cranial nerves III, IV, V (first and second divisions), and VI. The blood drainage of the orbit also traverses the cavernous sinus.

Table 17.1 Pituitary apoplexy pathophysiology and correlating clinical manifestations

Pathophysiology	Clinical manifestations
Leakage of blood or necrotic tissue into	
Subarachnoid space and/or basal cisterns	Features of subarachnoid hemorrhage or meningitis including hyperpyrexia, headache, nausea and/or vomiting, nuchal rigidity, and altered consciousness
Surrounding brain parenchyma	Altered consciousness and seizures
Pituitary damage	Hypopituitarism and resolution of preexisting hyper-functioning endocrinopathy
Pressure or compression on	
Cavernous sinus	Chemosis and proptosis
Cranial nerve III	Ptosis, mydriasis, diplopia due to medial rectus, superior rectus, and inferior oblique palsies
Cranial nerve IV	Head-tilt or diplopia due to superior oblique palsy
Cranial nerve V (first and second divisions)	Facial paresthesia and loss of corneal reflex
Cranial nerve VI	Diplopia due to lateral rectus palsy
Internal carotid and its branches	Hemiplegia, unilateral focal hemispheric signs, altered consciousness, and seizures
Hypothalamus	Hyperpyrexia, altered consciousness, impaired water balance, and sympathetic dysregulation
Optic tracts and/or chiasm	Impaired visual acuity and visual field defects
Sympathetic chain	Horner's syndrome: ptosis, miosis, anhidrosis, loss of ciliospinal reflex, and conjunctival erythema

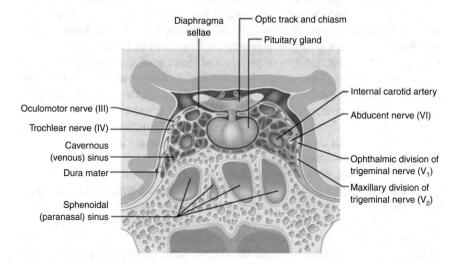

Fig. 17.2 Pituitary anatomy

Pituitary Blood Supply

The pituitary blood supply is derived through branches of the internal carotid arteries, the superior hypophyseal artery, a branch distal to the cavernous sinus, and the inferior hypophyseal artery, a branch at the cavernous sinus level. The neurohypophysis receives direct arterial blood from the inferior hypophyseal artery via an anastomotic arterial circle. In contrast, the adenohypophysis receives little to no direct systemic arterial blood supply from the internal carotid artery, but mainly via trabecular (loral) arteries, a branch of the superior hypophyseal artery that descends alongside the pituitary stalk [31, 32].

The pars distalis blood supply is delivered by long portal veins that connect a primary capillary plexus at the base of the hypothalamus, the median eminence, to a secondary capillary plexus of the pars distalis. These long portal veins descend along the ventral aspect of the pituitary stalk. The primary portal capillary plexus at the median eminence in turn receives arterial blood from the superior hypophyseal artery. The pars distalis also receives venous blood draining directly from the posterior pituitary through short portal vessels. Thus, the anterior pituitary receives most of its blood supply through the hypothalamus and posterior pituitary [33].

Pathogenesis

Pituitary apoplexy may occur in the setting of a rapidly growing pituitary tumor that outstrips its blood supply resulting in ischemic necrosis and hemorrhage [1, 15, 17]. Pituitary tumor growth may be responsible for disrupted tissue organization and vascularization at the parenchymal–pericapillary interface [34]. Furthermore, pituitary adenomas have a greater dependence on direct arterial blood than the normal gland [31, 35]. Despite the greater presence of direct arterial supply within adenomas, these small "twig" end arteries have little total effect on anterior pituitary perfusion compared to the portal venous system [32]. Therefore, pituitary apoplexy occurs due to the compromised vascular supply of a suddenly expanding large tumor, leading to ischemia, hemorrhage, and ultimately necrosis. However, this is unlikely to explain all cases of pituitary apoplexy [24], as the incidence of pituitary hemorrhage does not correlate with tumor size [29, 36].

Another potential mechanism is based on observations that increased intrasellar pressure due to coughing and sneezing has been associated with pituitary apoplexy in five patients [37]. As adenomas extend laterally, the cavernous sinus may gradually become occluded. Venous back pressure rises with repeated coughing and/or sneezing as a direct result of further increased tension in the cavernous sinus, leading to compromised adenoma arterial circulation. Subsequently, adenoma infarction and/or hemorrhage develop.

Ischemia, necrosis, and hemorrhage may also ensue within pituitary adenomas when an expanding pituitary neoplasm extends upward and compresses the infundibular and superior hypophyseal vessels against the diaphragmatic notch [38]. As a pituitary neoplasm grows, it compresses the normal gland, leading to expansion of the pituitary fossa, stretching the diaphragma sellae, and as space becomes limited the pituitary neoplasm must squeeze itself into the narrow channel that houses the hypophyseal stalk, ultimately resulting in distortion and impairment of infundibular circulation [38]. Concomitant hyperprolactinemia due to stalk compression, observed at high frequency with pituitary apoplexy, supports this theory [39–42]. However, angiography has demonstrated that vessels supplying adenomas often originate from the inferior hypophyseal artery [43]. Consequently, disruption of superior hypophyseal artery flow should not necessarily affect blood circulation to the enlarging adenoma. Ischemia and hemorrhage may also originate within the normal pituitary gland, either due to compression by the growing adenoma [24] or from disruption of superior hypophyseal artery flow that supplies the adenohypophysis [21].

Potential vascular risk factors for pituitary apoplexy in adenomas include decreased overall vascular density [44], newly formed immature blood vessels [45], and microscopic vascular injury with endothelial cell blebbing, modifications of the basal laminae, and changes in capillary permeability [34]. Difference in pituitary tumor immunological targets may also explain why some adenomas have a predilection toward apoplexy. Mou et al. analyzed 426 pituitary adenomas, 83 of which had undergone apoplexy [46]. Proliferating cell nuclear antigen (PCNA) expression was higher in patients with pituitary apoplexy for all hormonal subtypes except prolactin-secreting tumors, and growth-hormone-secreting and multi-hormonal adenomas with apoplexy had increased matrix metallopeptidase 9 (MMP-9) expression [46]. Differences in expression of angiogenesis factors may underlie distinctive mechanisms resulting in apoplexy in different hormonal subtypes.

Pathophysiology of the Clinical Manifestations

The typical presentation of pituitary apoplexy is characterized by sudden onset headache, followed within hours to days by nausea, vomiting, ocular palsies, decreased visual acuity or blindness, visual field defects, signs of meningeal irritation, and/or progressive alterations of consciousness [1, 21, 38, 47, 48]. Acute adrenal insufficiency is a major cause of mortality in these patients. Sudden headache is invariably the predominant and initial symptom, usually precedes visual symptoms [21], and is likely due to increased intrasellar pressure, mass effect, compression of neighboring structures and nerves within the cavernous sinus, and/or subarachnoid hemorrhage [29, 36, 49]. Likely mechanisms include referred pain due to stretching of dura and meningeal irritation secondary to subarachnoid hemorrhage [21, 50, 51]. Pituitary apoplexy also commonly presents with pyrexia induced by adrenal insufficiency, chemical meningitis, or hypothalamic dysregulation [1, 47]. Nausea and vomiting may be secondary to hypoadrenalism, hypothalamic injury or irritation, increased intracranial pressure, or meningeal irritation [47].

Altered mental status may present as mild stupor to coma, from insidious to abrupt, due to several possible pathophysiologic mechanisms. Although acute adrenal insufficiency may cause electrolyte abnormalities including hyponatremia and hypoglycemia, some patients continue to display alterations in mental status despite correction of electrolyte abnormalities and corticosteroid treatment. Dorsal tumor extension and hemorrhage with pressure on the hypothalamus or midbrain may also contribute [1, 21, 30, 38, 47]. Other mechanisms include obstructive hydrocephalus due to infiltration or displacement of the third ventricle by necrotic tissue or hemorrhage [36, 50], extensive brain edema with herniation of cerebellar tonsils [36, 52], or impaired cerebral circulation due to internal carotid artery vasospasm in the setting of subarachnoid hemorrhage or compression within the cavernous sinus [50, 53, 54].

Suprasellar extension and upward enlargement of the adenoma and hemorrhage may compress the optic pathways, diencephalon, and mesencephalon. Suprachiasmatic elevation with distention of optic nerves and chiasm leads to decreased visual acuity and visual field defects, including classical bitemporal hemianopsia. Hypothalamic involvement may lead to dysregulation of vital functions including hypotension, dysrhythmias, and disordered breathing, disturbances of temperature regulation, diabetes insipidus, or syndrome of inappropriate antidiuretic hormone [21, 30, 47]. Midbrain involvement may cause muscle tone changes, abnormal responses to visual and/or auditory stimuli, hiccups, and retraction nystagmus [21, 48, 55]. Pressure on nearby olfactory tracts may rarely cause anosmia [17].

Lateral tumor extension with pressure upon the cavernous sinus may cause variable symptoms consistent with the cavernous sinus syndrome [21, 30]. Involvement of cranial nerves III, IV, and VI may produce variable degrees and combinations of ocular palsies. Cranial nerve III palsy may be accompanied by ptosis and mydriasis depending on severity of nerve damage. Horner's syndrome with unilateral ptosis, miosis, and anhidrosis may present following damage to sympathetic fibers within the cavernous sinus [30], and compromise of the cavernous sinus venous plexus can lead to proptosis and chemosis [37, 56]. Compression of the first or second divisions of the trigeminal nerve may produce facial pain, altered facial sensation, and/or loss or decreased corneal reflex [1, 20, 38]. Hemispheric signs with possible addition of aphasia mimicking a cerebrovascular accident may also be induced by internal carotid artery compression, occlusion, or vasospasm [1, 15, 38, 47, 52, 57]. Venous stasis can also produce rhinorrhea or eyelid edema [21]. Extensive hemorrhage may extend into the subarachnoid space, surrounding brain parenchyma, and/or ventricles, with fever, photophobia, nausea, vomiting, meningeal signs, and altered mental status [3, 21, 36]. Hemorrhage into brain parenchyma and subsequent cortical irritation may induce seizures [47].

The acuity of pituitary apoplexy and degree of hemorrhage and edema within the sellar and parasellar region determine the nature and extent of presenting neurological symptoms. Generally, patients with pituitary tumors develop symptoms of mass compression after significant tumor growth due to adaptation of adjacent neurological structures to gradual tumor growth [58]. Alternatively, symptoms of pituitary apoplexy develop acutely due to rapid expansion of hemorrhage and/or infarction. While patients with histological evidence of hemorrhage have similar clinical presentations and hypopituitarism to those patients who exhibit infarction without hemorrhage, the severity of presenting clinical symptoms is greater, and neuro-ophthalmic clinical outcomes are less favorable in the former group [59]. These observed differences are likely due to slower rate of increase and overall decreased intrasellar pressure in lone-infarction pituitary apoplexy than in those with a hemorrhagic component [59]. This is in accordance with findings that microadenomas present less commonly with overt clinical features of pituitary apoplexy than macroadenomas, likely due their smaller size and relatively less extent of hemorrhage [60].

Pathophysiology of Hypopituitarism

Development of hypopituitarism may be due to preexisting deficiencies prior to apoplexy from a macroadenoma [2, 39] or occur rapidly from rapid increase of intrasellar pressure [61]. Most patients with pituitary apoplexy present with variable decreases in pituitary hormone function ranging from single hormone involvement to panhypopituitarism, while diabetes insipidus is relatively uncommon [2, 4, 5, 21, 24, 61, 62]. Differences in anterior and posterior pituitary blood supply may explain why transient or persistent anterior pituitary dysfunction is common, while there is relative sparing of antidiuretic hormone secretion [5]. While destruction of the adenohypophysis may lead to multiple pituitary hormone deficiencies, significant pituitary tissue loss is required prior to development of life-threatening endocrine abnormalities as survival has been estimated to occur with as little as 10% residual functional tissue [63].

Alterations of portal vessel blood flow can potentially disturb hypothalamic regulation of the anterior pituitary, and hypopituitarism may be due to impaired hypothalamic regulation of pituitary axis hormones, rather than a direct insult to the adenohypophysis [5]. Impaired delivery of hypothalamic releasing factors via the neurohypophyseal vasculature is a likely cause, as direct damage to the hypothalamus or median eminence derangements is rarely observed with pituitary apoplexy [5]. Given that adenomectomy may resolve macroadenoma-associated hypopituitarism, gradual compression of pituitary stalk and portal vessels by a growing macroadenoma may underlie pituitary failure [39]. Furthermore, urgent surgical decompression after pituitary apoplexy has been associated with rapid reversal of pituitary dysfunction [61]. The underlying mechanism of abrupt onset pituitary dysfunction may therefore likely be due to rapid increase in intrasellar contents causing compression of portal vessel circulation and pituitary stalk dysfunction during apoplexy, rather than adenohypophyseal destruction [61].

Increased intrasellar content and pressure may also cause progression of potentially reversible hypopituitarism during pituitary apoplexy [42, 64]. As intrasellar pressure increases, increased portal venous pressure may disrupt hypothalamic control of the anterior pituitary [42]. For example, valsalva maneuver with a positive airway pressure of only 30 mm H_2O has caused complete arrest of portal blood flow from the hypothalamus in Rhesus monkeys [65]. Intraoperative increases in intrasellar pressure of patients harboring pituitary tumors has been demonstrated to disrupt and even cause complete arrest of pituitary blood flow [66]. This theory is further supported by observations of higher recorded intrasellar pressures in patients who harbor macroadenomas and have hypopituitarism than in patients with macroadenomas and normal pituitary function [41]. Furthermore, higher elevated intrasellar pressures have been recorded with pituitary apoplexy [64] than with non-apoplectic macroadenomas [41]. Therefore, pituitary apoplexy results in greater, sudden increases of intrasellar pressure due to rapid increase in intrasellar contents with more abrupt cessation of portal vessel blood flow [64]. Hypopituitarism subsequently develops due to sudden decreased delivery of hypothalamic hormones and anterior pituitary perfusion [64].

Measurements of prolactin (PRL) levels may be used as a prognostic marker of pituitary function following pituitary apoplexy. Normally PRL may mildly increase in patients harboring non-PRL-secreting sellar masses due to a stalk effect, through disruption of the negative tonic hypothalamic control via dopamine. In contrast, low or suppressed serum PRL levels may indicate irreversible ischemic anterior pituitary necrosis due to loss of viable hormone producing cells [64]. Patients presenting with PRL levels less than 2.5 µg/L were less likely to recover or maintain pituitary function following surgical decompression than were patients with PRL levels greater than 3.5 µg/L [64]. Therefore, hypopituitarism may be reversible due to ischemia from decreased portal vessel blood flow [61], or irreversible with fulminate necrosis of the pituitary gland [64].

Epidemiology

Classical pituitary apoplexy is rare, with an incidence of approximately 1.2 per million per year [67]. Pituitary tumors account for 15% of all intracranial masses [68], with up to 90% due to adenomas [69–71]. Pituitary apoplexy develops in 9.5% of patients harboring asymptomatic non-functioning pituitary adenomas [72]. Hemorrhagic and necrotic changes have been reported in 9.5–28% of all surgically treated pituitary adenomas [19, 29, 36, 49, 73]. However, symptomatic pituitary apoplexy occurs in only 0.6–9.1% of patients harboring pituitary tumors [24, 29, 36, 50, 74–76].

Pituitary apoplexy most commonly occurs in middle-aged males in the fifth decade of life [2, 4, 24, 26, 50, 62, 75, 77], but it has been reported in a young 6-year-old child [78] and a 90-year-old male [79]. The frequency of pituitary apoplexy among different histological tumor types is similar to the distribution of pituitary tumor types in the population [21, 30]. However, there is often a low yield of tumor type identification by immunohistochemical staining due to extensive necrosis of most pathological specimens [2, 24, 26].

Recognition

Clinical History

Pituitary apoplexy is a clinical syndrome of sudden neurological, ophthalmologic, and endocrinological derangements that occur due to sudden tumor expansion and hemorrhage [1, 21, 30], normally evolving within hours to 2 days [48, 57]. Symptom manifestation is largely dependent on compression of neighboring neurovascular structures, extravasation of blood into the subarachnoid space of the basal cisterns, and/or partial to complete pituitary destruction. Pituitary apoplexy occurs in a small percentage of patients harboring pituitary tumors [24, 29, 36], and may be the first indication of the presence of a pituitary tumor [4, 24, 25, 62, 75, 79]. Severe attacks manifest with altered consciousness, hemiparesis, meningismus visual disturbances including loss of vision and visual field defects, and ocular palsies. Minor events are characterized by headache, nausea, vomiting, and vertigo. Major and minor symptoms are not exclusive, and usually overlap. Most common presenting symptoms are listed in Table 17.2. Occasionally patients present with sudden unexpected death [2, 12, 18, 29, 38, 57, 79, 82].

Headache is the most commonly observed symptom and is usually described as retro-orbital, frontal, or diffuse [2, 21, 24, 38, 75, 83]. Fever may be present in up to 20% of patients [24]. Blindness presents in up to 42% of patients [27]. Ocular palsy may be unilateral or bilateral, and involve any combination of the oculomotor nerves [2, 24, 84]. The oculomotor nerve is most commonly affected, followed by the abducens nerve [2, 25, 27, 57].

Table 17.2 Most common presenting symptoms and signs of pituitary apoplexy in 509 patients[a]

Symptom	Mean percentage (%)	Number of patients
Headache	87	509[b]
Ophthalmoplegia	61	370
Visual acuity deficit	57	469
Nausea and/or vomiting	54	436
Visual field defect	51	367
Photophobia	32	117
Meningismus	19	85
Hyperthermia	16	155
Altered mental status	15	470
Trigeminal neuralgia (V1 or V2)	7	76
Hemiparesis	4	84
Seizure	4	24

[a]The data presented in this table were generated from 16 published series [2, 4, 18, 24–27, 29, 50, 62, 75–77, 79–81]

[b]The following symptoms were not reported among all patients and/or among all series, except for headache

Patients with apoplexy may also rarely present with other neurological deficits including seizures [47] and Horner's syndrome [21, 30]. Unilateral facial pain or altered facial sensation with loss or decreased corneal reflex due to trigeminal nerve involvement occurs infrequently [1, 2, 20, 38]. Other nonspecific symptoms and signs include hiccups, anosmia, photophobia, eyelid edema, proptosis, abnormal pupillary reactions, retraction nystagmus, rhinorrhea, and epistaxis [21].

Symptoms and evidence of hypopituitarism are present prior to the apoplectic event in 20–62% of patients [2, 24, 29, 75]. The degree of hypopituitarism does not necessarily correlate with preoperative visual impairments [61]. Since pituitary apoplexy occurs most frequently with macroadenomas [36, 38, 57, 75], preexisting partial or complete hypopituitarism is an expected occurrence [39]. Menstrual disturbances and decreased libido due to decreased gonadal hormone secretion are often the most common clinical features suggesting preexisting hypopituitarism [2, 24, 27, 76]. Occasionally, pituitary apoplexy may result in regression of hyperfunctioning anterior pituitary states [3, 85, 86]. Hypocortisolism is of concern and can present with weakness, lightheadedness, nausea, vomiting, and abdominal pain. Signs of hypocortisolism include fever, tachycardia, hypovolemia, orthostatic vital signs, and hypotension refractory to intravenous fluids.

Initial Laboratory Assessment

Alterations of both electrolytes and pituitary function can occur. Hyponatremia, occurring in 12–44% of patients, may be due to the syndrome of inappropriate antidiuretic hormone secretion, hypocortisolism, and/or hypothyroidism [4, 18, 24, 62, 75, 87, 88]. Hypoglycemia may occur in the setting of hypocortisolism. Elevated leukocyte count may also be present, especially during the acute phase in up to 18% of patients [47, 62].

Up to 80% of patients have laboratory evidence of partial or complete hypopituitarism at presentation [4, 18, 25, 50, 61, 62, 77], including attenuated thyroid-stimulating hormone (TSH), adrenocorticotropic hormone (ACTH), follicle-stimulating hormone (FSH), luteinizing hormone (LH), and/or growth hormone (GH). Following pituitary apoplexy, 88% of patients are deficient in GH, 76% in LH, 66% in ACTH, 58% in FSH, and 42% in thyroid function [5]. PRL levels may also be either elevated or suppressed due to stalk effect or anterior pituitary destruction, respectively [64]. In contrast, diabetes insipidus is an uncommon finding of pituitary apoplexy, only occurring in 2–4% of patients [5].

High opening CSF pressure, elevated protein, increased red blood cell count, and/or xanthochromia [2, 38, 89, 90] may increase suspicion for alternative diagnoses, particularly subarachnoid hemorrhage and infectious meningitis. Pleocytosis may also be present, with either mixed [90] or neutrophilic predominance [91]. However, sterile CSF cultures are the norm [91–93], and serologic studies for infectious etiologies are negative [91].

Imaging Evaluation

Radiological evidence of pituitary apoplexy on computerized tomography (CT) or MRI includes sellar and/or suprasellar abnormalities consistent with hemorrhage and/or necrosis (see Fig. 17.3). CT findings suggesting hemorrhage evolve from a well-defined high-density mass with minimal to no enhancement at 1–2 weeks of presentation to intra-tumor low density areas with possible ring enhancement at greater than 2 weeks following pituitary apoplexy [21, 29, 90]. CT offers good reliability in detection of acute hemorrhage [90]. However, as blood density changes with hemoglobin degeneration, it can become difficult to distinguish subacute and chronic hematomas on CT scans from cystic degeneration, abscesses, and bland infarction [90]. Similarly, CT cannot readily distinguish pituitary infarction due to apoplexy from cysts or pituitary adenomas that have rim enhancement but have not undergone apoplexy [19, 90]. CT scan detection rates of 93% and 21% for pituitary tumor and hemorrhage/necrosis, respectively, were observed in 35 patients [24]. An apparently normal sella may be present in up to 14% of patients [2, 24, 26].

MRI is superior to CT, and tumor and hemorrhage/infarction detection rates of 100% and 88% have been observed in symptomatic cases of pituitary apoplexy, respectively [24]. Furthermore, MRI is often able to detect hemorrhage not initially

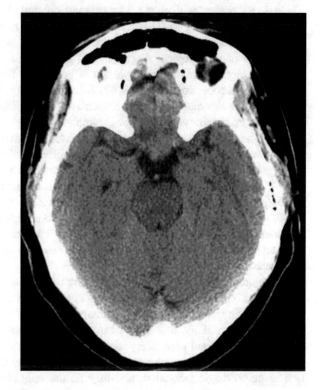

Fig. 17.3 Axial non-contrast-enhanced computed tomography imaging of the head demonstrates high density in the sella consistent with hemorrhage in a large pituitary macroadenoma due to apoplexy

detected by CT [18]. Increased detection rate of hemorrhage by MRI (84%) vs. CT (71%) was reported within apoplectic pituitary macroadenomas [75].

Pituitary apoplexy may present with hemorrhagic and nonhemorrhagic changes on T1-weighted images [20]. Intraparenchymal hemorrhage is typically hyperintense on T1-weighted images and hypointense on T2-weighted images during the acute phase, days 1–2, of pituitary apoplexy [20, 94, 95]. However, MRI may fail to demonstrate hemorrhage during this phase [96]. By days 3–15, during the subacute phase of hemorrhage, signal intensity changes occur due to degeneration of hemoglobin into methemoglobin, and both T1- and T2-weighted signals appear bright [94, 97]. After day 15, a fluid–fluid level may be observed in the mass due to sedimentation of blood products [20, 96]. Pituitary infarction without hemorrhage is described as low signal intensity with associated rim enhancement on T1- and T2-weighted MRI sequences [19, 90].

Etiologies

"Pituitary apoplexy" [1] applies to cases of pituitary hemorrhage and/or necrosis associated with symptoms and signs of compression of parasellar structures or meningeal irritation [21]. Therefore cases of pituitary hemorrhage and/or infarction, which do not present with classical acute neuro-ophthalmic clinical features of pituitary apoplexy, as with obstetrical hemorrhage [98] or asymptomatic hemorrhage, are considered separate entities. "Pituitary apoplexy" is a clinical rather than a radiological or pathological diagnosis and should be reserved for symptomatic cases. Symptomatic pituitary apoplexy has been most frequently associated with preexisting macroadenomas [21, 38, 57, 75]. Only a few cases of symptomatic pituitary apoplexy associated with microadenomas [99, 100], Rathke cleft cysts [18, 101, 102], craniopharyngiomas [55], lymphocytic hypophysitis [103, 104], and other non-adenomatous pituitary glands [20, 84, 105] have been reported.

Subclinical or asymptomatic pituitary apoplexy, defined as histopathological findings consistent with pituitary apoplexy without classical neuro-ophthalmic features, has been described in both macro- and microadenomas [29, 36, 49, 60, 106]. In 664 patients with pituitary adenomas, 9.5% of surgically treated adenomas had pathological evidence of hemorrhagic and/or necrotic degeneration while only 0.6% of patients had symptoms of classical pituitary apoplexy [36]. In 560 surgically resected adenomas, pituitary hemorrhage was present in 16.6% of cases, with clinical symptoms present in only 9.1% [29].

Asymptomatic pituitary hemorrhage and/or necrosis may present as a new headache or new onset endocrinopathy without other overt neurological or visual symptoms and be diagnosed incidentally on imaging or pathology [100, 106]. Due to lack of headache specificity, it is difficult to attribute episodes of headache to hemorrhagic foci discovered in pituitary adenomas of patients with previous hemorrhage. Occasionally, changes in anterior pituitary function may develop following infarction or hemorrhagic infarction, and may be the only sign of this event. Due to smaller relative size of microadenomas, infarction or hemorrhage of microadenomas will less commonly produce the classical clinical features of pituitary apoplexy, except for hypopituitarism [60]. Regardless, due to improved imaging techniques, asymptomatic or subclinical pituitary hemorrhage and/or infarction are likely being diagnosed earlier in presentation and with increasing frequency.

Precipitating Factors

Although pituitary apoplexy is most often a spontaneous vascular event [21, 107], it has been associated with numerous pathological conditions, medications, and dynamic pituitary testing (see Table 17.3). Although pituitary apoplexy presents similarly whether there is an associated risk factor present or not, patients with associated risk factors may present more frequently with altered mental status and worse visual prognosis, as well as more difficult disease to diagnose [79]. Since up to 80% of cases of pituitary apoplexy occur spontaneously without a prior history of pituitary tumor [4, 51, 107], many of these associated conditions are usually

Table 17.3 Precipitating factors in pituitary apoplexy	*Pathologic conditions*
	Acute hypotension
	Hypertension
	Diabetes mellitus
	Coagulopathy
	Pregnancy
	Head trauma
	Major surgical procedures (e.g., CABG)
	Transient changes in intracranial pressure
	Angiography
	Coughing and/or sneezing
	Lumbar puncture
	Pneumoencephalography
	Positive pressure ventilation
	Medications
	Anticoagulant
	Antiplatelet
	Clomiphene
	Dopamine agonist, initiation or withdrawal
	Dynamic pituitary function tests
	Estrogen therapy
	Gonadotropin-releasing hormone agonist
	Isosorbide dinitrate
	Pituitary irradiation
	Thrombolytic

regarded as precipitating factors retrospectively, after the catastrophic event has already occurred. Furthermore, the role of these potential risk factors in pituitary apoplexy in regard to pathophysiology, prognosis, and management is not completely understood [79].

Conditions that have been associated with pituitary apoplexy include sudden head trauma [2, 18, 75, 76, 108, 109], arterial hypertension [20, 24, 25, 50, 62, 110], diabetes mellitus [27, 110, 111], acute hypotension due to any cause including sepsis [83], coagulopathies including thrombocytopenia [36, 50], and high estrogen states including pregnancy [2, 18, 24]. Pituitary apoplexy has also been described after various surgical procedures [79, 112–114], most commonly coronary artery bypass [26, 79, 115–119]. Transient changes in intracranial pressure due to coughing or sneezing [37, 76], positive pressure ventilation [120], angiography [52, 57, 121], and pneumoencephalography [82, 122] have also been considered potential precipitating events.

Medical treatments have also been reported to precipitate pituitary apoplexy and increase the risk of such events. These include anticoagulants [2, 36, 50, 75, 123], antiplatelet medications [24, 124], thrombolytics [79, 124], clomiphene [125], gonadotropin-releasing hormone (GnRH) agonists [126–128], initiation or discontinuation of dopamine agonists [27, 29, 76, 129, 130], and pituitary radiation therapy [1, 17, 36, 48, 131, 132]. Development of pituitary apoplexy occurring soon after dynamic pituitary testing with GnRH, thyrotropin-releasing hormone, corticotropin-releasing hormone, chlorpromazine, and triple bolus test has also been reported [133–139].

Differential Diagnosis

Pituitary apoplexy is often misdiagnosed due to nonspecific symptoms and signs that mimic other common medical emergencies. Patients may present to different clinical specialties causing delays in diagnosis and appropriate treatment, unless the condition is recognized early. Diagnosis can be difficult since the apoplectic event is often the first indication of the presence of a pituitary tumor [4, 21, 24, 62, 75, 79], despite symptoms consistent with previously undiagnosed pituitary hormone dysfunction prior to the catastrophic event [29]. Therefore, heightened clinical acumen and suspicion is critical to early diagnosis and treatment to prevent significant morbidity and rarely mortality.

The differential diagnosis of pituitary apoplexy includes several intracranial and systemic pathologic entities (see Table 17.4). Most commonly, subarachnoid hemorrhage due to a ruptured intracranial aneurysm or meningitis are initially considered diagnoses [21, 51]. Headache, photophobia, stiff neck, and oculomotor palsy may mimic subarachnoid hemorrhage from a ruptured intracranial aneurysm [1, 29, 37, 57]. Alternatively fever, lethargy, photophobia, and meningismus may indicate bacterial or viral meningoencephalitis [37, 55, 57, 76, 89, 91]. Findings of a pituitary mass on brain imaging and CSF findings of neutrophilic pleocytosis with signs

Table 17.4 Differential
diagnosis of pituitary
apoplexy

Brain stem infarction
Carotid-cavernous fistula
Cavernous sinus thrombosis
Cerebral metastasis
Cerebrovascular accident
Cluster headache
Diabetic oculomotor palsy
Encephalitis
Hypertensive encephalopathy
Intracerebral hematoma/hemorrhage
Meningitis
Migraine
Optic neuritis
Subarachnoid hemorrhage from aneurysmal rupture
Temporal arteritis
Transtentorial herniation
Vertebrobasilar insufficiency
Viral gastritis

consistent with infectious meningitis have also been misinterpreted for a coexisting pituitary abscess [91]. Cavernous sinus thrombosis may be mistakenly diagnosed due to ocular palsies and periorbital edema caused by compression of cranial nerves and venous plexus, respectively, within the cavernous sinus [37, 56]. Pituitary apoplexy presenting with hemiplegia mimicking a cerebrovascular accident may also confound the diagnosis [37, 52, 76]. Headache and third cranial nerve palsy have also been incorrectly attributed to a primary or metastatic brain tumor [76, 83]. Occasionally, headache can be insidious and may mimic migraine or other forms of chronic headache [76, 140, 141]. Systemic shock with circulatory collapse secondary to sudden arrest of pituitary ACTH secretion or hypothalamic damage has also been observed [1, 37]. Due to the wide spectrum of symptomatology and presentations, it can be quite challenging to properly diagnose pituitary apoplexy during the acute presentation. However, with the advent of more reliable and detailed MRI, time to proper diagnosis has decreased and even asymptomatic cases are now being diagnosed with increasing frequency.

Management and Outcomes

Initial Assessment

Pituitary apoplexy is often misdiagnosed on early presentation and varies widely in duration and severity. Significant morbidity and mortality are often due to failure to recognize the condition and initiate appropriate interventions. Treatment is aimed at decreasing local compression that compromises adjacent neurologic and vascular structures. Once a suspicion of pituitary apoplexy is made, even prior to imaging confirmation, acute medical management of pituitary apoplexy with intravenous corticosteroids is critical for obtaining favorable clinical outcomes [21].

Acute management of pituitary apoplexy includes close observation and early endocrine, neurosurgical, and ophthalmologic consultations. Detailed history and physical examination should be undertaken, with focus on symptoms and signs of neuro-ophthalmologic derangements and hypopituitarism. Bedside visual acuity and field testing should be performed, followed by formal tests by an ophthalmologist. Baseline Snellen chart test and Goldmann perimetry or Humphrey visual field analyzer examinations may help guide clinical decision-making for either a surgical or conservative approach and document clinical responsiveness to treatment with repeat follow-up assessments throughout the hospitalization.

Baseline laboratory assessments include urgent analysis of electrolytes, renal function, liver function including clotting screen, and complete blood cell count. Electrolyte abnormalities, including hyponatremia and hypoglycemia, should be assessed and corrected. Fluid balance should be monitored closely as diabetes insipidus and inappropriate secretion of antidiuretic hormone may become apparent following corticosteroid treatment.

Endocrine Assessment

Endocrinological laboratory evaluation, with emphasis on adrenal function, should be performed to determine baseline hypothalamic–pituitary axis function in hemodynamically stable patients with serum ACTH and 8 A.M. serum cortisol evaluation. Initially, corticosteroid replacement with intravenous dexamethasone is preferable as it will not interfere with the serum cortisol assay, although hydrocortisone may be preferred afterward due to its favorable physiological properties. Hemodynamically unstable patients should have immediate initiation of intravenous hydrocortisone after baseline assessment of serum cortisol and ACTH regardless of time of day. There is limited utility in performing a cosyntropin stimulation test in the setting of acute secondary adrenal insufficiency.

Baseline testing should include PRL, TSH, free T4 (FT4), insulin-like growth factor 1 (IGF-1), GH, LH, FSH, and testosterone in men or estradiol in women. Intact gonadal function may be assumed by the presence of normal menses in premenopausal females. Although it is important to assess for thyrotropin deficiency, initiation of thyroid hormone replacement is not mandatory prior to contemplated surgery, and baseline GH function is also not critical for survival as replacement therapy is not acutely indicated. Monitoring PRL is important as patients with prolactin-secreting adenomas and clinically stable presentations may be successfully treated conservatively with intravenous fluids, corticosteroids, and dopamine agonist therapy without the need for surgery [24, 75, 77, 142]. One patient was reported with complete resolution of visual field deficit and ocular nerve palsy with administration of bromocriptine in treatment of an apoplectic macroprolactinoma, with follow-up MRI demonstrating decreased tumor burden [142]. Assessment of PRL levels may also help determine prognosis and responsiveness to decompressive surgery, as patients with elevated PRL not due to PRL-secreting tumors are more likely to have reversible hypopituitarism [64].

Radiological Assessment

When pituitary apoplexy is suspected, patients should have urgent brain MRI performed, preferably with a focused pituitary MRI. The use of neuroimaging studies to verify the diagnosis of pituitary apoplexy has evolved over the past several decades [77]. Even with high-quality CT scans, a diagnosis of pituitary apoplexy may be missed in up to 60% of patients unless physicians are aware of other CT findings, besides hemorrhage, that indicate pituitary apoplexy [90]. MRI is the diagnostic modality of choice in the evaluation of pituitary apoplexy [18, 24, 25, 51, 62]. In retrospective series, up to 60% of patients have MRI as the primary neuroimaging investigation, without CT to aid in diagnosis [4, 77]. With greater accessibility of MRI scans, and improvements in imaging resolution, the dependence on prior radiological studies and CSF analysis as a means to diagnosis has decreased. In fact, CSF findings often complicate reaching a proper diagnosis. Incidental findings of pituitary pathology may be discovered on CT or MRI during evaluation of nonspecific symptoms such as headache [70, 143], raising suspicion for pituitary apoplexy while potentially decreasing time to diagnosis and initiation of proper treatment. However, with diagnostic MRI improvements, incidental findings of subclinical or asymptomatic pituitary hemorrhage is also likely increasing in frequency.

MRI exhibits its multiplanar capability to characterize the extent of pituitary hemorrhage and necrosis in fine detail and evaluate effects of expanding pituitary mass on neighboring neurovascular structures [20, 24]. As MRI features of blood components evolve over time, hemorrhage age may be better estimated [20, 96], and cystic or degenerative changes from previous hemorrhage are better differentiated [94, 143]. Furthermore, MRI has demonstrated good ability to correlate images with surgical findings [96].

Although MRI has been unable to predict the severity of visual symptoms based on imaging findings of mass size or optic tract/chiasm involvement [20, 25], there is evidence that the presence of sphenoid sinus thickening may indicate less favorable neurological and endocrinological outcomes [77]. Furthermore, the ability to correlate MRI findings with pathological findings of pituitary apoplexy has profound effects on determining prognosis [28]. In a retrospective study, 22 patients with confirmed ischemic necrosis without hemorrhage on pathological examination had a more benign course with less severe visual symptoms and neurologic deficits than did 37 patients with hemorrhage on pathology [59]. A follow-up study demonstrated MRI findings correlated with histopathological diagnosis in approximately 80% of 26 subjects [28]. Therefore, in most cases, MRI can predict the nature of pituitary apoplexy and possibly guide the type and timing of therapy [28]. Furthermore, baseline MRI prior to any neurosurgical procedure will often guide the neurosurgical approach during surgical decompression.

Despite limitations of CT scanning to clearly delineate hemorrhage during subacute and chronic stages, it is still the most commonly used imaging modality in emergency situations in the evaluation of acute neurological deficits. Emergency rooms rarely begin evaluation of neurological changes with MRI scans. CT can be valuable during the acute period in demonstration of hemorrhage, during the first 24–48 h of symptoms [19]. Furthermore, the presentation of a patient with signs and symptoms consistent with pituitary apoplexy and discovery of any pituitary pathology on head CT, including evidence of a cyst, should alert a suspecting physician of this diagnosis [83]. Clinicians should still suspect pituitary apoplexy when patients present with sudden onset headache, visual alterations, ocular palsies, and altered mental status despite a normal head CT scan [51]. Although MRI is preferred, when it is not available or contraindicated, head CT scans may be acceptable as the initial diagnostic imaging examination.

Treatment and Outcomes

Steroid Therapy

Recognition of acute secondary adrenal insufficiency, if present, is critical, and prompt life-saving empiric intravenous corticosteroid therapy should be initiated to avert adrenal crisis and may also serve to improve visual outcomes [21]. Patients with hemodynamic instability or other symptoms or signs consistent with acute hypocortisolemia should be treated with corticosteroids prior to confirmatory laboratory tests. Other indications for steroid therapy include altered level of consciousness, reduced visual acuity, or severely restricted visual fields. Patients with suboptimal 8 A.M. cortisol levels, less than 18–20 µg/dL, should also be considered for corticosteroid therapy. Since some patients may not develop signs of adrenal insufficiency until surgery or during stress [55], empiric corticosteroids are indicated during the acute time period, especially if surgery is being considered.

As many patients with pituitary apoplexy are unable to tolerate oral medications due to altered mental status, nausea, and/or vomiting, intravenous hydrocortisone is preferred. A recommended hydrocortisone formulation during the acute phase is 200 mg of hydrocortisone bolus followed by 2–4 mg/h by continuous infusion or 50–100 mg injections every 6 h [144]. Once the patient is stabilized and can tolerate oral medication, hydrocortisone should be quickly tapered and standard oral maintenance doses of 15–30 mg/day may be initiated.

Surgical Versus Conservative Management

Traditionally, emergent surgical treatment within hours to several days of presentation has been advocated [47, 61, 74, 145]. Surgery provides an opportunity for direct and immediate sellar decompression with reversal of neurological, visual, and endocrine abnormalities and can potentially decrease the chance of continued neoplastic viability. Transsphenoidal surgery is the preferred route with low associated morbidity and mortality, favorable neuro-ophthalmic results [2, 18, 21, 57], and occasional restoration of normal pituitary function [61]. Transsphenoidal decompression can improve visual acuity in 88%, visual field defects in 95%, and ocular paresis in 100% of patients presenting with pituitary apoplexy [2].

Craniotomy carries higher morbidity rates than does transsphenoidal surgery, but an intracranial approach may be necessary in cases of severe suprasellar extension of hemorrhage, small sella with a large suprasellar mass, or poorly aerated sphenoid sinus [18, 21, 146], or when transsphenoidal surgery is unsuccessful in improving symptoms or removing significant amounts of hemorrhagic and/or necrotic tissue [50]. Currently, there is general consensus that emergent decompressive surgery under steroid cover is the definitive treatment of pituitary apoplexy in patients with sudden, severe diminishing level of consciousness, hypothalamic dysfunction, and/or visual acuity/field defects [2, 4, 12, 18, 21, 24, 27, 30, 51, 76]. Rapid diagnosis based on clinical grounds and imaging, steroid replacement, and transsphenoidal decompression offers excellent results [57]. While it is evident that complete blindness at presentation has a poor prognosis [4, 18, 26], it is difficult to decipher from the literature whether severe or rapid-onset symptoms should be used to mandate surgical intervention.

Retrospective studies have demonstrated similar outcomes in visual and endocrine function in patients managed conservatively or by timely surgical intervention [25, 26, 62]. Patients with visual acuity loss, visual field cuts, and/or ophthalmoplegia without complete blindness have been observed to have similar visual outcomes with either medical or surgical management [26]. There is evidence that rapid initiation of high-dose corticosteroids without surgical intervention can improve symptoms of pituitary apoplexy, sometimes within a few days [37, 76, 82, 115]. Therefore, there is a divergence of views regarding the role of surgery versus conservative management since it is unclear which management option offers the best outcome for patients, especially those with less severe presentations.

Perioperative and postoperative surgical complications, morbidity, and mortality should be considered in management decisions for pituitary apoplexy. These include cerebrospinal leaks, meningitis, cardiac arrest, cerebrovascular accidents, and postoperative pain [25, 76]. Visual acuity may also worsen following surgery [2], possibly due to residual tumor bleeding [87], and surgical reintervention should be considered. The risk of worsening hypopituitarism that may develop following surgical removal of anterior pituitary tissue should also be considered [3, 5]. Diabetes insipidus occurs more commonly postoperatively, and it is transient in up to 50% of patients and permanent in 6–30% of patients [5, 24–26, 61, 75].

Timing of Surgery

The timing of surgery is important for obtaining favorable outcomes. Emergent surgery is critical in patients with deteriorating clinical status and/or severe hypothalamic dysfunction given the high mortality rate despite optimal treatment [38].

Several retrospective studies have demonstrated that the optimal time period for decompressive surgery in patients who present with unilateral or bilateral blindness is within 1 week of development of symptoms [2, 24, 87, 106, 147]. Optic nerves appear to be able to withstand ischemia due to compression for up to 5–7 days, even if patients present with unilateral or even bilateral blindness [147].

A retrospective analysis of 37 patients demonstrated that surgery within 7 days of pituitary apoplexy onset resulted in significant improvement of visual acuity deficits, while further delay of surgery had less favorable results [2]. A significant difference was not observed for visual field deficit or ocular palsy improvement among the different surgical timeframes [2]. Surgery within 8 days led to higher rates of improvements of visual acuity deficits (88%), visual field deficits (95%), and ocular paresis (100%) than did surgery performed after this time frame [24]. Visual acuity improved within 24 h of transsphenoidal surgery in four of five patients, and in 50% of total eyes, who initially presented with near or complete visual loss when transsphenoidal surgery was performed within 7 days [147]. Alternatively, three patients who presented with complete bilateral blindness remained without observable improvement on Snellen test when surgery was performed after 10 days [147].

Deferral of surgical intervention for longer than 1 week in patients with neurological and visual deterioration is not advocated, unless comorbidities are the cause of delay [2, 24, 75, 87]. In one study, conservative medical management in seven patients with deferral of surgery to 8.7 days from onset of apoplectic symptoms due to associated medical conditions and/or coagulopathies resulted in less favorable visual outcomes and greater need for hormone replacement than in six patients without associated medical illnesses who underwent surgery within 3.5 days [87]. Patients with complicated medical histories may still benefit from timely surgery, although it is likely that older age, associated comorbidities, and coagulation disorders contribute to less favorable clinical outcomes [87].

Several retrospective studies observed no differences in outcomes among surgically managed patients regardless of whether surgery is performed within 1 week or later [25, 62, 76]. Nevertheless, if surgery has been delayed and more than a week has passed, surgery may still be considered, as there are cases of significant visual improvement after delayed surgical decompression from 2 weeks to several months after the initial event [2, 3, 24]. Ultimately, visual outcomes are more affected by optic disc appearance rather than by severity of initial visual acuity deficit or length of visual history [76].

Outcomes of Visual Function

Routine early transsphenoidal decompression has demonstrated improved visual acuity and visual field deficits in 41 of 46 and 60 of 65 patients, respectively, reviewed in retrospective studies [2, 18, 24, 25, 61, 62, 147]. Although such studies demonstrate high success with surgical management, other retrospective reviews report similar results with conservative management (see Table 17.5).

Table 17.5 Selected retrospective studies showing neuro-ophthalmic outcomes after surgery or conservative management of pituitary apoplexy

Studies	Number of patients		Key findings
	Total	Surgically treated	
Arafah et al. [61]	8	8	Complete or partial VF recovery in 7/7 and complete OP resolution in 4/4 patients
Onesti et al. [18]	16	16	Ophthalmic improvement in 13/16 patients; blindness had poor prognosis
McFadzean et al. [76]	15	9	Similar VA improvement in patients treated surgically and conservatively; similar VA outcome in patients undergoing surgery within 7 days of onset or later
Bonicki et al. [80]	39	19	Full ophthalmic recovery in 14/19 surgically treated patients; clinical improvement in 16 conservatively managed patients without severe ophthalmic signs at presentation
Bills et al. [2]	37	36	Better VA (but not VF or OP) outcome in patients undergoing surgery within 7 days of symptom onset
Maccagnan et al. [27]	12	5	Favorable ophthalmic recovery in most conservatively managed patients but five patients with severe VA at presentation and deferred surgical management had less favorable VA outcomes
Da Motta et al. [22]	16	10	Higher rates of ophthalmic improvement in surgically treated patients; higher rate of mortality in conservatively managed patients
Randeva et al. [24]	35	31	Better VA and VF (but not OP) outcomes in patients undergoing surgery within 8 days of onset of symptoms
Biousse et al. [79]	30	27	Less favorable VA and VF outcomes in patients with associated precipitating factors compared to those without precipitating factors despite similar time lag for diagnoses and surgery
Ayuk et al. [25]	33	15	No observed difference in visual recovery with surgery performed within or after 8 days
Sibal et al. [62]	45	27	VA, VF, and OP improvement in both surgical and conservative-treated groups; no difference in visual outcomes in patients undergoing surgery within 7 days or after 7 days
Agrawal et al. [147]	8	8	Greater resolution of complete blindness with surgery within 7 days than after 10 days
Lubina et al. [75]	40	34	VF and OP recovery in 81% and 71% of patients, respectively
Semple et al. [4]	62	58	Improved VA and VF in 76% and 79% of patients, respectively; blindness at presentation had poor prognosis
Chuang et al. [87]	13	13	Surgery in patients without comorbidities resulted in more favorable visual and endocrine function than in patients with associated comorbidities
Gruber et al. [26]	30	10	Similar ophthalmic outcomes in surgical and conservatively managed patients; complete blindness had poor prognosis
Liu et al. [77]	28	25	Improvement of visual function in 9/9 and OP in 8/8 surgically managed patients

Adapted with permission from Table 7 Sibal et al. [62]
VA visual acuity, *VF* visual fields, *OP* ocular palsy

The need for emergent surgery in patients with mild symptoms is also challenged by evidence of spontaneous resolution of neurological and visual symptoms following pituitary apoplexy [3]. Generally, conservative management may be considered in carefully selected cases. Several earlier retrospective studies demonstrated successful outcomes with conservative medical management in patients with stable or nonprogressive neuro-ophthalmic deficits [3, 55, 99, 132]. Later retrospective studies have reconfirmed such findings in patients presenting with absent, stable, or resolving neuro-ophthalmic symptoms and signs [25, 26, 62].

One non-randomized prospective trial of 12 patients reported the importance of carefully selecting patients prior to decision for conservative management [27]. Resolution or improvement of neuro-ophthalmic symptoms was observed in seven patients managed conservatively with intravenous dexamethasone, only two of whom had mild visual blurring [27]. Surgery was performed on five patients who either did not improve within 1 week of conservative management or had symptoms that worsened with tapering of dexamethasone [27]. Four of five patients who required surgery had either unilateral or bilateral blindness upon initial presentation, and one developed unilateral blindness due to tumor recurrence that required another surgical intervention [27]. Recovery of visual function was minimal in two, partial in one, and complete in only two patients, one of whom had a recurrent tumor [27].

Conservative management of 18 of 33 patients with pituitary apoplexy led to resolution of visual field defects in all six patients with these symptoms [25]. In a retrospective analysis of 30 patients, 10 surgically and 20 conservatively managed patients had similar visual outcomes when complete blindness was not a presenting symptom [26]. While these studies demonstrate that conservative management may be undertaken successfully, such favorable outcomes usually occur in patients with mild visual acuity loss, who do not have unilateral or bilateral blindness at presentation, or who do not experience acute visual deterioration. Generally, decompressive surgery is more effective than conservative management for decreased visual acuity caused by pituitary apoplexy. Patients managed by conservative therapy should be monitored diligently for signs of clinical deterioration and for indications that would require a surgical approach, including worsening visual deficits, decreasing level of consciousness, and development of hemiparesis [25, 26].

Outcomes of Ocular Palsies

There is controversy whether surgical decompression affects outcomes of ocular paresis. Ocular paresis is more likely to resolve from apoplexy than any other visual symptoms [21]. Some authors advocate surgical decompression in patients with ocular paresis, even if decreased level of consciousness or other visual defects are not present [24]. Higher rates (74%) of complete resolution of ocular paresis were observed in patients undergoing surgery within 8 days than in patients who underwent surgery after 8 days (42%), although these results were not significant [24].

Most studies demonstrate that ocular paresis without significant visual compromise does not appear to be an absolute indication for surgery [2, 25–27]. Timing of surgery did not affect improvement of ocular paresis in 36 patients managed with transsphenoidal decompression, with significant increase in eye movements noted in two patients who had surgery delayed by 3 months [2]. In a study of 33 patients, 100% of 18 conservatively managed and 63% of 15 surgically managed patients had full recovery of ocular palsies [25]. Similarly, in patients who presented with visual defects, but without complete blindness paresis, ocular paresis resolved completely in 83% and partially resolved in 17% of 12 conservatively managed patients [26]. In a prospective study, conservative management with intravenous dexamethasone resulted in significant improvement of ophthalmoplegia even with the presence of mild visual blurring upon initial evaluation [27].

Dopamine agonist therapy may decrease tumor mass effects and rapidly restore function of compressed vessels in patients harboring PRL-secreting adenomas with apoplexy. Several cases of apoplectic macroprolactinomas presenting with headache and oculomotor nerve palsy reported paresis resolution of symptoms within 48 h of initiation [77, 142]. Given such favorable rapid results, prompt initiation of dopamine agonist therapt in addition to intravenous corticosteroids may be administered at time of diagnosis, prior to obtaining results of PRL levels [142].

Outcomes of Hypopituitarism

Hypopituitarism, whether partial or complete, is a prominent feature of apoplexy and likely contributes to the morbidity and mortality of this disease [3, 5, 21, 38, 47, 61]. Hypopituitarism may be transient or permanent following pituitary apoplexy, with return of function occurring from weeks to months after the initial event [3, 4, 57, 61]. More than 50% of patients ultimately require hormone replacement [2, 3, 5, 24, 50, 61, 148]. Postoperative hypopituitarism occurred in 86% of 33 patients with at least one hormone dysfunction who underwent transsphenoidal surgery within 3 days of admission [75]. Similarly, 83% of 62 patients required hormone replacement [4].

However, there is no clear consensus on whether surgical treatment improves pituitary function outcomes. An increased incidence of hormonal deficiencies was reported with conservative management [27]. Emergent surgical surgery within 3 days after onset of symptoms restored endocrine function, assessed by return of ACTH secretion, in 11 of 15 patients within 3 days of surgery [51]. Transsphenoidal decompressive surgery resulted in resolution of hypopituitarism with return of normal adrenal, thyroidal, and gonadal function in the immediate postoperative period in 86%, 67%, and 50% of eight patients, respectively [61], although findings have not been repeated in larger studies [25]. Earlier surgery has also been suggested to decrease the occurrence of long-term hormone replacement therapy as those undergoing surgery within 6 days of admission had lower hormone replacement requirements [24] compared to those who had surgery within 7.7 of admission [2].

Advocates of conservative management maintain no difference in long-term hypopituitarism rates between surgically managed and carefully selected conservatively managed patients [25, 62]. Eighteen conservatively managed patients presenting with absent or improving visual deficits had similar rates of hypocortisolism, hypothyroidism, and hypogonadism compared with 15 surgically managed patients who underwent transsphenoidal surgery with a median time of 4 days, without significant deleterious effects on visual function [25]. Indications for surgery included worsening visual deficits, decreased level of consciousness, or development of hemiparesis [25]. Similar long-term hormone replacement rates were observed, with requirements of corticosteroid therapy in 60% and 68%, testosterone in 86% and 82% of males, and thyroxine in 70% and 68%, among 10 surgically and 20 medically managed patients, respectively [26]. Although advocates of timely surgical treatment argue that conservatively managed patients may have decreased rates of pituitary dysfunction had they been treated surgically given their less severe initial presentation, this approach has not been substantiated since the degree of hypopituitarism and visual impairments at presentation and postoperatively do not necessarily correlate [61]. Diabetes insipidus is a relatively rare consequence of pituitary apoplexy with an incidence of 4% for transient and 2% for persistent diabetes insipidus [5]. However, diabetes insipidus occurs commonly after surgery, with permanent dysfunction present in as many as 11–30% of patients [2, 25, 26].

Postoperative Care

Patients managed surgically should be monitored carefully for any of the aforementioned surgical complications. Hourly fluid intake and output should be carefully followed and if diabetes insipidus is suspected, hourly sodium, serum creatinine, and serum osmolalities should be monitored. Daily laboratory assessments of complete blood count, electrolytes, and renal function should also be followed during the immediate postoperative period. Visual acuity, visual fields, and extraocular eye movements should be assessed within 48 h of surgery, followed by formal tests prior to discharge. Development of worsening visual symptoms should prompt an urgent MRI and neurosurgical reevaluation.

Since many patients may not have undergone preoperative endocrine function assessments, evaluation of steroid reserve and thyroid functions are essential prior to hospital discharge. Measurements of 8 A.M. serum cortisol should be undertaken on postoperative days 2 and 3. If the patient is already receiving hydrocortisone, the cortisol measurement should be performed at least 12 h after the last dose of corticosteroid dose by omitting the evening dose. Results of 8 A.M. cortisol levels will determine postoperative hydrocortisone requirements. TSH and FT4 should be assessed prior to discharge and thyroid replacement hormone should be initiated if deficient, although TSH and FT4 may be falsely normal during acute pituitary damage. Euthyroid sick syndrome may also confound diagnosis.

Long-Term Management

Long-term endocrine reassessments are essential since anterior pituitary function may fully or partially recover [3, 5, 106]. Decreased requirement for endocrine replacement therapy was observed in 78% at 3-month follow-up and in 26% at 2-year follow-up in 22 patients who presented with acute classical pituitary apoplexy [106]. Each case should be individualized, and timing of follow-up interval assessments is based on symptoms and clinical signs.

Patients with chronic secondary adrenal insufficiency should be continued on maintenance hydrocortisone therapy of 15–30 mg/day, and during times of illness, such as pneumonia, they should be treated with stress dose corticosteroid treatment. Such patients should also wear emergency wrist bracelets indicating their disease.

Hypothyroidism should be monitored by measurements of FT4 4–8 weeks following pituitary apoplexy. There is little utility in monitoring TSH in patients with secondary hypothyroidism. Maintenance of regular menses in premenopausal women implies an intact pituitary–gonadal axis; otherwise, LH, FH, and estradiol may be measured. Men should be screened for secondary hypogonadism with evaluation of FSH, LH, and total testosterone levels, especially if decreased libido or erectile dysfunction is present. PRL levels should also be monitored, especially if pituitary apoplexy occurs in a PRL-secreting adenoma, as supra-physiologic PRL levels can cause hypogonadism. GH function may also be monitored with IGF-1 levels, although GH is rarely replaced. Annual laboratory endocrine function tests should be performed to regularly assess for return or further loss of pituitary function.

Follow-up radiological imaging is essential since recurrent apoplexy has been reported in both medically [25, 48, 84] and surgically managed patients [2, 24, 25, 27, 149]. Residual tumor tissue may be observed in up to 37% of operated cases [75]. Therefore, it is prudent to follow patients with serial MRI scans over several years for evidence of tumor recurrence after transsphenoidal surgery, especially since late tumor occurrence up to 3 years after the apoplectic episode has been reported [3, 24–26]. Prophylactic radiotherapy is not recommended prior to adenoma recurrence, as it may precipitate further unnecessary hemorrhagic necrosis [17, 47, 48].

Mortality

Significant morbidity and mortality occur due to delay of medical and surgical interventions or failure to diagnose pituitary apoplexy [1, 17]. Historically, mortality was attributed to lack of medical treatment of hypopituitarism, specifically corticosteroid replacement therapy [12, 17]. Fatalities in the modern medical era typically occur due to massive subarachnoid hemorrhage [50, 150], extensive hypothalamic involvement [5, 12, 50], or from secondary systemic complications, such as myocardial infarction or respiratory distress [47, 52].

Death, although now rare [12], still remains a concern despite early diagnosis in both surgically [50, 75] and conservatively managed patients [22, 26]. Patients with severe or declining clinical status on presentation, including progression to coma, have high mortality rates regardless of surgical and medical treatments [38]. Higher mortality rate have also been reported in nonsurgically treated patients [22].

However, there is some controversy as conservative management with high-dose intravenous dexamethasone has been adequate in over 50% of patients, and patient mortality was not increased by delaying surgery by 1 week from initial presentation [27]. Patients with non-functioning pituitary adenomas have similar survival rates whether pituitary apoplexy is present or not [67]. Nevertheless, with early diagnosis and rapid initiation of endocrinological management and modern neurosurgical techniques, mortality has decreased from a rate of 61% in the 1950s [17] to 6.7% in the 1980s [21].

Conclusion

Pituitary apoplexy commonly presents as a neurosurgical emergency with sudden onset, severe headache accompanied by nausea, vomiting, fever, loss of visual acuity or blindness, visual field defects, ophthalmoplegia, meningismus, alterations of mental status, hypopituitarism, and sometimes bizarre neurological deficits. Symptoms develop from hemorrhage and/or infarction of the pituitary with surrounding mass compression of parasellar structures. Diagnosis is confirmed by radiological imaging, with MRI as diagnostic modality of choice (see Fig. 17.4).

Important initial investigations include assessments of intact neurological status and visual field acuity and fields. Acute pituitary insufficiency should be assumed until excluded by endocrinological laboratory tests, and empiric corticosteroid replacement therapy is vital to outcomes of mortality and morbidity. Although rare cases of spontaneous recovery have been reported, pituitary apoplexy may potentially follow a fatal course if not diagnosed early and treated promptly with medical and/or surgical treatment. Definitive management is transsphenoidal decompression and pituitary tumor removal under corticosteroid cover, although conservative management, with corticosteroids and dopamine agonists, may be successful in selected groups of patients.

Ultimately, decisions for emergent surgery or conservative management should be addressed by a multidisciplinary team, including specialists in neurosurgery, ophthalmology, and endocrinology (see Fig. 17.5). Patients presenting with severe alterations of consciousness and visual acuity including blindness should be managed by timely surgery, preferably by transsphenoidal decompression, within 1 week of development of symptoms. Equally, patients with sudden, worsening, severe neurological and visual deterioration should have expedited surgery. Alternatively, patients with absent, stable, or improving visual symptoms and normal mental status may be successfully managed conservatively, despite the presence of ophthalmoplegia (Fig. 17.5).

Visual improvement and resolution of ocular palsies usually appear following either surgery or medical intervention, and long-term anterior pituitary function is usually poor regardless of therapy and multiple hormone deficits persist in most patients [2, 24, 75]. Due to the unpredictable clinical course of pituitary apoplexy, prompt surgical decompression may be considered even though results suggest

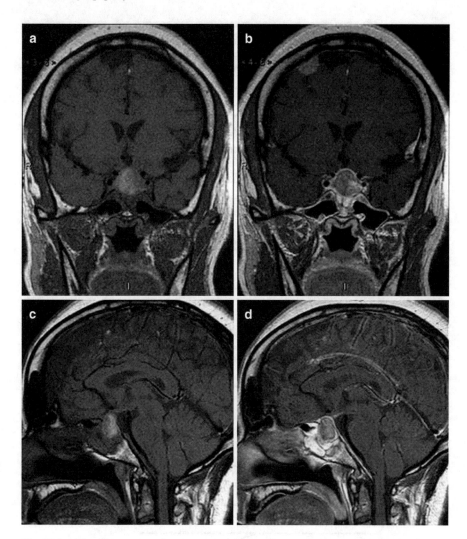

Fig. 17.4 Magnetic resonance imaging T1-weighted sequences in the coronal (**a**) and sagittal (**c**) planes demonstrate acute infarction of a pituitary macroadenoma with expansion of the sella. High T1 signal intensity is consistent with hemorrhage. Post-contrast coronal (**b**) and sagittal (**d**) T1-weighted sequences demonstrate heterogeneous enhancement with clival epidural hematoma

favorable outcomes with conservative management [51, 75]. Especially in conditions of visual acuity and field compromise, waiting for absorption of hemorrhagic areas and spontaneous resolution of these signs is potentially risky. It may not be possible to predict which physical conditions will remain stable or which continue to deteriorate [51]. Furthermore, clinicians should be aware of the preselection bias in data supporting conservative management. Most patients treated with conservative management in such studies often lack altered mental status, and visual deficits were absent, stable, or improving [25, 27, 75].

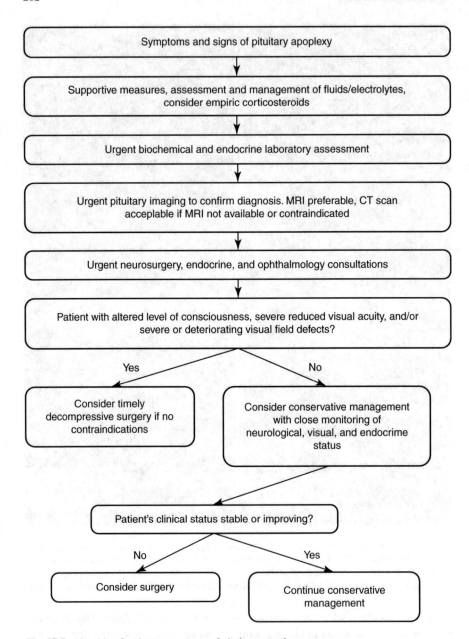

Fig. 17.5 Algorithm for the management of pituitary apoplexy

Overall, treatment strategies should be individualized and determined by the severity of clinical presentation and disease course. Long-term management should include reevaluations of hypothalamic–pituitary axis function, visual acuity and fields, and serial MRI studies to prevent long-term neurological or endocrinological deficits and screen for tumor recurrence.

References

1. Brougham M, Heusner AP, Adams RD. Acute degenerative changes in adenomas of the pituitary body—with special reference to pituitary apoplexy. J Neurosurg. 1950;7(5):421–39.
2. Bills DC, Meyer FB, Laws ER Jr, et al. A retrospective analysis of pituitary apoplexy. Neurosurgery. 1993;33(4):602–8; discussion 608–609.
3. Pelkonen R, Kuusisto A, Salmi J, et al. Pituitary function after pituitary apoplexy. Am J Med. 1978;65(5):773–8.
4. Semple PL, Webb MK, de Villiers JC, Laws ER Jr. Pituitary apoplexy. Neurosurgery. 2005;56(1):65–72; discussion 72–73.
5. Veldhuis JD, Hammond JM. Endocrine function after spontaneous infarction of the human pituitary: report, review, and reappraisal. Endocr Rev. 1980;1(1):100–7.
6. Bailey P. Pathological report of a case of akromegaly, with special reference to the lesions in the hypophysis cerebri and in the thyroid gland; and a case of hemorrhage into the pituitary. Philadelphia Med J. 1898;1:789–92.
7. Bleibtreu L. Ein Fall von Akromegalie (Zerstörung der Hypophysis durch Blutung). Munch Med Wochenschr. 1905;52:2079–80.
8. Coxon RV. A case of haemorrhage into a pituitary tumour simulating rupture of an intracranial aneurysm. Guys Hosp Rep. 1943;92:89–93.
9. Dingley LA. Sudden death due to a tumour of the pituitary gland. Lancet. 1932;2:183–4.
10. Kux E. Über ein bösartiges Pinealom und ein bösartiges fötales Adenom der Hypophyse. Beitr Path Anat. 1931;87:59–70.
11. Voss O. Beitrag zur Hirnblutung an der Schädelbasis. Intrakranielle basale Blutungen. Dtsch Z Chir. 1938;250:727–35.
12. Lange M, Woenckhaus M, Segiet W, Oeckler R. A rare fatal course of disease in a patient with spontaneous pituitary apoplexy. Case report and literature review. Neurosurg Rev. 1999;22(2–3):163–9.
13. Dott NM, Bailey P, Cushing H. A consideration of the hypophysial adenomata. Br J Surg. 1925;13:314–66.
14. Sosman MC. The roentgen therapy of pituitary adenomas. J Am Med Assoc. 1939;113:1282–5.
15. List CF, Williams JR, Balyeart GW. Vascular lesions in pituitary adenomas. J Neurosurg. 1952;9(2):177–87.
16. Tönnis W, Oberdisse K, Weber E. Bericht über 264 operierte Hypophysenadenome. Acta Neurochir. 1953;3(2):113–30.
17. Uihlein A, Balfour WM, Donovan PF. Acute hemorrhage into pituitary adenomas. J Neurosurg. 1957;14(2):140–51.
18. Onesti ST, Wisniewski T, Post KD. Clinical versus subclinical pituitary apoplexy: presentation, surgical management, and outcome in 21 patients. Neurosurgery. 1990;26(6):980–6.
19. Ostrov SG, Quencer RM, Hoffman JC, Davis PC, Hasso AN, David NJ. Hemorrhage within pituitary adenomas: how often associated with pituitary apoplexy syndrome? AJR Am J Roentgenol. 1989;153(1):153–60.
20. Piotin M, Tampieri D, Rufenacht DA, et al. The various MRI patterns of pituitary apoplexy. Eur Radiol. 1999;9(5):918–23.
21. Cardoso ER, Peterson EW. Pituitary apoplexy: a review. Neurosurgery. 1984;14(3):363–73.
22. da Motta LA, de Mello PA, de Lacerda CM, Neto AP, da Motta LD, Filho MF. Pituitary apoplexy. Clinical course, endocrine evaluations and treatment analysis. J Neurosurg Sci. 1999;43(1):25–36.
23. Laws ER. Pituitary tumor apoplexy: a review. J Intensive Care Med. 2008;23(2):146–7.
24. Randeva HS, Schoebel J, Byrne J, Esiri M, Adams CB, Wass JA. Classical pituitary apoplexy: clinical features, management and outcome. Clin Endocrinol. 1999;51(2):181–8.
25. Ayuk J, McGregor EJ, Mitchell RD, Gittoes NJ. Acute management of pituitary apoplexy—surgery or conservative management? Clin Endocrinol. 2004;61(6):747–52.

26. Gruber A, Clayton J, Kumar S, Robertson I, Howlett TA, Mansell P. Pituitary apoplexy: retrospective review of 30 patients—is surgical intervention always necessary? Br J Neurosurg. 2006;20(6):379–85.
27. Maccagnan P, Macedo CL, Kayath MJ, Nogueira RG, Abucham J. Conservative management of pituitary apoplexy: a prospective study. J Clin Endocrinol Metab. 1995;80(7):2190–7.
28. Semple PL, Jane JA, Lopes MB, Laws ER. Pituitary apoplexy: correlation between magnetic resonance imaging and histopathological results. J Neurosurg. 2008;108(5):909–15.
29. Wakai S, Fukushima T, Teramoto A, Sano K. Pituitary apoplexy: its incidence and clinical significance. J Neurosurg. 1981;55(2):187–93.
30. Reid RL, Quigley ME, Yen SS. Pituitary apoplexy. A review. Arch Neurol. 1985;42(7):712–9.
31. Baker HL Jr. The angiographic delineation of sellar and parasellar masses. Radiology. 1972;104(1):67–78.
32. Stanfield JP. The blood supply of the human pituitary gland. J Anat. 1960;94:257–73.
33. Page RB. Pituitary blood flow. Am J Phys. 1982;243(6):E427–42.
34. Schechter J. Ultrastructural changes in the capillary bed of human pituitary tumors. Am J Pathol. 1972;67(1):109–26.
35. Schechter J, Goldsmith P, Wilson C, Weiner R. Morphological evidence for the presence of arteries in human prolactinomas. J Clin Endocrinol Metab. 1988;67(4):713–9.
36. Mohr G, Hardy J. Hemorrhage, necrosis, and apoplexy in pituitary adenomas. Surg Neurol. 1982;18(3):181–9.
37. Dawson BH, Kothandaram P. Acute massive infarction of pituitary adenomas. A study of five patients. J Neurosurg. 1972;37(3):275–9.
38. Rovit RL, Fein JM. Pituitary apoplexy: a review and reappraisal. J Neurosurg. 1972;37(3):280–8.
39. Arafah BM. Reversible hypopituitarism in patients with large nonfunctioning pituitary adenomas. J Clin Endocrinol Metab. 1986;62(6):1173–9.
40. Arafah BM, Kailani SH, Nekl KE, Gold RS, Selman WR. Immediate recovery of pituitary function after transsphenoidal resection of pituitary macroadenomas. J Clin Endocrinol Metab. 1994;79(2):348–54.
41. Arafah BM, Prunty D, Ybarra J, Hlavin ML, Selman WR. The dominant role of increased intrasellar pressure in the pathogenesis of hypopituitarism, hyperprolactinemia, and headaches in patients with pituitary adenomas. J Clin Endocrinol Metab. 2000;85(5):1789–93.
42. Lees PD, Pickard JD. Hyperprolactinemia, intrasellar pituitary tissue pressure, and the pituitary stalk compression syndrome. J Neurosurg. 1987;67(2):192–6.
43. Powell DF, Baker HL Jr, Laws ER Jr. The primary angiographic findings in pituitary adenomas. Radiology. 1974;110(3):589–95.
44. Turner HE, Nagy Z, Gatter KC, Esiri MM, Harris AL, Wass JA. Angiogenesis in pituitary adenomas and the normal pituitary gland. J Clin Endocrinol Metab. 2000;85(3):1159–62.
45. Hirano A, Tomiyasu U, Zimmerman HM. The fine structure of blood vessels in chromophobe adenoma. Acta Neuropathol. 1972;22(3):200–7.
46. Mou C, Han T, Zhao H, Wang S, Qu Y. Clinical features and immunohistochemical changes of pituitary apoplexy. J Clin Neurosci. 2009;16(1):64–8.
47. Epstein S, Pimstone BL, De Villiers JC, Jackson WP. Pituitary apoplexy in five patients with pituitary tumours. Br Med J. 1971;2(5756):267–70.
48. Weisberg LA. Pituitary apoplexy. Association of degenerative change in pituitary adenoma with radiotherapy and detection by cerebral computed tomography. Am J Med. 1977;63(1):109–15.
49. Mohanty S, Tandon PN, Banerji AK, Prakash B. Haemorrhage into pituitary adenomas. J Neurol Neurosurg Psychiatry. 1977;40(10):987–91.
50. Dubuisson AS, Beckers A, Stevenaert A. Classical pituitary tumour apoplexy: clinical features, management and outcomes in a series of 24 patients. Clin Neurol Neurosurg. 2007;109(1):63–70.
51. Verrees M, Arafah BM, Selman WR. Pituitary tumor apoplexy: characteristics, treatment, and outcomes. Neurosurg Focus. 2004;16(4):E6.
52. Rosenbaum TJ, Houser OW, Laws ER. Pituitary apoplexy producing internal carotid artery occlusion. Case report. J Neurosurg. 1977;47(4):599–604.

53. Cardoso ER, Peterson EW. Pituitary apoplexy and vasospasm. Surg Neurol. 1983;20(5):391–5.
54. Pozzati E, Frank G, Nasi MT, Giuliani G. Pituitary apoplexy, bilateral carotid vasospasm, and cerebral infarction in a 15-year-old boy. Neurosurgery. 1987;20(1):56–9.
55. Lloyd MH, Belchetz PE. The clinical features and management of pituitary apoplexy. Postgrad Med J. 1977;53(616):82–5.
56. Seyer H, Kömpf D, Fahlbusch R. Optomotor palsies in pituitary apoplexy. Neuro-Ophthalmology. 1992;12(4):217–24.
57. Ebersold MJ, Laws ER Jr, Scheithauer BW, Randall RV. Pituitary apoplexy treated by trans-sphenoidal surgery. A clinicopathological and immunocytochemical study. J Neurosurg. 1983;58(3):315–20.
58. Trumble HC. Pituitary tumours; observations on large tumours which have spread widely beyond the confines of the sella turcica. Br J Surg. 1951;39(153):7–24.
59. Semple PL, De Villiers JC, Bowen RM, Lopes MB, Laws ER Jr. Pituitary apoplexy: do histological features influence the clinical presentation and outcome? J Neurosurg. 2006;104(6):931–7.
60. Findling JW, Tyrrell JB, Aron DC, Fitzgerald PA, Wilson CB, Forsham PH. Silent pituitary apoplexy: subclinical infarction of an adrenocorticotropin-producing pituitary adenoma. J Clin Endocrinol Metab. 1981;52(1):95–7.
61. Arafah BM, Harrington JF, Madhoun ZT, Selman WR. Improvement of pituitary function after surgical decompression for pituitary tumor apoplexy. J Clin Endocrinol Metab. 1990;71(2):323–8.
62. Sibal L, Ball SG, Connolly V, et al. Pituitary apoplexy: a review of clinical presentation, management and outcome in 45 cases. Pituitary. 2004;7(3):157–63.
63. Sheehan HL. Atypical hypopituitarism. Proc R Soc Med. 1961;54(1):43–8.
64. Zayour DH, Selman WR, Arafah BM. Extreme elevation of intrasellar pressure in patients with pituitary tumor apoplexy: relation to pituitary function. J Clin Endocrinol Metab. 2004;89(11):5649–54.
65. Antunes JL, Muraszko K, Stark R, Chen R. Pituitary portal blood flow in primates: a Doppler study. Neurosurgery. 1983;12(5):492–5.
66. Kruse A, Astrup J, Cold GE, Hansen HH. Pressure and blood flow in pituitary adenomas measured during transsphenoidal surgery. Br J Neurosurg. 1992;6(4):333–41.
67. Nielsen EH, Lindholm J, Bjerre P, et al. Frequent occurrence of pituitary apoplexy in patients with non-functioning pituitary adenoma. Clin Endocrinol. 2006;64(3):319–22.
68. Terada T, Kovacs K, Stefaneanu L, Horvath E. Incidence, pathology, and recurrence of pituitary adenomas: study of 647 unselected surgical cases. Endocr Pathol. 1995;6(4):301–10.
69. Famini P, Maya MM, Melmed S. Pituitary magnetic resonance imaging for sellar and parasellar masses: ten-year experience in 2598 patients. J Clin Endocrinol Metab. 2011;96(6):1633–41.
70. Freda PU, Wardlaw SL, Post KD. Unusual causes of sellar/parasellar masses in a large trans-sphenoidal surgical series. J Clin Endocrinol Metab. 1996;81(10):3455–9.
71. Valassi E, Biller BM, Klibanski A, Swearingen B. Clinical features of nonpituitary sellar lesions in a large surgical series. Clin Endocrinol. 2010;73(6):798–807.
72. Arita K, Tominaga A, Sugiyama K, et al. Natural course of incidentally found nonfunctioning pituitary adenoma, with special reference to pituitary apoplexy during follow-up examination. J Neurosurg. 2006;104(6):884–91.
73. Rolih CA, Ober KP. Pituitary apoplexy. Endocrinol Metab Clin N Am. 1993;22(2):291–302.
74. Kaplan B, Day AL, Quisling R, Ballinger W. Hemorrhage into pituitary adenomas. Surg Neurol. 1983;20(4):280–7.
75. Lubina A, Olchovsky D, Berezin M, Ram Z, Hadani M, Shimon I. Management of pituitary apoplexy: clinical experience with 40 patients. Acta Neurochir. 2005;147(2):151–7; discussion 157.
76. McFadzean RM, Doyle D, Rampling R, Teasdale E, Teasdale G. Pituitary apoplexy and its effect on vision. Neurosurgery. 1991;29(5):669–75.
77. Liu JK, Couldwell WT. Pituitary apoplexy in the magnetic resonance imaging era: clinical significance of sphenoid sinus mucosal thickening. J Neurosurg. 2006;104(6):892–8.
78. Tiwary CM. Thrombocytopenia and pituitary necrosis associated with rubella. Proc R Soc Med. 1969;62(9):908–9.

79. Biousse V, Newman NJ, Oyesiku NM. Precipitating factors in pituitary apoplexy. J Neurol Neurosurg Psychiatry. 2001;71(4):542–5.
80. Bonicki W, Kasperlik-Zaluska A, Koszewski W, Zgliczynski W, Wislawski J. Pituitary apoplexy: endocrine, surgical and oncological emergency. Incidence, clinical course and treatment with reference to 799 cases of pituitary adenomas. Acta Neurochir. 1993;120(3–4):118–22.
81. Takeda N, Fujita K, Katayama S, Akutu N, Hayashi S, Kohmura E. Effect of transsphenoidal surgery on decreased visual acuity caused by pituitary apoplexy. Pituitary. 2010;13(2):154–9.
82. Sachdev Y, Gopal K, Garg VK, Mongia SS. Pituitary apoplexy (spontaneous pituitary necrosis). Postgrad Med J. 1981;57(667):289–93.
83. Watt A, Pobereskin L, Vaidya B. Pituitary apoplexy within a macroprolactinoma. Nat Clin Pract Endocrinol Metab. 2008;4(11):635–41.
84. Conomy JP, Ferguson JH, Brodkey JS, Mitsumoto H. Spontaneous infarction in pituitary tumors: neurologic and therapeutic aspects. Neurology. 1975;25(6):580–7.
85. Dunn PJ, Donald RA, Espiner EA. Regression of acromegaly following pituitary apoplexy. Aust NZ J Med. 1975;5(4):369–72.
86. Rigolosi RS, Schwartz E, Glick SM. Occurrence of growth-hormone deficiency in acromegaly as a result of pituitary apoplexy. N Engl J Med. 1968;279(7):362–4.
87. Chuang CC, Chang CN, Wei KC, et al. Surgical treatment for severe visual compromised patients after pituitary apoplexy. J Neuro-Oncol. 2006;80(1):39–47.
88. Ebner FH, Hauser TK, Honegger J. SIADH following pituitary adenoma apoplexy. Neurol Sci. 2010;31(2):217–8.
89. Jassal DS, McGinn G, Embil JM. Pituitary apoplexy masquerading as meningoencephalitis. Headache. 2004;44(1):75–8.
90. Post MJ, David NJ, Glaser JS, Safran A. Pituitary apoplexy: diagnosis by computed tomography. Radiology. 1980;134(3):665–70.
91. Huang WY, Chien YY, Wu CL, Weng WC, Peng TI, Chen HC. Pituitary adenoma apoplexy with initial presentation mimicking bacterial meningoencephalitis: a case report. Am J Emerg Med. 2009;27(4):517.e1–4.
92. Bjerre P, Lindholm J. Pituitary apoplexy with sterile meningitis. Acta Neurol Scand. 1986;74(4):304–7.
93. Haviv YS, Goldschmidt N, Safadi R. Pituitary apoplexy manifested by sterile meningitis. Eur J Med Res. 1998;3(5):263–4.
94. Bonneville F, Cattin F, Marsot-Dupuch K, Dormont D, Bonneville JF, Chiras J. T1 signal hyperintensity in the sellar region: spectrum of findings. Radiographics. 2006;26(1):93–113.
95. Rogg JM, Tung GA, Anderson G, Cortez S. Pituitary apoplexy: early detection with diffusion-weighted MR imaging. AJNR Am J Neuroradiol. 2002;23(7):1240–5.
96. Kurihara N, Takahashi S, Higano S, et al. Hemorrhage in pituitary adenoma: correlation of MR imaging with operative findings. Eur Radiol. 1998;8(6):971–6.
97. Lazaro CM, Guo WY, Sami M, et al. Haemorrhagic pituitary tumours. Neuroradiology. 1994;36(2):111–4.
98. Sheehan HL, Murdoch R. Post-partum necrosis of the anterior pituitary: pathological and clinical aspects. J Obstet Gynaecol Br Emp. 1938;45(3):456–88.
99. Jeffcoate WJ, Birch CR. Apoplexy in small pituitary tumours. J Neurol Neurosurg Psychiatry. 1986;49(9):1077–8.
100. Randall BR, Couldwell WT. Apoplexy in pituitary microadenomas. Acta Neurochir. 2010;152(10):1737–40.
101. Binning MJ, Liu JK, Gannon J, Osborn AG, Couldwell WT. Hemorrhagic and nonhemorrhagic Rathke cleft cysts mimicking pituitary apoplexy. J Neurosurg. 2008;108(1):3–8.
102. Pawar SJ, Sharma RR, Lad SD, Dev E, Devadas RV. Rathke's cleft cyst presenting as pituitary apoplexy. J Clin Neurosci. 2002;9(1):76–9.
103. Dan NG, Feiner RI, Houang MT, Turner JJ. Pituitary apoplexy in association with lymphocytic hypophysitis. J Clin Neurosci. 2002;9(5):577–80.

104. Lee MS, Pless M. Apoplectic lymphocytic hypophysitis. Case report. J Neurosurg. 2003;98(1):183–5.
105. Cooperman D, Malarkey WB. Pituitary apoplexy. Heart Lung. 1978;7(3):450–4.
106. Liu ZH, Chang CN, Pai PC, et al. Clinical features and surgical outcome of clinical and sub-clinical pituitary apoplexy. J Clin Neurosci. 2010;17(6):694–9.
107. Nawar RN, AbdelMannan D, Selman WR, Arafah BM. Pituitary tumor apoplexy: a review. J Intensive Care Med. 2008;23(2):75–90.
108. Holness RO, Ogundimu FA, Langille RA. Pituitary apoplexy following closed head trauma. Case report. J Neurosurg. 1983;59(4):677–9.
109. Uchiyama H, Nishizawa S, Satoh A, Yokoyama T, Uemura K. Post-traumatic pituitary apoplexy—two case reports. Neurol Med Chir (Tokyo). 1999;39(1):36–9.
110. Sussman EB, Porro RS. Pituitary apoplexy: the role of atheromatous emboli. Stroke. 1974;5(3):318–23.
111. Brennan CF, Malone RG, Weaver JA. Pituitary necrosis in diabetes mellitus. Lancet. 1956;271(6932):12–6.
112. Abbott J, Kirkby GR. Acute visual loss and pituitary apoplexy after surgery. BMJ. 2004;329(7459):218–9.
113. Goel V, Debnath UK, Singh J, Brydon HL. Pituitary apoplexy after joint arthroplasty. J Arthroplasty. 2009;24(5):826.e7–10.
114. Yahagi N, Nishikawa A, Matsui S, Komoda Y, Sai Y, Amakata Y. Pituitary apoplexy following cholecystectomy. Anaesthesia. 1992;47(3):234–6.
115. Armstrong MR, Douek M, Schellinger D, Patronas NJ. Regression of pituitary macroadenoma after pituitary apoplexy: CT and MR studies. J Comput Assist Tomogr. 1991;15(5):832–4.
116. Absalom M, Rogers KH, Moulton RJ, Mazer CD. Pituitary apoplexy after coronary artery surgery. Anesth Analg. 1993;76(3):648–9.
117. Alzetani A, Fisher C, Costa R, Ohri SK. Ptosis postcardiac surgery: a case of pituitary apoplexy. Ann Thorac Surg. 2002;73(1):300–1.
118. Cooper DM, Bazaral MG, Furlan AJ, et al. Pituitary apoplexy: a complication of cardiac surgery. Ann Thorac Surg. 1986;41(5):547–50.
119. Thurtell MJ, Besser M, Halmagyi GM. Pituitary apoplexy causing isolated blindness after cardiac bypass surgery. Arch Ophthalmol. 2008;126(4):576–8.
120. Barber SG. Airways insufficiency and pituitary failure. Br Med J. 1979;1(6177):1564.
121. Reichenthal E, Manor RS, Shalit MN. Pituitary apoplexy during carotid angiography. Acta Neurochir. 1980;54(3–4):251–5.
122. Tsitsopoulos P, Andrew J, Harrison MJ. Pituitary apoplexy and haemorrhage into adenomas. Postgrad Med J. 1986;62(729):623–6.
123. Nourizadeh AR, Pitts FW. Hemorrhage into pituitary adenoma during anticoagulant therapy. JAMA. 1965;193:623–5.
124. Fuchs S, Beeri R, Hasin Y, Weiss AT, Gotsman MS, Zahger D. Pituitary apoplexy as a first manifestation of pituitary adenomas following intensive thrombolytic and antithrombotic therapy. Am J Cardiol. 1998;81(1):110–1.
125. Walker AB, Eldridge PR, MacFarlane IA. Clomiphene-induced pituitary apoplexy in a patient with acromegaly. Postgrad Med J. 1996;72(845):172–3.
126. Chanson P, Schaison G. Pituitary apoplexy caused by GnRH-agonist treatment revealing gonadotroph adenoma. J Clin Endocrinol Metab. 1995;80(7):2267–8.
127. Morsi A, Jamal S, Silverberg JD. Pituitary apoplexy after leuprolide administration for carcinoma of the prostate. Clin Endocrinol. 1996;44(1):121–4.
128. Sinnadurai M, Cherukuri RK, Moses RG, Nasser E. Delayed pituitary apoplexy in patient with advanced prostate cancer treated with gonadotrophin-releasing hormone agonists. J Clin Neurosci. 2010;17(9):1201–3.
129. Alhajje A, Lambert M, Crabbe J. Pituitary apoplexy in an acromegalic patient during bromocriptine therapy. Case report. J Neurosurg. 1985;63(2):288–92.

130. Biller BM, Molitch ME, Vance ML, et al. Treatment of prolactin-secreting macroadenomas with the once-weekly dopamine agonist cabergoline. J Clin Endocrinol Metab. 1996;81(6):2338–43.
131. Jacobi JD, Fishman LM, Daroff RB. Pituitary apoplexy in acromegaly followed by partial pituitary insufficiency. Arch Intern Med. 1974;134(3):559–61.
132. Wright RL, Ojemann RG, Drew JH. Hemorrhage into pituitary adenomata. Report of two cases with spontaneous recovery. Arch Neurol. 1965;12:326–31.
133. Arafah BM, Taylor HC, Salazar R, Saadi H, Selman WR. Apoplexy of a pituitary adenoma after dynamic testing with gonadotropin-releasing hormone. Am J Med. 1989;87(1):103–5.
134. Bernstein M, Hegele RA, Gentili F, et al. Pituitary apoplexy associated with a triple bolus test. Case report. J Neurosurg. 1984;61(3):586–90.
135. Korsic M, Lelas-Bahun N, Surdonja P, Besenski N, Horvat S, Plavsic V. Infarction of FSH-secreting pituitary adenoma. Acta Endocrinol. 1984;107(2):149–54.
136. Otsuka F, Kageyama J, Ogura T, Makino H. Pituitary apoplexy induced by a combined anterior pituitary test: case report and literature review. Endocr J. 1998;45(3):393–8.
137. Rotman-Pikielny P, Patronas N, Papanicolaou DA. Pituitary apoplexy induced by corticotrophin-releasing hormone in a patient with Cushing's disease. Clin Endocrinol. 2003;58(5):545–9.
138. Silverman VE, Boyd AE III, McCrary JA III, Kohler PO. Pituitary apoplexy following chlorpromazine stimulation. Arch Intern Med. 1978;138(11):1738–9.
139. Vassallo M, Rana Z, Allen S. Pituitary apoplexy after stimulation tests. Postgrad Med J. 1994;70(824):444–5.
140. Dodick DW, Wijdicks EF. Pituitary apoplexy presenting as a thunderclap headache. Neurology. 1998;50(5):1510–1.
141. Silvestrini M, Matteis M, Cupini LM, Troisi E, Bernardi G, Floris R. Ophthalmoplegic migraine-like syndrome due to pituitary apoplexy. Headache. 1994;34(8):484–6.
142. Brisman MH, Katz G, Post KD. Symptoms of pituitary apoplexy rapidly reversed with bromocriptine. Case report. J Neurosurg. 1996;85(6):1153–5.
143. Kyle CA, Laster RA, Burton EM, Sanford RA. Subacute pituitary apoplexy: MR and CT appearance. J Comput Assist Tomogr. 1990;14(1):40–4.
144. Rajasekaran S, Vanderpump M, Baldeweg S, et al. UK guidelines for the management of pituitary apoplexy. Clin Endocrinol. 2011;74(1):9–20.
145. Robinson JL. Sudden blindness with pituitary tumors. Report of three cases. J Neurosurg. 1972;36(1):83–5.
146. Wilson CB, Dempsey LC. Transsphenoidal microsurgical removal of 250 pituitary adenomas. J Neurosurg. 1978;48(1):13–22.
147. Agrawal D, Mahapatra AK. Visual outcome of blind eyes in pituitary apoplexy after transsphenoidal surgery: a series of 14 eyes. Surg Neurol. 2005;63(1):42–6; discussion 46.
148. Lewin IG, Mohan J, Norman PF, Gibson RA, Francis JR. Pituitary apoplexy. BMJ. 1988;297(6662):1526–7.
149. Ahmed M, Rifai A, Al-Jurf M, Akhtar M, Woodhouse N. Classical pituitary apoplexy presentation and a follow-up of 13 patients. Horm Res. 1989;31(3):125–32.
150. Wohaibi MA, Russell NA, Ferayan AA, Awada A, Jumah MA, Omojola M. Pituitary apoplexy presenting as massive subarachnoid hemorrhage. J Neurol Neurosurg Psychiatry. 2000;69(5):700–1.

Chapter 18
Ovarian Hyperstimulation Syndrome (OHSS)

Robert L. Barbieri

Précis

1. Clinical setting: Abdominal bloating and distention, intravascular volume depletion, ascites, hemoconcentration, and oliguria *following a fertility intervention involving the administration of exogenous follicle stimulating hormone (FSH).*
2. Diagnosis:

    (a) History: Abdominal bloating, distention, abdominal and/or pelvic pain, acute weight gain, and shortness of breath. A recent fertility intervention involving the administration of exogenous FSH. Young age, polycystic ovary syndrome, or low body mass. A previous history of OHSS.

    (b) Physical examination: Abdominal distention, weight gain, evidence for ascites (flank dullness), or pleural effusion (dullness to percussion, decreased breath sounds).

    (c) Laboratory values: Hemoconcentration (Hct >50%), elevated BUN and creatinine, elevated liver function tests.

    (d) Imaging: Bilateral ovarian enlargement, peritoneal fluid or ascites on ultrasound, pleural effusions on ultrasound.

    (e) Treatment: Close monitoring of hemodynamic status and renal function. Paracentesis to resolve the abdominal compartment syndrome. Administration of albumin or hydroxyethyl starch to improve renal function and urine output. Treatment with cabergoline to reduce ovarian vascular endothelial growth factor (VEGF) production. Thrombosis prophylaxis to reduce the risk of thromboembolism.

R. L. Barbieri (✉)
Department of Obstetrics and Gynecology, Brigham and Women's Hospital, Harvard Medical School, Boston, MA, USA
e-mail: rbarbieri@partners.org

© Springer Nature Switzerland AG 2021   209
L. Loriaux, C. Vanek (eds.), *Endocrine Emergencies*, Contemporary Endocrinology,
https://doi.org/10.1007/978-3-030-67455-7_18

The most dangerous complications of OHSS are renal failure, hypovolemic shock, thrombosis, stroke, acute respiratory distress, ovarian torsion, ovarian rupture, and death.

Ovarian hyperstimulation syndrome (OHSS) is the presence of the combination of *ovarian enlargement* due to hormone-secreting *luteinized ovarian cysts* and an associated vascular dysfunction manifested by *increased capillary permeability*, resulting in the accumulation of fluid in the peritoneal and pleural cavity, and hemoconcentration.

Definition and Staging of OHSS There is no established uniform definition of OHSS [1]. One staging system for OHSS is presented in Table 18.1 [2]. Most staging systems regard *mild* OHSS, which includes abdominal discomfort and distention, along with variably enlarged ovaries, as a normal physiological consequence of ovarian hyperstimulation regimens that stimulate the growth of multiple ovarian follicles. *Severe* OHSS is a serious problem characterized by marked fluid shifts into the extravascular compartment and renal dysfunction. Mathur and colleagues have championed the division of OHSS into early and late cases. Early cases of OHSS present 3–7 days after follicle luteinization [3]. Late cases of OHSS present 12–17 days after luteinization. Early cases of OHSS are associated with excessive ovarian stimulation and the events surround luteinization. Late cases of OHSS are associated with singleton and multiple gestations with continuing stimulation of the ovary by rising levels of hCG from the trophoblast tissue. Late cases of OHSS are more severe and difficult to anticipate based on events during the follicular phase of the stimulated cycle [3].

Table 18.1 Ovarian hyperstimulation syndrome staging system

Category	Description
Mild	
Grade 1	Abdominal distention and discomfort, abdominal pain
Grade 2	Features of grade 1 *plus* nausea, vomiting, and diarrhea
	Ovaries are 5–12 cm in diameter
Moderate	
Grade 3	Features of *mild* OHSS *plus* sonographic evidence of ascites
Severe	
Grade 4	Features of *moderate* OHSS *plus* clinical evidence of ascites or hydrothorax or breathing difficulties
Grade 5	All of the above *plus* hemoconcentration or diminished renal perfusion and function or coagulation abnormalities

Adapted from Ovarian Hyperstimulation Syndrome Staging (Golan et al. [2])

Pathophysiology

In most cases of OHSS, the inciting cause is fertility treatment involving the sequential administration of exogenous FSH to stimulate multiple follicle growth followed by administration of a hormone to induce luteinization of the large follicles. Occasionally, OHSS may occur following clomiphene ovulation induction, during the agonist phase of GnRH agonist monotherapy [4, 5] or following monotherapy with an anti-estrogen such as tamoxifen [6]. Rarely a spontaneous pregnancy may cause OHSS [7].

A goal of many fertility treatments, such as in vitro fertilization (IVF) and FSH-intrauterine insemination (FSH-IUI), is to stimulate the growth and luteinization (IVF) or ovulation (FSH-IUI) of *multiple* follicles. In a typical IVF cycle, exogenous FSH is administered at a dose sufficient to stimulate the development of approximately ten or more large follicles. When the follicles are sufficiently mature, a luteinizing hormone is administered to cause luteinization of the granulosa and theca cells in the follicles. Hormones that can be used to trigger luteinization of mature follicles include recombinant human LH (rLH), human chorionic gonadotropin (hCG), or a GnRH agonist, which triggers the release of endogenous LH from the pituitary gland. These hormones trigger luteinization of the follicle, shifting the granulosa cells from estradiol production to progesterone and estradiol synthesis. They also stimulate the oocyte to resume meiotic division in order to prepare it for fertilization. The sequential ovarian stimulation regimen of FSH followed by a luteinization trigger is termed a controlled ovarian hyperstimulation (COH) or controlled ovarian stimulation (COS) cycle. In COH and COS cycles, hCG is the most commonly used hormone to trigger luteinization of the follicles.

Luteinized granulosa cells, stimulated by hCG or LH, secrete vascular endothelial growth factor (VEGF). In turn, VEGF increases endothelial permeability [8–10]. In model systems of ovarian hyperstimulation, increased capillary permeability caused by excessive VEGF secretion from luteinized follicles can be blocked by the administration of an inhibitor of VEGF, such as Flt-1 Fc [11].

In a COH cycle, the multiple luteinized cysts secrete large quantities of VEGF, which cause a marked increase in capillary permeability resulting in fluid shift from the intravascular to extravascular space. Circulating concentrations of VEGF are positively correlated with the risk of developing OHSS and the severity of the syndrome. Other proteins, which may play an auxiliary role in the development of OHSS, include interleukin-6, the renin-angiotensin system, the kinin-kallikrein system, selectins, IGF-1, epidermal growth factor, transforming growth factors alpha and beta, basic fibroblast growth factor, platelet-derived growth factor, and interleukin-1 beta.

During fertility treatment, OHSS most often occurs after luteinization triggered by hCG (early cases occur 3–7 days after the administration of the luteinization trigger). Compared to endogenous or recombinant LH, hCG has a much longer half-life (>24 h for hCG versus <20 min for LH). Compared to LH, hCG has a higher affinity for the LH receptor and a longer duration of intracellular effect [12]. Interestingly, GnRH agonist stimulation of ovulatory events, by causing the endogenous pituitary release of LH, is associated with lower ovarian production of VEGF. In contrast, hCG administration is associated with greater ovarian production of VEGF [13]. As noted below, one approach to reducing the risk of developing OHSS, following the use of FSH to stimulate multiple follicle growth, is to trigger ovulation with a GnRH agonist or rLH rather than hCG.

Among women, there is great variability in the magnitude of ovarian follicle response to a fixed dose of FSH. The size of the woman's ovarian follicle pool is an important predictor of response to FSH. Women with large numbers of responsive antral follicles, such as young women and women with polycystic ovary syndrome (PCOS), respond more vigorously to a given dose of FSH than women with a small number of antral follicles, such as women >40 years of age and those with premature loss of ovarian follicles due to alkylating chemotherapy or multiple ovarian surgeries. Genetic mutations in proteins that regulate ovarian follicle growth may modulate the risk of developing OHSS by sensitizing the ovary to the stimulatory effects of FSH. Bone morphogenetic protein 15 (BMP15) is an important regulator of ovarian follicle development in sheep and mice. Certain alleles of BMP15 appear to be associated with increased ovarian response to FSH and an increased risk of OHSS [14, 15].

The ovary contains high concentrations of dopamine, and the theca-lutein cells of the corpus luteum contain dopamine receptors [16]. In human granulosa cells, cabergoline, a dopamine agonist, inhibits VEGF production. Women with PCOS are at increased risk for developing OHSS when treated with the sequential combination of FSH and a luteinizing hormone. Follicles from women with PCOS appear to have reduced ovarian dopamine concentration and decreased concentration of dopamine receptors suggesting that reduced dopamine tone permits increased VEGF secretion in these women [17]. As noted below, cabergoline treatment appears to have a beneficial effect on women with OHSS.

Rare causes of OHSS include an FSH secreting pituitary tumor or genetic mutations in the FSH receptor [18]. The most common FSH receptor mutation associated with OHSS (FSHR D567N) results in the expression of a permissive FSH receptor that binds not only FSH but also LH, hCG, and TSH. Women with FSH receptor mutations typically develop OHSS when they become pregnant due to excessive ovarian stimulation of the FSH receptor by placental hCG.

OHSS is associated with the accumulation of large amounts of fluid in the peritoneal cavity and occasionally in the pleural space. In women with OHSS, intra-abdominal pressure is often elevated, creating an *abdominal compartment syndrome*. In patients with mild and severe OHSS, the intra-abdominal pressure has been reported to be 13 and 40 mmHg, respectively [19]. Intra-abdominal pressure greater than 16 mmHg can cause reduced renal blood flow, decreased urine output, decreased cardiac output, increased systemic vascular resistance, and coagulopathy. Paracentesis performed early and often in the course of OHSS can reduce intra-abdominal pressure and prevent the complications associated with the abdominal compartment syndrome.

Epidemiology   Moderate and severe forms of OHSS have been reported to occur in approximately 4% and 0.5%, respectively, of women undergoing ovarian stimulation for IVF [20]. In a consecutive case series of 214,219 US women undergoing assisted reproductive treatment (ART), moderate and severe OHSS developed in 0.7% and 0.3% of the women, respectively, but under-reporting may have occurred [21]. Mild forms of OHSS occur in about 30% of ART cycles.

The most important pretreatment risk factors for developing OHSS include the following: (1) a previous history of OHSS, (2) age <30 years, and (3) diagnosis of polycystic ovary syndrome. The most important risk factors identified during an ovarian stimulation cycle include the following: (1) elevated circulating estradiol, >3500 pg/mL, (2) rapidly rising estradiol, (3) large number of follicles, for example >20 follicles, and (4) use of hCG to stimulate luteinization [22]. On a positive note, OHSS is more likely to occur in women who become pregnant during their fertility treatment, likely because of the continued stimulation of ovarian VEGF secretion by hCG secreted from trophoblast cells. Women who become pregnant with multiple gestations, which are associated with higher levels of circulating hCG, are also more likely to develop OHSS.

Clinical Presentation

Most cases of OHSS occur following ovarian stimulation with fertility medications. Women with mild OHSS typically present with lower abdominal pain, discomfort and distention, bloating, mild nausea, and occasionally vomiting. Women with moderate and severe forms of OHSS present with rapid weight gain, shortness of breath and tachypnea, reduced urine output, orthostatic hypotension, and tachycardia. The differential diagnosis includes ovarian hemorrhage, ovarian torsion, pelvic infection, intra-abdominal hemorrhage, ectopic pregnancy, and appendicitis.

Clinical examination should include sequential measurement of body weight, abdominal circumference, and pelvic ultrasound to measure ovarian size and check for the presence of ascites. Laboratory tests that are useful include hemoglobin/hematocrit concentration, creatinine, electrolytes, and liver function tests. Follow-up evaluation every 2–3 days is adequate to assess the progress of the condition. If a woman reports increasing and severe pain, abdominal distention, shortness of breath, and reduced urine output, immediate clinical reevaluation is warranted. Early cases of OHSS (3–7 days after administration of a luteinizing agent) tend to resolve within 1–2 weeks if pregnancy does not occur. Late cases of OHSS (presenting 12–17 days after administration of LH or hCG) are often associated with an ongoing pregnancy and may persist for weeks.

Women with severe OHSS should be considered for hospitalization. Specific conditions that may require intensive unit care include adult respiratory distress syndrome, renal failure, or thromboembolism. Severe OHSS is associated with hematocrit >50% and hyponatremia in about 50% of cases. Oliguria is present in about 30% of women with severe OHSS. Abnormal liver function tests are present in about 30% of women with OHSS. Severe OHSS may occasionally be associated with pulmonary dysfunction including pneumonia, respiratory distress syndrome, and pulmonary embolism [23]. Chest X-ray is indicated to assess women for pleural effusion and coincident pulmonary infection.

Severe OHSS is associated with increased plasma levels of D-dimer, increased thrombin-antithrombin III complex, and decreased protein S activity [24]. Rarely, severe OHSS may cause arterial and venous thrombosis [25]. When the CNS is involved in the thrombotic process, the results can be devastating [26, 27]. Thrombosis can also occur in arteries supplying the limbs, rarely requiring amputation [28].

Prevention of OHSS

Selection of Stimulation Regimens Based on Risk Stratification

Prior to the initiation of a cycle of ovarian stimulation, higher circulating levels of antimullerian hormone (AMH) and a higher basal ovarian antral follicle count are associated with an increased risk of developing OHSS [29]. Therefore, it is possible to stratify women into high and low risk groups for the development of OHSS. It is known that certain ovarian stimulation protocols are associated with a higher risk of OHSS and other protocols with a lower risk of OHSS. For example, the risk of developing OHSS is lower with an ovarian stimulation protocol that uses FSH injections, GnRH antagonist to suppress a premature LH surge, and a GnRH agonist analog to trigger luteinization by stimulating the pituitary to release endogenous LH [30, 31]. In contrast, the risk of developing OHSS is greater with an ovarian stimulation protocol that uses a long downregulation regimen with GnRH agonist analog started in the luteal phase of the cycle preceding the treatment cycle (to suppress a premature LH surge), FSH injections, and hCG to trigger luteinization. Using this information, it has been proposed that women with high AMH (>29 pM), who are at higher risk of OHSS, receive the ovarian stimulation protocol that is associated with a lower risk of OHSS (FSH, GnRH antagonist, GnRH agonist) and women with normal AMH (16–29 pM), who are at a lower risk of developing OHSS receive a standard protocol (long-cycle downregulation GnRH agonist analog, FSH injections, hCG) [32].

Why not treat all women with the protocol associated with the lowest risk of OHSS? Many clinicians believe that the protocol with the lowest risk of OHSS, which utilizes a GnRH antagonist plus a GnRH agonist to trigger luteinization, is associated with lower pregnancy rates than the standard long downregulation protocol with a GnRH agonist or protocols that use a GnRH antagonist plus hCG to trigger luteinization [33]. Experienced clinicians are concerned that the stimulation protocols associated with a low risk of developing OHSS increase the risk of the "empty follicle syndrome," where no oocytes can be retrieved at the time of oocyte harvest. Therefore, the use of the GnRH antagonist plus a GnRH agonist to trigger luteinization might best be limited to those women at the highest risk of OHSS and women who have experienced OHSS in a previous cycle.

Another option for reducing the risk of OHSS is to stratify women into high and low risk groups for OHSS and then give the women at high risk for OHSS, lower doses of FSH [34]. In a similar manner, if the treatment cycle appears to have resulted in excessive stimulation, the luteinization trigger can be switched from a standard dose of hCG to a low dose of hCG [35] or to switch, mid-cycle, to a GnRH antagonist plus GnRH agonist for luteinization protocol [36].

Coasting   A very elevated level of estradiol (>3000 pg/mL) and/or the presence of a marked excess of growing antral follicles (>20 follicles >12 mm in diameter) are risk factors for developing OHSS. It is likely that the presence of a very elevated level of estradiol is a predictor for excessive ovarian production of VEGF following luteinization. Since estradiol levels are somewhat predictive of the risk of developing OHSS, one approach to prevention is to stop administering daily FSH when estradiol exceeds some predetermined threshold, such as 3000 pg/mL. Without continuing FSH stimulation, granulosa production of estradiol will decrease during the following days. When circulating estradiol reaches a lower level, such as 2000 pg/mL, a luteinizing stimulus is administered, and the cycle proceeds. A major advantage of coasting is that the treatment cycle is not abandoned, and for IVF cycles, in contrast to cryopreservation of all embryos, it allows the transfer of fresh embryos [37]. Coasting for more than 3 days may reduce oocyte quality and pregnancy rates. Some experts recommend that after 3 days coasting should be abandoned, and the cycle should proceed with cryopreservation of all the embryos [38]. In a systematic review of four randomized trials, there was no evidence that coasting reduced the risk of moderate or severe OHSS. However, in the review, coasting was associated with the retrieval of fewer oocytes [39].

Colloid Infusion at the Time of Oocyte Retrieval   Women with an estradiol >3000 pg/mL on the day of triggering luteinization are at increased risk for OHSS. In one trial, women with an estradiol >3000 pg/mL, or >20 follicles on the day of hCG administration, were randomized to receive 500 mL of 6% hydroxyethyl starch or 50 mL of 20% human albumin or 500 mL of 0.9% NaCl at the time of oocyte retrieval [40]. The rate of moderate or severe OHSS was 19%, 10%, and 6% in the groups receiving saline, albumin, or hydroxyethyl starch, respectively.

Cryopreserving All Embryos and Delaying Embryo Transfer to Another Cycle

The goal of fertility treatments is to achieve a pregnancy. In programs involving the administration of FSH to stimulate multiple follicle development followed by the administration of an agent to trigger ovulation, the pregnancy rate is positively correlated with the magnitude of the ovarian response. Within a corridor of safety, the greater the number of follicles stimulated, the greater the pregnancy rate. Clinicians who are highly focused on achieving a pregnancy recognize the increased risk of OHSS but want to achieve the highest pregnancy rate possible. Sometimes FSH stimulation results in the development of a great excess of mature ovarian follicles, thereby putting the patient at a risk of OHSS. One option to prevent OHSS in these cases is to retrieve the oocytes, fertilize the oocytes with sperm, and then freeze all the oocytes at an early embryonic stage [41], or after the embryos have developed for a few days in vitro. The embryo transfer is then cancelled for the stimulation cycle complicated by a high risk of OHSS.

The "freeze all" approach reduces the risk of severe and late onset OHSS, but mild or moderate early onset OHSS may still occur. In one study, women with circulating estradiol >3500 pg/mL had all their embryos cryopreserved after oocyte retrieval and fertilization. The outcomes in this experimental group were compared with a group of historical controls with a similar estradiol concentration, but who had their embryos transferred to the uterus. In this study, 60% of the historical controls with an estradiol >3500 pg/mL who had embryos transferred and became pregnant had OHSS compared to 6% of the women who had all their embryos cryopreserved [42]. Following a "freeze all" cycle, the patient is prepared for a cryopreserved embryo transfer in a subsequent cycle. In large IVF programs, this approach is used in about 2% of all initiated cycles [43]. In the "freeze all" cycle following oocyte retrieval, the patient may be treated with agents to reduce VEGF and estradiol production by the ovary (GnRH antagonist, dopamine agonist, and/or aromatase inhibitor) in order to further reduce the risk of OHSS [44].

Cabergoline As noted above, excess ovarian production of VEGF causes increased vascular permeability and plays a central role in the development of OHSS. Ovarian theca-lutein cells contain dopamine receptors, and the dopamine agonist, cabergoline, appears to reduce VEGF production from these cells [16]. Clinical trials report that cabergoline, initiated at the time of hCG administration, in women at high risk reduces the severity of OHSS. For example, in one trial, women with >20 growing follicles >12 mm in diameter were randomized to receive cabergoline 0.5 mg daily or a placebo daily for 8 days starting on the day of hCG administration. Hemoconcentration and ascites were significantly reduced by cabergoline compared to placebo. MRI scanning documented reduced vascular permeability in the women receiving cabergoline [45]. A meta-analysis reported that women at risk treated with cabergoline had a reduced incidence of OHSS (OR 0.41, 95% CI 0.25–0.66), and a trend to a reduced severity of OHSS. Cabergoline treatment did not reduce clinical pregnancy rate [46]. A standard prevention dose of cabergoline is to administer 0.5 mg daily for 8 days beginning on the day of hCG administration.

The dopamine agonist, quinagolide, when administered at doses of 50, 100, or 200 µg daily for 17–21 days starting on the day of hCG administration reduced the incidence and severity of OHSS in women at high risk of OHSS ($\geq$20 follicles $\geq$110 mm in diameter) [47]. Quinagolide is not approved for use in the United States.

Treatment of OHSS

Women with mild OHSS and many women with moderate OHSS can be managed as ambulatory patients. Pain can be managed with narcotics. Nonsteroidal anti-inflammatory drugs should not be used to treat pain in women with OHSS because they can reduce renal function [48]. Nausea may be treated with agents consistent with the possibility of a developing pregnancy, such as prochlorperazine, metoclopramide, or cyclizine. Strenuous exercise and sexual intercourse should be avoided by women with OHSS because of the risk of torsion or ovarian rupture and hemorrhage. hCG injections to support the luteal phase should not be given to women with established OHSS.

Women with severe OHSS should be considered for hospitalization. Specific conditions that may require intensive unit care include adult respiratory distress syndrome, renal failure, or thromboembolism. Increasing abdominal pain, oliguria, weight gain, increased abdominal circumference, and shortness of breath suggest worsening OHSS. In the hospital, hydration and cardiopulmonary function should be assessed frequently. Abdominal examination should include an assessment for peritoneal signs, presence of ascites (flank dullness), and paralytic ileus. Diuretics should not be used in women with OHSS because they may further reduce intravascular volume unless hemodynamic monitoring is instituted. Women with hemoconcentration and oliguria may benefit from the administration of 6% hydroxyethylstarch or albumin (see below). Paracentesis (see below) may help reduce symptoms, reduce intra-abdominal pressure, and increase renal perfusion.

Thromboprophylaxis should be administered to all hospitalized women with OHSS. Compression stockings and prophylactic heparin (5000 unit sc twice daily) are commonly used because they permit the patient to ambulate. If the patient is at bed rest, an intermittent pneumatic compression device may be used.

Paracentesis As noted above, leaky vessels and the accumulation of fluid in the peritoneal cavity can result in an *abdominal compartment syndrome* causing decreased cardiac output, reduced renal blood flow, and decreased urine output. In non-randomized case series, aggressive and early paracentesis has been reported to be successful in the outpatient management of OHSS [49]. Based on modeling the cost-effectiveness of outpatient paracentesis versus in-patient management of OHSS, early aggressive outpatient paracentesis was reported to result in lower costs [50].

Paracentesis can be initiated for symptom control in patients with moderate or severe OHSS. Paracentesis can be performed either through a transvaginal route or through a standard lateral abdominal wall approach historically used to treat ascites caused by liver disease. In both cases, paracentesis is performed under ultrasound guidance. Gravity drainage or controlled vacuum suction can be used to remove the fluid. In most patients, 500–4500 mL of fluid is removed during a paracentesis over the course of 30–60 min. When massive pleural effusion occurs, pleurocentesis may be performed, or a chest tube inserted [51].

Anticoagulation Some experts recommend full anticoagulation when the hematocrit rises above 50%. Heparin or enoxaparin administered through subcutaneous injection have both been utilized. If the patient is hospitalized, and not mobile, the use of an intermittent pneumatic compression device is recommended. If the patient is mobile, compression stockings may be preferred.

Colloid Infusion Colloid infusion may improve hemodynamic function in women with OHSS. In a systematic review of three trials, hydroxyethyl starch infusion was reported to be more effective in reducing the risk of developing severe OHSS than no treatment (OR 0.12, 95% CI 0.04–0.40) [52]. In a systematic review of eight trials, albumin infusion was reported to be modestly more effective than no treatment in reducing the risk of developing severe OHSS (OR 0.67, 95% CI 0.45–0.99) [52]. Building on these findings, investigators have reported that in cases of OHSS, hydroxyethyl starch 6% infusion is modestly more effective than albumin for increasing urine output, reducing the need for paracentesis, and reducing the length of hospitalization [53]. However, hydroxyethyl starch infusions have been reported to be associated with renal dysfunction and coagulopathy [54], causing some experts to prefer albumin infusions for the treatment of OHSS.

Recombinant Tissue Plasminogen Activator to Treat Thrombosis

Major arterial thrombosis is a devastating consequence of severe OHSS. In one case of OHSS causing thrombosis of the middle cerebral artery, intra-arterial infusion of recombinant tissue plasminogen activator was used to lyse the clot and facilitate neurological recovery [55].

Pregnancy Outcome

IVF pregnancy complicated by moderate or severe OHSS has an increased risk of spontaneous abortion, venous thrombosis, gestational diabetes, pregnancy-induced hypertension, placental abruption, premature delivery, and low birthweight compared to IVF pregnancy not associated with OHSS [56, 57]. A pregnancy occurring following an IVF cycle complicated by OHSS is a high-risk pregnancy and should be monitored closely during the antepartum period.

References

1. Golan A. A modern classification of OHSS. Reprod Biomed Online. 2009;19:28–32.
2. Golan A, Ron-el R, Herman A, Soffer Y, Weinraub Z, Caspi E. Ovarian hyperstimulation syndrome: an update review. Obstet Gynecol Surv. 1989;44:430–40.

3. Mathur RS, Akande AV, Keay S, Hunt LP, Jenkins JM. Distinction between early and late ovarian hyperstimulation syndrome. Fertil Steril. 2000;73:901–7.
4. Yeh J, Barbieri RL, Ravnikar VA. Ovarian hyperstimulation syndrome associated with leuprolide suppression: a case report. J In Vitro Fert Embryo Transf. 1989;6:261–3.
5. Droesch K, Barbieri RL. Ovarian hyperstimulation syndrome associated with the use of the gonadotropin releasing hormone agonist: leuprolide acetate. Fertil Steril. 1994;62:189–90.
6. Baigent A, Lashen H. Ovarian hyperstimulation syndrome in a patient treated with tamoxifen for breast cancer. Fertil Steril. 2011;95:2429.e5–7.
7. Ayhan A, Tuncer ZS, Aksu AT. Ovarian hyperstimulation syndrome associated with spontaneous pregnancy. Hum Reprod. 1996;11:1600–1.
8. Chen SU, Chen RJ, Shieh JY, Chou CH, Lin CW, Lu HF, et al. Human chorionic gonadotropin up- regulates expression of myeloid cell leukemia-1 protein in human granulosa-lutein cells: implication of corpus luteum rescue and ovarian hyperstimulation syndrome. J Clin Endocrinol Metab. 2010;95:3982–92.
9. Levin ER, Rosen GF, Cassidenti DL, Yee B, Meldrum D, Wisot A. Role of vascular endothelial cell growth factor in ovarian hyperstimulation syndrome. J Clin Invest. 1998;102:1978–85.
10. Neulen J, Yan Z, Raczek S, Weindel K, Keck C, Weich HA. Human chorionic gonadotropin-dependent expression of vascular endothelial growth factor/vascular permeability factor in human granulosa cells: importance in ovarian hyperstimulation syndrome. J Clin Endocrinol Metab. 1995;80:1967–71.
11. Rodewald M, Herr D, Duncan WC, Fraser HM, Hack G, Konrad R, et al. Molecular mechanisms of ovarian hyperstimulation syndrome: paracrine reduction of endothelial claudin T by hCG in vitro is associated with increased endothelial permeability. Hum Reprod. 2009;24:1191–9.
12. Casper RF. Ovarian hyperstimulation: effects of GnRH analogues. Does triggering ovulation with gonadotropin-releasing hormone analogue prevent severe ovarian hyperstimulation syndrome. Hum Reprod. 1996;11:1144–6.
13. Cerrillo M, Pacheco A, Rodriguez S, Gomez R, Delgado F, Pellicer A, et al. Effect of GnRH agonist and hCG treatment on VEGF, angiopoietin-2 and VE-cadherin: trying to explain the link to ovarian hyperstimulation syndrome. Fertil Steril. 2011;95:2517–9.
14. Moron FJ, de Castro F, Royo JL, Montor L, Mira E, Saez ME, et al. Bone morphogenetic protein 15 (BMP15) alleles predict over-response to recombinant follicle stimulating hormone and iatrogenic ovarian hyperstimulation syndrome (OHSS). Pharmacogenet Genomics. 2006;16:485–95.
15. Hanevik HI, Hilmarsen HT, Skjelbred CF, Tanbo T, Kahn JA. A single nucleotide polymorphism in BMP-15 is associated with high response to ovarian stimulation. Reprod Biomed Online. 2011;23:97–104.
16. Ferrero H, Gaytan F, Delgado-Rosas F, Gaytan M, Gomez R, Simon C, et al. Dopamine receptor 2 activation inhibits VEGF secretion in granulosa luteinized cells. Hum Reprod. 2010;25(S1):i56–8.
17. Gomez R, Ferrero H, Delgado-Rosas F, Gaytan M, Morales C, Zimmerman RC, et al. Evidence for the existence of a low dopaminergic tone in polycystic ovarian syndrome: implications for OHSS development and treatment. J Clin Endocrinol Metab. 2011;96:2484–92.
18. Rodien P, Beau I, Vasseur C. Ovarian hyperstimulation syndrome (OHSS) due to mutations in the follicle stimulating hormone receptor. Ann Endocrinol. 2010;71:206–9.
19. Grossman LC, Michalakis KG, Browne H, Payson MD, Segars JH. The pathophysiology of ovarian hyperstimulation syndrome: an unrecognized compartment syndrome. Fertil Steril. 2010;94:1392–8.
20. Delvigne A. Epidemiology of OHSS. Reprod Biomed Online. 2009;19:8–113.
21. Luke B, Brown MB, Morbeck DE, Hudson SB, Coddington CC, Stern JE. Factors associated with ovarian hyperstimulation syndrome (OHSS) and its effect on assisted reproductive technology treatment and outcome. Fertil Steril. 2010;94:1399–404.
22. Delvigne A, Rozenberg S. Epidemiology and prevention of ovarian hyperstimulation syndrome (OHSS): a review. Hum Reprod Update. 2002;8:559–77.

23. Abramov Y, Elchalal U, Schenker JG. Pulmonary manifestations of severe ovarian hyper-stimulation syndrome: a multicenter study. Fertil Steril. 1999;71:645–51.
24. Yoshi F, Ooki N, Shinohara Y, Uehara K, Mochimaru F. Multiple cerebral infarctions associated with ovarian hyperstimulation syndrome. Neurology. 1999;53:225–30.
25. Chan WS. The ART, of thrombosis: a review of arterial and venous thrombosis in assisted reproductive technology. Curr Opin Obstet Gynecol. 2009;21:207–18.
26. Jing Z, Yanping L. Middle cerebral artery thrombosis after IVF and ovarian hyperstimulation: a case report. Fertil Steril. 2011;95:2435.e13–5.
27. Man BL, Hui AC. Cerebral venous thrombosis secondary to ovarian hyperstimulation syndrome. Hong Kong Med J. 2011;17:155–6.
28. Mancini A, Milrdi D, DiPietro ML, Giacchi E, Spagnolo AG, Donna VD, De Marinis L, Jensen L. A case of forearm amputation after ovarian stimulation for in vitro fertilization-embryo transfer. Fertil Steril. 2001;76:198–200.
29. Broer SL, Dolleman M, Opmeer BC, Fauser BC, Mol BW, Broekmans FJ. AMH and AFC as predictors of excessive response in controlled ovarian hyperstimulation: a meta-analysis. Hum Reprod Update. 2011;17:46–54.
30. Al-Inany HG, Yousssef MA, Aboulghar M, Broekmans F, Sterrenburg M, Smit J, et al. Gonadotropin-releasing hormone antagonists for assisted reproductive technology. Cochrane Database Syst Rev. 2011;(5):CD001750.
31. Humaidan P, et al. GnRH agonist for triggering the final oocyte maturation: time for a change in practice? Hum Reprod Update. 2011;17:51–24.
32. Yates AP, Rustamov O, Roberts SA, Lim HY, Pemberton PW, Smith A, et al. Anti-mullerian hormone-tailored stimulation protocols improve outcomes whilst reducing adverse effects and costs of IVF. Hum Reprod. 2011;26:2353–62.
33. Youssef MA, van der Veen F, Al-Inany HG, Griesinger G, Mochtar MH, Aboulfoutouh I, et al. Gonadotropin releasing hormone agonist versus hCG for oocyte triggering in antagonist assisted reproductive technology cycles. Cochrane Database Syst Rev. 2011;(10):CD008046.
34. Oliveness F, Howies CM, Borini A, Germond M, Tew G, Wikland M, et al. Individualizing FSH dose for assisted reproduction using a novel algorithm: the CONSORT study. Reprod Biomed Online. 2011;22(S1):S73–82.
35. Lin H, Wang W, Li Y, Chen X, Yang D, Zhang Q. Triggering final oocyte maturation with reduced doses of hCG or IVF/ICSI: a prospective randomized and controlled study. Eur J Obstet Gynecol Reprod Biol. 2011;159:143–7.
36. Martinez F, Rodriguez DB, Buxaderas R, Tur R, Mancini F, Coroleu B. GnRH antagonist rescue of a long-protocol IVF cycle and GnRH agonist trigger to avoid ovarian hyperstimulation syndrome: three case reports. Fertil Steril. 2011;95:2432.e17–9.
37. Delvigne A, Rozenberg S. Preventive attitude of physicians to avoid OHSS in IVF patients. Hum Reprod. 2001;16:2491–5.
38. Ulug U, Bahcecci M, Erden HF, Shalev E, Ben-Shlomo I. The significance of coasting duration during ovarian stimulation for conception in assisted fertilization cycles. Hum Reprod. 2002;17:310–3.
39. D'Angelo A, Brown J, Amso NN. Coasting for preventing ovarian hyperstimulation syndrome. Cochrane Database Syst Rev. 2011;(6):CD002811.
40. Gokmen O, Ugur M, Ekin M, Keles G, Turan C, Oral H. Intravenous albumin versus hydroxy-ethyl starch for the prevention of ovarian hyperstimulation in an in vitro fertilization programme: a prospective randomized controlled study. Eur J Obstet Gynecol Reprod Biol. 2001;96:187–92.
41. Griesinger G, Berndt H, Schultz L, Depenbusch M, Schultze-Mosgau A. Cumulative live birth rates after GnRH agonist triggering of final oocyte maturation in patients at risk of OHSS: a prospective clinical cohort study. Eur J Obstet Gynecol Reprod Biol. 2010;149:190–4.
42. Wada I, Matson PL, Troup SA, Morroll DR, Hunt L, Lieberman BA. Does elective cryopreservation of all embryos from women at risk of ovarian hyperstimulation syndrome reduce the incidence of this condition? BJOG. 1993;100:265–9.

43. Sills ES, McLoughlin LJ, Genton MG, Walsh DJ, Coull GD, Walsh AP. Ovarian hyperstimulation syndrome and prophylactic human embryo cryopreservation: analysis of reproductive outcome following thawed embryo transfer. J Ovarian Res. 2008;1:7.
44. Rollene NL, Amols MH, Hudson SB, Coddington CC. Treatment of ovarian hyperstimulation syndrome using a dopamine agonist and gonadotropin releasing hormone antagonist: a case series. Fertil Steril. 2009;92:1169.e15–7.
45. Alvarez C, Marti-Bonmati L, Novella-Maestre E, Sanz R, Gomez R, Fernandez-Sanchez M, Simon C, Pellicer A. Dopamine agonist cabergoline reduces hemoconcentration and ascites in hyperstimulated women undergoing assisted reproduction. J Clin Endocrinol Metab. 2007;92:2931–7.
46. Youssef MA, van Wely M, Hassan MA, Al-Inany HG, Mochtar M, Khattab S, van der Veen F. Can dopamine agonists reduce the incidence and severity of OHSS in IVF/ICSI treatment cycles? A systematic review and meta-analysis. Hum Reprod Update. 2010;16:459–66.
47. Busso C, Fernandez-Sanchez M, Garcia-Velasco JA, Landeras J, Ballesteros A, Munoz E, Gonzalez S, Simon C, Arce JC, Pellicer A. The non-ergot derived dopamine agonist quinagolide in prevention of early ovarian hyperstimulation syndrome in IVF patients: a randomized, double-blind placebo- controlled trial. Hum Reprod. 2010;25:995–1004.
48. Balasch J, Carmona F, Llach J, Arroyo V, Jove I, Vanrell JA. Acute prerenal failure and liver dysfunction in a patient with severe ovarian hyperstimulation syndrome. Hum Reprod. 1990;5:348–51.
49. Smith LP, Hacker MR, Alper MM. Patients with severe ovarian hyperstimulation syndrome can be managed safely with aggressive outpatient transvaginal paracentesis. Fertil Steril. 2009;92:1953–9.
50. Csokmay JM, Yauger BJ, Henne MB, Armstrong AY, Queenan JT, Segars JH. Cost analysis model of outpatient management of ovarian hyperstimulation syndrome with paracentesis: tap early and often versus hospitalization. Fertil Steril. 2010;93:167–73.
51. Ceyhan ST, Goktolga U, Karasahin E, Alanbay I, Duru NK. Continuous vaginal and bilateral thoracic fluid drainage for management of severe ovarian hyperstimulation syndrome. Gynecol Endocrinol. 2008;24:505–7.
52. Youssef AFM, Al-Inany HG, Evers LHJ, Aboulghar M. Intravenous fluids for the prevention of severe ovarian hyperstimulation syndrome. Cochrane Database Syst Rev. 2010;(2):CD001302.
53. Abramov Y, Fatum M, Abrahamov D, Schenker JG. Hydroxyethylstarch versus human albumin for the treatment of severe ovarian hyperstimulation syndrome: a preliminary report. Fertil Steril. 2001;75:1228–30.
54. Bayer O, Reinhart K, Sakr Y, Kabisch B, Kohl M, Riedermann NC, et al. Renal effects of synthetic colloids and crystalloids in patients with severe sepsis: a prospective sequential comparison. Crit Care Med. 2011;39:1335–42.
55. Elford K, Leader A, Wee R, Stys PK. Stroke in ovarian hyperstimulation syndrome in early pregnancy treated with intra-arterial rt-PA. Neurology. 2002;59:1270–2.
56. Abramov Y, Elchalal U, Schenker JG. Obstetric outcome of in-vitro fertilized pregnancies complicated by severe ovarian hyperstimulation syndrome: a multicenter study. Fertil Steril. 1998;70:1070–5.
57. Courbiere B, Oborski V, Braunstein D, Desparoir A, Noizet A, Gamerre M. Obstetric outcome of women with in vitro fertilization pregnancies hospitalized for ovarian hyperstimulation syndrome: a case–control study. Fertil Steril. 2011;95:1629–32.

Chapter 19
Ambiguous Genitalia in the Newborn

Selma F. Witchel and Walter L. Miller

Précis

1. Clinical setting: Development of the external genitalia is atypical and examination does not allow for accurate determination as to whether the infant is a girl or a boy.
2. Diagnosis:

    (a) History: Family history of genetic disorders, infertility, infant deaths, and disorders of puberty should be obtained. Other questions include virilization of mother during pregnancy and exposures to androgens and anti-androgens.
    (b) Physical examination: The external genitalia should be inspected for symmetry. Location of gonads and urethral meatus should be ascertained. Length and diameter of the phallus should be determined. The distance from the anus to the posterior fourchette or scrotum should be measured. A thorough physical examination to assess for other anomalies should be performed.
    (c) Laboratory evaluation: Karyotype with fluorescence in situ hybridization (FISH) probes for the Y chromosome should be obtained. Depending on the physical examination, an ACTH stimulation test with measurement of 17-hydroxyprogesterone, 11-deoxycortisol, and cortisol should be obtained. Basal LH, FSH, testosterone, dihydrotestosterone, anti-Müllerian hormone, inhibin B, plasma renin activity, and 21-deoxycortisol should be considered.

S. F. Witchel (✉)
Division of Pediatric Endocrinology, UPMC Children's Hospital of Pittsburgh,
University of Pittsburgh, Pittsburgh, PA, USA
e-mail: witchelsf@upmc.edu

W. L. Miller
Department of Pediatrics, Center for Reproductive Sciences, University of California,
San Francisco, San Francisco, CA, USA
e-mail: wlmlab@ucsf.edu

© Springer Nature Switzerland AG 2021
L. Loriaux, C. Vanek (eds.), *Endocrine Emergencies*, Contemporary Endocrinology,
https://doi.org/10.1007/978-3-030-67455-7_19

Serum electrolytes may be normal during the first few days of life even among infants with salt-losing congenital adrenal hyperplasia. Genetic testing can include a microarray or whole exome sequencing.

(d) Imaging studies: Pelvic ultrasound is extremely useful to assess for uterine development. Gonads may or may not be visualized on ultrasound. Failure to visualize gonads does not indicate absence of gonads.

3. Initial assessment and treatment: Specific medical management depends on the underlying disorder. The multidisciplinary team should meet with the parents to explain that their infant has a disorder affecting the complex system that directs genital development. Sex assignment and naming of the infant should be deferred until adequate information is available.

Clinical Issues

The birth of a child with genital ambiguity, also known as a difference of sex development or DSD, is not a medical emergency. Initially, such infants appear healthy with normal cardiopulmonary function. Electrolyte and glucose concentrations are typically normal at the time of delivery. For infants with adrenal insufficiency accompanied by mineralocorticoid deficiency, the features of adrenal failure (hyperkalemia, hyponatremia, acidosis, hypotension, and hypoglycemia) are typically not seen until 5–10 days of age.

The immediate emergency is social. The standard question starting with the prenatal ultrasound is "are you having a boy or a girl?" This standard question reflects society's intransigently dichotomous Manichean obsession of classifying people by their sex. Thus, following the physical examination and review of the pregnancy history, the next step in the evaluation of an infant with a DSD is to speak to the family, congratulate them on the baby's birth, and reassure them about all the good news about the baby. It is critical to avoid guesses or presumptive diagnoses. Instead, explain to the parents that, as embryos, girls and boys start out looking the same, that the processes involved in genital development (internal and external structures) are complex, and that a definitive diagnosis will likely be available within the next 3–7 days depending on the laboratory infrastructure. Parents remain anxious, but are grateful and appreciative when physicians are honest, caring, and state that "We don't know if your baby is a boy or a girl, but we know how to find out, we know how to deal with this situation, and everything will work out." The next step is to call the best pediatric endocrinologist available.

A DSD may be suspected prenatally based on fetal ultrasound findings. In some instances, the fetal karyotype differs from that suggested by the appearance of the fetal genitalia. More recently, noninvasive prenatal screening (NIPS) is being performed; this test examines fetal (placental) cell-free DNA in the mother's circulation. NIPS results may also differ from that inferred from the appearance of the fetal genitalia. When genital ambiguity is evident on the infant's exam or discordant results from NIPS/genetic testing are obtained, consultation with a multidisciplinary DSD team should be arranged immediately. Members of this team should include pediatric endocrinologists, pediatric urologists/surgeons, geneticists, neonatologists, radiologists, behavioral health specialists, and pediatric nurse educators. Some pediatric hospitals have ongoing committees to help with the decision-making and management of children with DSDs.

A Word about "Sex" and "Gender"

Sex pervades our popular culture, music, literature, advertising, and personal interactions. Yet, much of the contemporary American public remains surprisingly squeamish about the word "sex." Instead, applications for drivers' licenses and airline reservations typically ask one to check a genteel box labeled "Gender" as "M" or "F." People are catalogued into two binary groups – male or female. "Sex" is a biological concept that can be defined at various levels: genetic (presence or absence of the SRY gene), karyotypic, gonadal, hormonal, and anatomic. By contrast, "gender" refers to one's sense of self. This is a psychological concept that only an individual can delineate. Rats, cats, dogs, and people have a biological sex, but gender identity is uniquely human. Only people express gender identity. For most individuals, biological sex and gender identity are congruent. It is increasingly recognized that some individuals experience a "disconnect" between their biological sex and gender identity. This chapter is limited to "sex" and will not discuss "gender identity."

Embryology

DSDs are defined as external genital development that differs from normal male or female appearance. DSDs encompass a broad range of congenital conditions with diverse pathogenesis in which genetic, chromosomal, hormonal, or anatomic sex is atypical. Consensus conferences have refined the terminology and categorization of DSDs to provide descriptive names reflecting the genetic etiology [1]. In some instances, such as bladder or cloacal exstrophy, external genital development can be altered due to non-endocrine malformation syndromes.

Normal sexual development entails two sequential processes: *sex determination* and *sexual differentiation*. Sex determination entails the regulated temporal-spatial expression and interactions of specific genes and gene products that ultimately govern gonadal structure and function. This process reflects the outcome of a binary switch that directs the embryonic gonads to become either testes or ovaries [2]. Sexual differentiation refers to the processes by which the presence or absence of hormones secreted by the gonads mediate the differentiation of the embryonic structures into the more familial postnatal structures.

Understanding the mechanisms involved in sex determination and sex differentiation is essential in the evaluation of infants with DSD. This knowledge drives the choice of initial laboratory studies. In addition, this knowledge helps explain the DSD and the diagnostic process to the parents.

The gonads, internal genital ducts, and external genital structures develop from bipotential embryologic tissues. In the male zygote, the sex-determining region on the Y chromosome (*SRY*) gene, located on the Y chromosome, encodes the testis-determining factor, which is the initial switch in sexual differentiation. The presence or absence of the Y chromosome sets the developmental trajectory of the undifferentiated gonad to become a testis or an ovary, respectively. While there are rare cases of 46,XX males in whom the *SRY* gene has been transferred to another chromosome, the *karyotype* is a rapid, reliable surrogate to ascertain the presence of the *SRY* gene. In the presence of the *SRY* gene, the embryonic bipotential testis differentiates into a testis. Ovarian development requires both the absence of the *SRY* gene and the actions of other specific genes including *FOXL2*, *WNT4*, and *RSPO1* [3]. The gonads, internal genital ducts, and external genital structures develop from bipotential embryologic tissues. By 4–6 weeks of gestation, the urogenital ridges have developed as outgrowths of coelomic epithelium. Hormones and transcription factors direct the urogenital ridges to develop into the gonads, adrenal cortex, kidneys, internal genital structures, and external genitalia [4–6].

Testicular hormones are required for male sexual differentiation. In contrast, the fetal ovary is hormonally quiescent and ovarian hormones are not needed for the development of the female reproductive structures, as evidenced by the normal internal and external reproductive anatomy in 45,X females with Turner syndrome who lack functioning ovaries. Thus, much of the discussion regarding the causes of DSD centers on the testis and its products.

The early human embryo has transient structures (Wolffian and Müllerian ducts, urogenital sinus, genital tubercle, urethral folds, and labioscrotal swellings), which are precursors (anlage) of adult reproductive structures. The Wolffian (male) ducts originate as the excretory duct of the mesonephros. Testosterone secreted by the fetal testes stabilizes the Wolffian ducts so that they develop into the epididymis, vas deferens, ejaculatory duct, and seminal vesicle. In the absence of testosterone and presence of the transcription factor, COUP-TFII, the Wolffian ducts regress, as occurs in the normal female fetus [7, 8]. The Müllerian ducts are the precursors of the female reproductive structures (fallopian tubes, uterus, cervix, and upper 1/3 of the vagina). In the male fetus, testicular Sertoli cells secrete anti-Müllerian hormone (AMH), also known as Müllerian inhibitory hormone (MIH). AMH acts through specific receptors in Müllerian duct cells to induce their apoptosis. Thus, males lack Müllerian structures. In the absence of AMH, the Müllerian structures persist and differentiate in the female fetus.

The genital tubercle, urethral folds, and labioscrotal swellings give rise to the external genital structures. In the absence of androgens, as in a typical 46,XX female, the genital tubercle becomes the clitoris, the urethral folds become the labia minora, and the labioscrotal folds become the labia majora. In male development between 7 and 13 weeks, dihydrotestosterone (DHT) induces the urethral folds to fuse to form the corpus spongiosum and penile urethra, the genital tubercle develops into the corpora cavernosa of the penis, and the labioscrotal folds fuse to form the scrotum in the male fetus. Two pathways exist for DHT synthesis: (1) genital skin converts circulating testosterone to DHT and (2) DHT is produced in the testis and adrenal by an alternative pathway [9]. The testes descend from their original location near the kidneys through the abdomen and into the scrotum. Insulin-like peptide 3 (INSL3) is required for transabdominal testicular descent. Testicular descent into the scrotum requires the action of testosterone and is usually complete by 32 weeks gestation [10].

The bipotential external genital structures are sensitive to androgens at different times during development; these structures are sensitive to androgens regardless of the sex of the fetus or the source of the androgens. The androgen-induced labioscrotal fusion is unidirectional, from posterior to anterior providing a "bio-assay" of first trimester fetal androgen action [11]. Thus, first trimester exposure of a female fetus can lead to varying degrees of labioscrotal fusion, whereas later exposure (after 20 weeks) may result in isolated clitoromegaly. As virtually all DSD is genetic and occurs during the first trimester, the physical exam of the infant with DSD should emphasize the extent of labioscrotal fusion.

Both the adrenal and the testis express the enzymes needed for androgen biosynthesis, so that either gland can be the source of androgens. The fetal adrenal secretes very little cortisol until later in the third trimester with the exception of transient cortisol production between 8 and 12 weeks post-conception. This small amount of cortisol suppresses secretion of fetal pituitary ACTH and adrenal androgen precursors to prevent virilization of a female fetus [12].

Pathophysiology of DSD

Updated classifications of DSD have discarded the older terminology that some regard as pejorative (female pseudohermaphrodite, male pseudohermaphrodite, and true hermaphrodite) and substituted descriptive terminology, e.g., 46,XX DSD; 46,XY DSD; ovotesticular DSD; 46,XX testicular DSD; and 46,XY complete gonadal dysgenesis [1]. In general, two broad categories can be considered: (1) abnormalities in sex determination such as sex chromosome anomalies and gene mutations that interrupt or disrupt normal gonadogenesis and (2) abnormalities of sex differentiation resulting in abnormal development of the somatic sex structures (genital ducts, urogenital sinus, and external genitalia). Genital ambiguity is common, affecting 1:2000 to 1:4500 newborns [13]. Cryptorchidism affects approximately 3% of liveborn males. Newer genetic techniques such as whole exome sequencing have detected multiple genomic alterations associated with DSD. These discoveries add to the body of knowledge regarding the differentiation of the gonads and reproductive structures (Table 19.1).

Table 19.1 Classification of disorders of sex development associated with ambiguous genitalia

I. Disorders of sex determination (gonadal differentiation)
A. 46,XY gonadal dysgenesis
B. 45,X/46,XY gonadal dysgenesis
C. 46,XX (+SRY) Male
D. 46,XX (-SRY) Male
E. Ovotesticular DSD
II. 46,XX DSD
A. Androgen-induced
1. Fetal-placental disorders
(a) Congenital virilizing adrenal hyperplasias (*CYP21A2, CYP11B1, POR*)
(b) Glucocorticoid receptor (*NR3C1*)
(c) Aromatase deficiency (*CYP19A1*)
2. Maternal source
(a) Ingestion
(i) Testosterone and related steroids
(ii) Synthetic oral progestagens
(b) Virilizing ovarian or adrenal tumor
(c) Virilizing luteoma of pregnancy
B. Genetic
1. *FOXL2*
2. *RSPO1*
3. *WNT4*
III. 46,XY DSD
A. Testicular unresponsiveness to hCG and LH (Leydig cell agenesis or hypoplasia)
B. Defects in steroidogenesis
1. Enzyme deficits affecting synthesis of both adrenal and gonadal steroids
(a) StAR deficiency (congenital lipoid adrenal hyperplasia)
(b) Cholesterol side chain cleavage (P450scc) deficiency
(c) 3β-Hydroxysteroid dehydrogenase-2 deficiency
(d) P450c17 (17α-hydroxylase/17,20-lyase) deficiency
(e) P450 oxidoreductase deficiency
2. Enzyme defects primarily affecting testosterone biosynthesis by the testes
(a) 17β-Hydroxysteroid dehydrogenase-3 deficiency
(b) 5α-Reductase-2 deficiency
C. Defects in androgen action (androgen receptor defects)
D. Non-syndromic 46,XY DSD
1. Testicular regression syndrome
2. Genetic
(a) *CBX2*
(b) *DHH*
(c) *MAMLD1*
(d) *MAP3K1*

Table 19.1 (continued)

(e) *NROB1* (DAX1)
(f) *NR5A1* (SF1)
(g) *SOX8*
(h) *SRY*
(i) *WWOX*
E. Syndromic 46,XY
1. *ARX*
2. *ATRX* syndrome (XH2 mutation)
3. *CDKN1C* (IMAGe syndrome)
4. *DHCR7* (Smith-Lemli-Opitz syndrome)
5. *KAT6B* (genitopatellar syndrome)
6. *SOX9* (campomelic dysplasia)
7. *ZEB2* (Mowat-Wilson syndrome)
F. Defects in synthesis, secretion, or response to AMH
1. Persistent Müllerian duct syndrome (in otherwise normal men)
(a) *AMH*
(b) *AMHR*
G. Environmental chemicals (endocrine disrupters)
IV. Syndromic 46,XX or 46,XY
A. WT1 (Denys-Drash, Fraser, and Meacham syndromes)
B. GLI3 (Pallister-Hall syndrome)
C. HOXA13 (hand-foot-genital syndrome)
D. CHD7 (CHARGE syndrome)
E. VATER syndrome
V. Disorders of genitourinary tract development
A. Cloacal/bladder exstrophy
B. Penoscrotal transposition

46,XX DSD

Patients with 46,XX DSD have disorders of sexual differentiation. Disorders of female sex determination, such as 45,X Turner syndrome, do not result in a DSD phenotype because a functional ovary is not needed for female sexual differentiation. Most patients with 46,XX DSD are genetic females with ovaries. These female infants have experienced varying degrees of masculinization of the urogenital sinus and external genitalia secondary to intrauterine androgen exposure. The virilizing forms of congenital adrenal hyperplasia (CAH) are the most common causes of XX,DSD, accounting for approximately one-half of all cases of ambiguous external genitalia [14]. This group of autosomal recessive disorders, due to mutations in genes involved in adrenal steroidogenesis, results in inappropriate adrenal secretion of androgenic hormones [14].

The most common form of CAH is 21-hydroxylase deficiency (21OHD), which accounts for over 90% of cases with an incidence of approximately 1:15,000 live births. This form of CAH is due to mutations in the *CYP21A2* gene located at chromosome 6p21.33 within the histocompatibility locus. The genetics, pathophysiology, and management of 21-hydroxylase deficiency are well characterized [15]. Depending on the severity of the *CYP21A2* mutation, patients may experience severe salt-wasting 21OHD, in which aldosterone synthesis is deficient, or simple virilizing 21OHD in which overt salt loss is not severe. Both salt-wasting and simple virilizing 21OHD cause 46,XX DSD. The hyponatremia, hyperkalemia, and acidosis associated with salt-wasting 21OHD are generally not observed until 5–10 days of life. Hence, normal electrolytes prior to this time may not be informative. The mild non-classic 21OHD does not cause DSD and is not associated with salt-wasting [16].

Other disorders of steroidogenesis associated with 46,XX DSD include 11β-hydroxylase deficiency (*CYP11B1* gene), P450 oxidoreductase (*POR* gene) deficiency, and, very rarely aromatase (*CYP19A1* gene) deficiency [17]. 11β-hydroxylase deficiency is the second most common form of CAH in the United States and Europe. This enzyme deficiency, often associated with hypertension in older children and adults, is paradoxically associated with salt loss in the newborn. POR deficiency can cause both 46,XX and 46,XY DSD, but it is not associated with adrenal insufficiency in the newborn [17]. Rare disorders associated with 46,XX DSD include maternal androgen-secreting tumors and environmental exposures.

Because 21OHD is common and salt loss can be fatal, all 50 states and most industrialized countries have instituted newborn screening programs for 21OHD based on elevated 17-hydroxyprogesterone (17OHP) levels [18, 19]. Values of 17OHP can be spuriously elevated when obtained before 24 hours of age, in preterm infants, and in stressed infants. Unfortunately, newborn screening programs fail to identify all affected infants; both false-positive and false-negative results can occur. For this reason, some regions mandate a second blood test [20]. In addition, newborn 17OHP values may be elevated in patients with 11β-hydroxylase deficiency, 3β-hydroxysteroid dehydrogenase deficiency, and P450 oxidoreductase deficiency. If the clinical circumstances suggest 21OHD with non-diagnostic 17OHP concentrations, a careful ACTH stimulation test with measurement of all relevant steroid precursors (not just cortisol and 17OHP) is needed. If available, measuring 21-deoxycortisol concentrations offers greater specificity to diagnose 21OHD [21].

46,XY DSD

Patients with 46,XY DSD may have disordered sex determination or disordered sexual differentiation leading to undervirilization. Disordered sex determination is characterized by abnormal gonadal differentiation. Disordered sexual differentiation is characterized by testicular development with abnormal hormone synthesis or action [22]. Etiologies of disordered sex determination causing 46,XY DSD include chromosomal aberrations and mutations in genes involved in testicular development. This category includes *SRY* gene mutations, sex chromosome anomalies (e.g., 45,X/46,XY mosaicism), structural abnormalities of the Y chromosome, or translocation of the *SRY* gene to an X chromosome or autosome. Mutations in the *WT1* gene cause Denys-Drash syndrome, which is associated with Wilms tumor [23]. Frasier syndrome, due to a specific splice site *WT1* mutation, is associated with an increased risk for gonadoblastoma [24]. Meacham syndrome, characterized by 46,XY gonadal dysgenesis, congenital diaphragmatic hernia, and congenital heart disease, is also due to *WT1* mutations [25]. Duplications of the DAX1 (*NR0B1*) gene are associated with male to female sex reversal. Heterozygous mutations in the *SRY*-related high-mobility group box (*SOX9*) gene are associated with campomelic dysplasia, and 46,XY DSD.

Defects in androgen synthesis or androgen action result in disordered sexual differentiation, undervirilization, and 46,XY DSD. These infants typically have normal Sertoli cell function, AMH secretion, and AMH action. Due to deficient androgen exposure, these infants have undervirilized external genitalia (e.g., perineoscrotal hypospadias, small phallus, and/or a short vaginal pouch without a uterus). The testes are typically palpable in the scrotum or inguinal area. Defects in androgen synthesis include mutations in the steroidogenic acute regulatory protein (*StAR* gene), the cholesterol side-chain cleavage enzyme (P450scc, *CYP11A1* gene), 17α-hydroxylase/17,20-lyase (P450c17, *CYP17A1* gene), the type 3 (testicular) 17β-hydroxysteroid dehydrogenase (*HSD17B3* gene), 5α-reductase type 2 (*SRD5A2* gene), and the 3α-hydroxysteroid dehydrogenases (*AKR1C2/4* genes). Mutations in the 7-dehydrocholestrol (*DHCR7* gene) cause Smith-Lemli-Opitz syndrome, which is characterized by multiple congenital anomalies including genital anomalies. Mutations in the LH receptor (*LHR*) gene are a rare cause of defective testicular steroidogenesis. Mutations in the androgen receptor (*AR*) gene cause varying degrees of androgen insensitivity; testosterone production is normal or increased, but target tissues cannot respond to androgens. The spectrum of androgen insensitivity ranges from complete to partial forms. In the complete form of androgen insensitivity syndrome, affected infants have normal female external genitalia, labial masses, and absence of a uterus. The phenotype in partial androgen insensitivity ranges from 46,XY DSD to phenotypically normal males with decreased fertility.

Other Disorders to Consider

Ovotesticular DSD is characterized by presence of both ovarian follicles and seminiferous tubules in the gonads. The patient's phenotype reflects the extent of gonadal function, which governs the development of the internal and external genital structures. Gonadal histology can include ovarian, testicular, ovotesticular, and dysgenetic patterns.

Other *malformation* disorders associated with abnormal external genital development include Aarskog-Scott, CHARGE, IMAGe, and VATER syndromes.

Bladder exstrophy is associated with abnormal genital-urinary tract development but is not due to an abnormality in sex development. Males with bladder exstrophy may have bifid penis and scrotum with a testis located on each side. Penoscrotal transposition in which the phallus is positioned between or behind the scrotum is another malformation syndrome due to abnormal genital tubercle development and delayed midline fusion of the urethral folds [26]. Cloacal exstrophy is a congenital malformation reflecting an abdominal wall defect with failed closure of the lower urinary tract. Additional anomalies involving the gastrointestinal tract, genitourinary tract, and skeleton may be present. Acute management for infants with bladder or cloacal exstrophy involves protection of the exposed mucosal surfaces [27].

Diagnosis

Clinical Setting

Because prenatal ultrasound examinations are routine, parents have often been told the (presumed) sex of their child and may have already selected a sex-specific name. The birth of a newborn with genital ambiguity is disconcerting and disrupts the family's plans. Infants with ambiguous genitalia are usually recognized in the delivery room or at the time of their initial examination. The approach to the infant with ambiguous genitalia needs to be systematic and involve a multidisciplinary team. The diagnostic evaluation focuses on etiology, appropriate sex assignment, and ascertainment of associated potentially life-threatening conditions such as mineralocorticoid deficiency.

The infant should be referred to "your baby" avoiding terms conveying a sex assignment. The parents need to be involved in the infant's evaluation and informed that the child's sex of rearing will be determined as rapidly as possible. The parents' level of understanding, cultural background, and religious views must be considered to enable them to participate in this process, have full disclosure, and to provide true "informed consent."

History

Information should be obtained concerning maternal exposures to androgens or androgen-modifying drugs (e.g., finasteride). Maternal virilization during pregnancy suggests a luteoma, aromatase deficiency, or POR deficiency. The family history may provide information about genetic disorders. Details should be sought regarding relatives with infertility or abnormal pubertal development and regarding other infants with genital ambiguity or neonatal deaths.

Physical Examination

A careful, knowledgeable physical examination of the genitalia is essential. Palpable gonads must be sought; gonads may be "hiding" in the inguinal canal. The urethral meatus must be located. The length and width of the phallus must be measured (both a clitoris and a penis are phalluses). Mean stretched penile length is 3.5 ± 0.4 cm for full-term infant boys and 2.5 ± 0.4 cm for males at 30 weeks gestation [28]. The pigmentation and rugation of the labioscrotal structures must be described. The potential presence of posterior labial fusion must be quantitated by measurement of the ano-genital ratio. In normal girls, the distance from the base of the phallus to the posterior fourchette should be 2/3 of the distance from the base of the phallus to the anus [29]. The infant should be carefully examined to ascertain for other physical anomalies.

One specific form of gonadal dysgenesis is characterized by asymmetric external genital development; the karyotype is often 45,X/46,XY and features of Turner syndrome may be present. Gonadal asymmetry may also occur in ovotesticular disorder. The physical exam for infants with complete androgen insensitivity often reveals female external genitalia with labial masses. The presence of mid-line defects, renal anomalies, and syndactyly of the second and third toe prompts consideration of Smith-Lemli-Opitz syndrome.

Laboratory Evaluation

Several diagnostic algorithms have been published; no single evaluation protocol covers all circumstances. Each infant benefits from an individualized approach to the selection of diagnostic studies, guided by the history and physical examination. The karyotype should be immediately ordered since results are generally not available for several days. The chromosome studies should be supplemented with Y and X chromosome-specific FISH (fluorescence in situ hybridization) probes. Probes specific for the *SRY* gene can be used to ascertain for chromosomal rearrangements affecting the Yp region.

Infants with 21OHD have normal electrolytes for several days after birth, typically developing hyperkalemia, hyponatremia, and elevated plasma renin activity after 5–10 days. Initial bloodwork should include 17-OHP, testosterone, LH, FSH, AMH, electrolytes, plasma renin activity, and, if available, 21-deoxycortisol. Testosterone may be normal or elevated in infants with androgen insensitivity. Simultaneous measurements of testosterone and DHT are needed to diagnose 5α-reductase deficiency. To assess for CAH, ACTH stimulation testing must be done with measurement of all steroids in the glucocorticoid and androgen pathways. This should be performed after 24 hours of age to permit clearance of fetal steroids. Samples should be sent to a reference lab equipped for small assay volumes and utilizing HPLC/tandem mass spectrometric methods for steroid hormone determinations. Fetal adrenal steroids can cross-react in the clinical radioimmuno-assay making this type of analysis unreliable [30]. Rare defects in testicular steroidogenesis (e.g., 17β-HSD3 deficiency) will require an hCG stimulation test. The physiologic mini-puberty of infancy permits assessment of the newborn HPG axis in the second month of life [31]. The Genetic Testing Registry (GTR) sponsored by the National Center for Biotechnology Information provides disorder-specific information and serves as a volunteer registry of available genetic testing (https://www.ncbi.nlm.nih.gov/gtr/).

Imaging Studies

Sonographic studies to assess for the presence of a uterus can be helpful, with the caveat that the uterus may not be visualized in some normal newborn females. A uterus may be visualized in males with dysgenetic testes associated with decreased AMH secretion. Normal gonads can escape detection by ultrasound or MRI. The inability to detect gonads radiographically does not indicate that the gonads are absent. Sonography and MR imaging of the pelvis and perineum may identify the urogenital sinus when separate urethral and vaginal orifices cannot be identified by inspection. A renal sonogram is important to assess for anomalies of the urinary tract. Adrenal glands may or may not be enlarged in infants with virilizing CAH. Invasive urologic procedures such as cystoscopies are almost never indicated for diagnosis.

Treatment

The first interview with the parents should set a positive and optimistic tone to promote parental bonding with their infant. The emotional tone of this initial interaction is usually more meaningful than the factual information provided and is recalled by parents for many years. Initially, the parents need to hear that there has been a problem in the complex system that directs genital development, which makes it impossible to tell the sex of their child simply by examining the external genitalia. It is important to acknowledge that such development is not a consequence of anything that they, as parents, did or did not do. Respect for the parents, extended family, and their cultural viewpoints together with a willingness to repeat or defer detailed explanations are crucial. Sex assignment and naming of the infant should be deferred until the diagnostic evaluation has been completed. During this initial evaluation, a patient information publication of the Endocrine Society might be helpful for parents (https://pubmed.ncbi.nlm.nih.gov/21378218/) [32].

During the diagnostic evaluation, information needs to be obtained to assist the parents and healthcare professionals in determining the most appropriate sex of rearing. Usually this can be accomplished within a few days. In more complex instances, the diagnostic process may take longer. In situations in which it is impossible to identify the specific etiology, the general DSD category provides a basis for decision-making. These considerations include the extent of external and internal reproductive system development, evidence of gonadal functional (potential hormone secretion and fertility), and hormone responsiveness. In some instances, these factors are more relevant than the karyotype. Involvement of the multidisciplinary team comprised of pediatric endocrinologists, neonatologists, geneticists, pediatric urologists/surgeons, radiologists, and behavioral health professionals is essential. When consensus has been reached regarding a diagnostic category, available outcome information for that diagnosis should be reviewed. The primary healthcare professional, usually the pediatric endocrinologist, should present the results of all tests at one time with a definitive conclusion. Informing families of each result incrementally can exacerbate parental confusion and anxiety. Knowledge of the specific etiology including the details of the diagnosis enables planning therapeutic interventions and genetic counseling for future pregnancies. A written resource that might be helpful to families is the "Consortium on the Management of Disorders of Sex Development. Handbook for Parents" (https://dsdguidelines.org/files/parents.pdf).

Medical Management

Specific medical management depends on the underlying disorder. All children with genital ambiguity require long-term care by pediatric endocrinology, pediatric urology/surgery, behavioral health, and their primary care provider [33, 34].

The management of 21OHD has been reviewed recently [15]. Children with congenital adrenal hyperplasia or any other cause of adrenal insufficiency require glucocorticoid, and often mineralocorticoid replacement therapy. The typical glucocorticoid dose for newborn infants is approximately 25 mg/m^2/day hydrocortisone (Cortef®) divided into three daily doses; this should be reduced after the first month and adjusted frequently as the child gets older. Infants require higher mineralocorticoid doses than older children or adults; 9α-fludrocortisone (Florinef®) at 0.1–0.3 mg daily is generally sufficient. Newborns with salt-losing CAH need sodium supplementation. Both hydrocortisone and 9α-fludrocortisone are available only as tablets. The tablets are crushed and administered orally. Hydrocortisone suspensions are unstable leading to variable dosing and should be avoided. Parents of children with CAH need to learn how to administer parenteral hydrocortisone sodium succinate in case of medical emergencies; parents should keep injectable hydrocortisone (e.g., Solu-Cortef®) and appropriate needles/syringes at home.

Surgical Management

Surgical treatment is rarely necessary in the immediate newborn period. In rare instances, diagnostic laparoscopy and gonadal biopsy may be necessary to evaluate internal genital structures and obtain tissue for histological examination. Extremely virilized infants with female gender of rearing, i.e., infant girl with 21OHD, may benefit from feminizing genitoplasty and repair of the common urogenital sinus [15]. This surgery should be performed only by highly skilled pediatric urologists and surgeons with appropriate attention to anatomic structures to preserve erectile function and clitoral innervation and following a shared decision-making process involving parents and health care providers [35]. Contemporary reports favor repair before age 1 year as the neonatal exposure to placental estrogens reduces scarring [36]. Hypospadias repair is often performed in stages and involves surgical urethral reconstructive and repair of associated chordee. For children with dysgenetic gonads, gonadectomy may be necessary at some future time because of the risk for malignant degeneration. In all cases, a skilled and experienced pediatric surgeon or urologist is essential [37].

Complications

Infants with unrecognized classical salt-losing 21OHD can die due to mineralocorticoid and glucocorticoid deficiencies. Extremely virilized 46,XX infants with 21OHD can resemble male infants with bilateral undescended testes and have been assigned to a male sex at birth. The availability and use of newborn screening for 21OHD has greatly decreased the occurrence of these complications [15, 19].

Prognosis

The goal for a child with genital ambiguity is thorough and accurate diagnosis followed by appropriate regular medical and surgical management. The overall goal is that the child experiences normal growth and development and is a productive member of society. Long-term outcome concerns include internal and external genital anatomy, pubertal development, fertility, gender identity, psychosexual adjustment, mental health, healthy relationships, and risk for gonadal malignancy arising in dysgenetic gonads. Available data are inconsistent regarding long-term outcome for children with DSDs.

References

1. Lee PA, Nordenström A, Houk CP, Ahmed SF, Auchus R, Baratz A, Baratz Dalke K, Liao LM, Lin-Su K, Looijenga LH 3rd, Mazur T, Meyer-Bahlburg HF, Mouriquand P, Quigley CA, Sandberg DE, Vilain E, Witchel S, Global DSD Update Consortium. Global disorders of sex development update since 2006: perceptions, approach and care. Horm Res Paediatr. 2016;85(3):158–80. https://doi.org/10.1159/000442975. Epub 2016 Jan 28. Review. Erratum in: Horm Res Paediatr. 2016;85(3):180. Koopman, Peter [added]. Horm Res Paediatr. 2016;86(1):70.

2. Biason-Lauber A. Control of sex development. Best Pract Res Clin Endocrinol Metab. 2010;24:163–86.
3. Biason-Lauber A, Chaboissier MC. Ovarian development and disease: the known and the unexpected. Semin Cell Dev Biol. 2015;45:59–67.
4. Park SY, Jameson JL. Minireview: transcriptional regulation of gonadal development and differentiation. Endocrinology. 2005;146:1035–42.
5. Capel B. Vertebrate sex determination: evolutionary plasticity of a fundamental switch. Nat Rev Genet. 2017;18:675–89.
6. Yatsenko SA, Witchel SF. Genetic approach to ambiguous genitalia and disorders of sex development: what clinicians need to know. Semin Perinatol. 2017;41:232–43.
7. Zhao F, Franco HL, Rodriguez KF, Brown PR, Tsai MJ, Tsai SY, Yao HH. Elimination of the male reproductive tract in the female embryo is promoted by COUP-TFII in mice. Science. 2017;357:717–20.
8. Swain A. Ductal sex determination. Science. 2017;357:648.
9. Flück CE, Meyer-Böni M, Pandey AV, et al. Why boys will be boys: two pathways of fetal testicular androgen biosynthesis are needed for male sexual differentiation [published correction appears in Am J Hum Genet. 2011 Aug 12;89(2):347]. Am J Hum Genet. 2011;89:201–18.
10. Rodprasert W, Virtanen HE, Mäkelä JA, Toppari J. Hypogonadism and cryptorchidism. Front Endocrinol (Lausanne). 2020;10:906.
11. Fischer MB, Ljubicic ML, Hagen CP, et al. Anogenital distance in healthy infants: method-, age- and sex-related reference ranges. J Clin Endocrinol Metab. 2020;105(9):2996–3004.
12. Goto M, Piper Hanley K, Marcos J, et al. In humans, early cortisol biosynthesis provides a mechanism to safeguard female sexual development. J Clin Invest. 2006;116:953–60.
13. Hughes IAN-FC, Thomas B, Cohen-Kettenis PT. Consequences of the ESPE/LWPES guidelines for diagnosis and treatment of disorders of sex development. Best Pract Res Clin Endocrinol Metab. 2007;21(3):351–65.
14. Miller WL, Auchus JR. The molecular biology, biochemistry, and physiology of human steroidogenesis and its disorders. Endocr Rev. 2011;32:81–151.
15. Speiser PW, Arlt W, Auchus RJ, et al. Congenital adrenal hyperplasia due to steroid 21-hydroxylase deficiency: an endocrine society clinical practice guideline [published correction appears in J Clin Endocrinol Metab. 2019 Jan 1;104(1):39–40]. J Clin Endocrinol Metab. 2018;103:4043–88.
16. Carmina E, Dewailly D, Escobar-Morreale HF, et al. Non-classic congenital adrenal hyperplasia due to 21-hydroxylase deficiency revisited: an update with a special focus on adolescent and adult women. Hum Reprod Update. 2017;23:580–99.
17. Miller WL. Rare defects in adrenal steroidogenesis. Eur J Endocrinol. 2018;179:R125–41. https://doi.org/10.1530/EJE-18-0279.
18. Therrell BL Jr, Berenbaum SA, Manter-Kapanke V, et al. Results of screening 1.9 million Texas newborns for 21-hydroxylase-deficient congenital adrenal hyperplasia. Pediatrics. 1998;101(4 Pt 1):583–90.
19. White PC. Neonatal screening for congenital adrenal hyperplasia. Nat Rev Endocrinol. 2009;5:490–8.
20. Held PK, Shapira SK, Hinton CF, Jones E, Hannon WH, Ojodu J. Congenital adrenal hyperplasia cases identified by newborn screening in one- and two-screen states. Mol Genet Metab. 2015;116:133–8.
21. Miller WL. Congenital adrenal hyperplasia: time to replace 17OHP with 21-deoxycortisol. Horm Res Paediatr. 2019;91:416–20.
22. Grinspon RP, Bergadá I, Rey RA. Male hypogonadism and disorders of sex development. Front Endocrinol (Lausanne). 2020;11:211.
23. Pelletier J, Bruening W, Li FP, Haber DA, Glaser T, Housman DE. WT1 mutations contribute to abnormal genital system development and hereditary Wilms' tumour. Nature. 1991;353(6343):431–4.
24. Barbaux S, Niaudet P, Gubler MC, et al. Donor splice-site mutations in WT1 are responsible for Frasier syndrome. Nat Genet. 1997;17:467–70.

25. Suri M, Kelehan P, O'neill D, et al. WT1 mutations in Meacham syndrome suggest a coelomic mesothelial origin of the cardiac and diaphragmatic malformations. Am J Med Genet A. 2007;143A(19):2312–20.
26. Grinspon RP, Rey RA. When hormone defects cannot explain it: malformative disorders of sex development. Birth Defects Res C Embryo Today. 2014;102:359–73.
27. Woo LL, Thomas JC, Brock JW. Cloacal exstrophy: a comprehensive review of an uncommon problem. J Pediatr Urol. 2010;6:102–11.
28. Feldman KW, Smith DW. Fetal phallic growth and penile standards for newborn male infants. J Pediatr. 1975;86(3):395–8.
29. Callegari C, Everett S, Ross M, Brasel JA. Anogenital ratio: measure of fetal virilization in premature and full-term newborn infants. J Pediatr. 1987;111:240–3.
30. Shackleton CH. Clinical steroid mass spectrometry: a 45-year history culminating in HPLC-MS/MS becoming an essential tool for patient diagnosis. J Steroid Biochem Mol Biol. 2010;121(3–5):481–90.
31. Grumbach MM. A window of opportunity: the diagnosis of gonadotropin deficiency in the male infant. J Clin Endocrinol Metab. 2005;90(5):3122–7.
32. Achermann JC, Eugster E, Shulman DI. Ambiguous genitalia. J Clin Endocrinol Metab. 2011;96(3):33A, 34A.
33. Auchus RJ, Witchel SF, Leight KR, et al. Guidelines for the Development of Comprehensive Care Centers for Congenital Adrenal Hyperplasia: Guidance from the CARES Foundation Initiative. Int J Pediatr Endocrinol. 2010;2010:275213.
34. Witchel SF. The medical home concept and congenital adrenal hyperplasia: a comfortable habitat! Int J Pediatr Endocrinol. 2010;2010:561526.
35. Sandberg DE, Gardner M, Kopec K, Urbanski M, Callens N, Keegan CE, Yashar BM, Fechner PY, Shnorhavorian M, Vilain E, Timmermans S, Siminoff LA. Development of a decision support tool in pediatric Differences/Disorders of Sex Development. Semin Pediatr Surg. 2019;28(5):150838.
36. Braga LH, Pippi Salle JL. Congenital adrenal hyperplasia: a critical appraisal of the evolution of feminizing genitoplasty and the controversies surrounding gender reassignment. Eur J Pediatr Surg. 2009;19:203–10.
37. Mouriquand PD, Gorduza DB, Gay CL, et al. Surgery in disorders of sex development (DSD) with a gender issue: If (why), when, and how? J Pediatr Urol. 2016;12(3):139–49.

Chapter 20
Porphyrias: Acute Manifestations

Akshata Moghe and Karl E. Anderson

Précis

1. Acute porphyria:
   (a) Clinical setting: An acute illness characterized by abdominal and other pain, mental symptoms, and motor neuropathy.
   (b) Diagnosis:
      i. History: A family history is uncommon due to variable penetrance. Symptoms are more common in women and rare before puberty. Central nervous system abnormalities may include agitation, disorientation, hallucinations and seizures. The abdominal pain is usually constant and severe and often associated with ileus. A peripheral motor neuropathy can cause weakness beginning in the upper extremities, and can progress to quadriparesis, respiratory paralysis and involvement of cranial nerves. Neurological findings may be misdiagnosed as Guillain-Barre syndrome.
      ii. Physical examination: Tachycardia and hypertension are common. Examination of the abdomen shows little tenderness or other findings since the abdominal symptoms are neuropathic. Bowel sounds are usually decreased. Neurological findings may include initial hyperreflexia, progressing to loss of muscle strength, decreased reflexes and sensory loss.

A. Moghe
University of Pittsburgh Medical Center, Pittsburgh, PA, USA

K. E. Anderson (✉)
Preventive Medicine and Population Health, University of Texas Medical Branch, Galveston, TX, USA
e-mail: kanderso@utmb.edu

© Springer Nature Switzerland AG 2021
L. Loriaux, C. Vanek (eds.), *Endocrine Emergencies*, Contemporary Endocrinology,
https://doi.org/10.1007/978-3-030-67455-7_20

     iii. Laboratory studies: The key laboratory finding is a marked increase in urinary porphobilinogen (PBG). This establishes the presence of one of three most common acute porphyrias and allows treatment to be started as soon as possible. Hyponatremia may result from the syndrome of inappropriate secretion of antidiuretic hormone (SIADH).

   (c) Treatment: The treatment for an acute porphyric crisis is hemin (lyophilized hematin) 3–4 mg/kg body weight, as an intravenous infusion once a day for 4 days. Carbohydrate loading can be used for less severe attacks.

2. Protoporphyric crisis:
   (a) Clinical setting: Acute onset of jaundice and abdominal pain with markedly abnormal liver function tests in a patient with a history of nonblistering photosensitivity.

   (b) Diagnosis:
     i. History: A family history is often absent. Longstanding nonblistering photosensitivity may not have been diagnosed previously as due to protoporphyria.
     ii. Physical examination: Evidence of liver failure, with few skin manifestations. Peripheral motor neuropathy may develop late in the course.
     iii. Laboratory studies: Protoporphyria is diagnosed by marked elevation in erythrocyte protoporphyrin which is predominantly metal-free and not chelated with zinc. Other abnormalities include mild hypochromic anemia and findings of advanced liver disease.

   (c) Treatment: A combination of plasmapheresis, erythrocyte transfusions, hemin, cholestyramine, ursodeoxycholic acid and vitamin E may achieve remission or bridge the patient to liver transplantation.

Introduction

Porphyrias result from altered activity of enzymes in the heme biosynthetic pathway. The genes encoding all eight enzymes in the heme biosynthetic pathway have been sequenced, and multiple mutations have been found in each of the porphyrias. Because these disorders are heterogeneous at the molecular level, different mutations are to be expected in unrelated families [1]. As shown in Fig. 20.1, a type of porphyria has been associated with each of the eight enzymatic steps in the heme biosynthetic pathway. With one exception, these diseases are due to heritable mutations affecting a specific enzyme. Porphyria cutanea tarda is due to an acquired tissue-specific inhibition of the fifth enzyme in the pathway, and the majority of patients do not have mutations of this enzyme [2, 3].

As shown in Table 20.1, porphyrias are classified as erythropoietic or hepatic, depending on whether overproduction of heme pathway intermediates occurs in the bone marrow or liver. In addition, they are classified based on clinical features. The

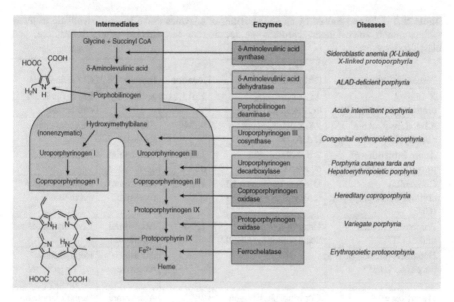

Fig. 20.1 Intermediates and enzymes of the heme biosynthetic pathway and the major diseases of porphyrin metabolism that have been associated with altered activity of specific enzymes. The initial and last three enzymes are mitochondrial, and the other four are cytosolic. Heme is synthesized from glycine and succinyl coenzyme A. Intermediates in the pathway include δ-aminolevulinic acid (an amino acid used exclusively for heme synthesis), porphobilinogen (a pyrrole), and hydroxymethylbilane (a linear tetrapyrrole). Uroporphyrinogen III cosynthase catalyzes closure of hydroxymethylbilane, with inversion of one of the pyrroles, to form a porphyrin macrocycle, uroporphyrinogen III (nonenzymatic closure occurs without inversion of this pyrrole, forming uroporphyrinogen I, which is not metabolized beyond coproporphyrinogen I.) The next two enzymes result in decarboxylation of six of the eight side chains of uroporphyrinogen III, with sequential formation of heptacarboxyl porphyrinogen, hexacarboxyl porphyrinogen, pentacarboxyl porphyrinogen, tetracarboxyl porphyrinogen (coproporphyrinogen III), tricarboxyl porphyrinogen (harderoporphyrinogen), and dicarboxyl porphyrinogen (protoporphyrinogen IX). The final two enzymes catalyze oxidation of protoporphyrinogen IX to protoporphyrin IX and insertion of ferrous iron into the porphyrin macrocycle to form heme (iron protoporphyrin IX). With the exception of protoporphyrin IX, all porphyrin intermediates are in their reduced forms (hexahydroporphyrins or porphyrinogens). Chemical structures of two intermediates are shown: porphobilinogen and protoporphyrin. (From Anderson [76], with permission)

acute porphyrias are characterized by neuropathic manifestations and the cutaneous porphyrias by skin photosensitivity resulting from activation of porphyrins by light with generation of activated oxygen species that damage the skin. Effective treatments differ among the different types of porphyria, as summarized in Table 20.2.

Although heme is required in all tissues for many vital hemoproteins, the bone marrow and liver are most active in heme synthesis. Heme is used in the bone marrow primarily for hemoglobin and in the liver for synthesis of cytochrome P-450 enzymes (CYPs). Hepatic heme biosynthesis is regulated primarily by activity of the ubiquitous form of δ-aminolevulinic acid (ALA) synthase (ALAS1), which is the initial and rate-limiting enzyme, and is under sensitive feedback control by a

Table 20.1 Diseases caused by altered activities of enzymes in the heme biosynthetic pathway with common abbreviations, chromosome location of the affected genes, inheritance, and classifications

Disease (abbreviation)	Altered enzyme (abbreviation)	Gene location	Inheritance	Classifications
X-Linked protoporphyria (XLP)	ALA synthase, erythroid (ALAS2)[a]	Xp11.21	X-linked	Erythropoietic/ cutaneous
ALA dehydratase porphyria (ADP)	ALA dehydratase (ALAD)	9q34	Autosomal recessive	Hepatic/acute
Acute intermittent porphyria (AIP)	Porphobilinogen deaminase (PBGD)[b]	11q24.1 q24.2	Autosomal dominant	Hepatic/acute
Congenital erythropoietic porphyria (CEP)	Uroporphyrinogen III (co)synthase (UROS)	10q25.2 q26.3	Autosomal recessive	Erythropoietic/ cutaneous
Porphyria cutanea tarda(PCT)	Uroporphyrinogen decarboxylase (UROD)[c]	1p34	Autosomal dominant	Hepatic/cutaneous
Hepatoerythropoietic porphyria (HEP)			Autosomal recessive	Hepatic and erythropoietic/ cutaneous
Hereditary coproporphyria (HCP)	Coproporphyrinogen	3q12	Autosomal dominant	Hepatic/acute and cutaneous
Variegate porphyria (VP)	Protoporphyrinogen oxidase	1q22 or 23	Autosomal dominant	Hepatic/acute and cutaneous
Erythropoietic protoporphyria (EPP)	Ferrochelatase oxidase[d]	18q21.3 or 22	Autosomal recessive	Erythropoietic/ cutaneous

The **bolded** diseases are discussed in this chapter

ALA δ-aminolevulinic acid

[a]The X-linked variant of EPP is due to gain-of-function mutations of ALAS2. Loss-of-function mutations affecting this enzyme are found in X-linked sideroblastic anemia. Disease-causing mutations of ALAS1, the ubiquitous form of ALAS, which is encoded by a gene on chromosome 3p21, have not been described

[b]This enzyme is also known as hydroxymethylbilane synthase and formerly as uroporphyrinogen I synthase

[c]PCT results from an acquired inhibition of UROD to <20% of normal in the liver in the presence of multiple susceptibility factors. In ~80% of cases (type 1), there are no *UROD* mutations; ~20% are heterozygous for *UROD* mutations (type 2). HEP is the homozygous (or compound heterozygous) form of type 2 PCT

[d]>90% of EPP cases are due to *FECH* mutations. Inheritance was previously classified as autosomal dominant with variable penetrance but is now recognized as recessive at the molecular level, with inherited mutations affecting both *FECH* alleles. Most patients have a null mutation trans to a hypomorphic mutation, IVS3-48 T > C, that is common in the population but does not itself cause disease

regulatory "free" heme pool in hepatocytes. Disease-causing mutations of ALAS1 are not known [1].

This chapter will discuss the four acute porphyrias and EPP, with emphasis on diagnosis and management of their acute, life-threatening features. PCT, the most common porphyria, and congenital erythropoietic porphyria (CEP), which is very

Table 20.2 Clinical features including contributing factors and treatment of the three most common human porphyrias

	Presenting symptoms	Exacerbating factors	Screening tests	Treatment
Porphyria cutanea tarda[a]	Blistering skin lesions (chronic)	Iron, alcohol, estrogens, hepatitis C virus, halogenated hydrocarbons	Plasma (or urine) porphyrins	Phlebotomy, low-dose hydroxychloroquine
Acute intermittent porphyria[b]	Neurovisceral (acute)	Drugs (mostly P-450 inducers) Progesterone Dietary restriction	Porphobilinogen (urine)	Heme, glucose, givosiran
Erythropoietic protoporphyria	Painful skin and swelling (mostly acute)	Cirrhosis	Total erythrocyte protoporphyrin	β-Carotene, afamelanotide

[a]Porphyria cutanea tarda, the most common porphyria, is not discussed here because its manifestations are chronic and rarely emergent or life-threatening

[b]The same considerations pertain to the other three acute porphyrias (HCP, VP, ADP) except that HCP and VP can also cause skin lesions identical to those in porphyria cutanea tarda, and ADP does not significantly elevate porphobilinogen

rare, cause chronic blistering skin manifestations that are rarely emergent and will not be discussed.

Acute Porphyrias: AIP, HCP, VP, and ADP

The four acute hepatic porphyrias present with identical attacks of neurological symptoms and are due to deficiencies of different enzymes in the heme pathway (Table 20.1). Acute intermittent porphyria (AIP), hereditary coproporphyria (HCP), and variegate porphyria (VP) are autosomal dominant genetic disorders due to deficiencies of the third, sixth, and seventh enzymes in the pathway, respectively. They manifest most commonly in adult females. AIP is the most common acute porphyria. Porphyria due to an inherited deficiency of ALA dehydratase, the second enzyme in this pathway, is the fourth acute porphyria. It is very rare, with only eight documented cases in the literature. Features of ALAD porphyria (ADP) that differ from the other three acute porphyrias include autosomal recessive inheritance, occurrence in males in the cases reported to date, and some erythropoietic features [4]. Lead poisoning is an acquired form of ALAD deficiency (ADP) [1]. VP and less commonly HCP may also cause blistering skin lesions, either with or apart from the neurological manifestations. Although the skin lesions are identical to the skin findings in PCT, they do not respond to the same treatments.

Clinical Presentation

The acute porphyrias usually present after puberty, lasting for several days or longer and, with the exception of ADP, more commonly in women than men. These
disorders are almost never symptomatic before puberty, except in very rare homozygous cases of AIP, HCP, and VP. Symptoms are highly variable and nonspecific,
and the history and physical examination may not immediately suggest the diagnosis [5].

Pertinent History and Exam

A family history of porphyria may suggest the diagnosis of acute porphyria. But
usually there is no such history, because most relatives who have inherited mutations for AIP, HCP, or VP never have symptoms. These mutations occur in all populations, so race and country of origin are of little importance in suspecting the
diagnosis. Founder effects may increase prevalence in some populations. Most
notable is a high prevalence of VP in South Africans of Dutch ancestry. Patients
with symptoms may or may not have a history of similar manifestations in the
past [5].

A porphyric attack may begin with insomnia and anxiety and progress over hours
or days, with abdominal pain (the most common symptom); nausea; vomiting; constipation; less commonly diarrhea; pain in the extremities, head, neck, or chest;
muscle weakness; dysuria; and other symptoms of bladder dysfunction. Paresis may
develop especially with severe and prolonged attacks and is caused by peripheral
motor neuropathy, often accompanied by pain in the extremities, back, and chest.
Motor weakness typically affects more proximal muscles initially, most commonly
in the upper extremities, and may then progress to include respiratory and bulbar
paralysis. Paresis is usually symmetrical but can be asymmetrical and focal, and
cranial nerves can be affected. Sudden death may occur, presumably from elevated
catecholamines and cardiac arrhythmia. Anxiety and insomnia may be accompanied
by other central nervous system manifestations such as agitation, depression, disorientation, hallucinations, and paranoia. Hyponatremia is common in severe attacks
and may be due to inappropriate antidiuretic hormone secretion or a combination of
causes such as vomiting, diarrhea, poor intake, or excess renal sodium loss [6–8].
Seizures may be caused by hyponatremia or be a neurological manifestation of
porphyria itself [5]. Recurrent attacks tend to be similar in a given patient but may
vary depending on exacerbating factors. Some patients develop frequently recurring
attacks and chronic symptoms including pain and depression [5, 9].

A history of exposure to certain drugs known to cause attacks (Table 20.3) may
suggest the diagnosis and prompt diagnostic testing. Many such drugs are inducers
of hepatic CYPs. ALAS1 and CYP genes share upstream enhancer elements that
respond to inducing drugs and chemicals that interact with the pregnane X receptor

Table 20.3 Selected drugs considered unsafe and safe in the acute porphyrias

Unsafe	Safe
Alcohol	Acetaminophen
Barbiturates	Acetazolamide
	Allopurinol
Carbamazepine	Amiloride
Carisoprodol	Angiotensin-converting enzyme inhibitors
Clonazepam	Angiotensin receptor antagonists
Danazol	Aspirin
Diclofenac	Atropine
Ergots	Beta-adrenergic antagonists
Glutethimide	Bromides
Methyprylon	Cimetidine
Ethchlorvynol	Erythropoietin
Griseofulvin	Estrogens[a]
Hydralazine	
Mephenytoin	Gabapentin
Meprobamate (also mebutamate, tybutamate)	Gentamicin
Metoclopramide	Glucocorticoids
Nifedipine	
Phenytoin	Insulin
Primidone	Narcotic analgesics
Progesterone and synthetic progestins	Ofloxacin
Pyrazinamide	Penicillin and derivatives
Pyrazolones (aminopyrine, antipyrine)	Phenothiazines
Rifampin	Ranitidine
Succinimides (ethosuximide, methsuximide)	Streptomycin
Sulfonamide antibiotics	Tetracycline
Valproic acid	Vigabatrin

Evidence for classifying drugs is often limited, and updated information can be accessed at websites of the American Porphyria Foundation (https://porphyriafoundation.org/) and the European Porphyria Network (http://www.drugsporphyria.org/languages/UnitedKingdom/s1.php?l=gbr)
[a]There is little evidence that estrogens alone are harmful in acute porphyrias. They have been implicated as harmful mostly on the basis of experience with estrogen-progestin combinations and because they can exacerbate porphyria cutanea tarda

(PXR) [10]. Therefore, half-normal activity of an enzyme in the heme biosynthetic pathway resulting from a mutation inherited from one parent can become limiting in the liver when there is exposure to drugs or hormones that induce ALAS1 and CYPs. Attacks are also provoked by reduced calorie intake (as in crash dieting to lose weight), infections, and major surgery [11]. Induction of ALAS1 by fasting is mediated by the peroxisome proliferator-activated receptor γ coactivator 1α (PGC-1α), now recognized as an important link between nutritional status and acute porphyrias [12]. Onset after puberty and more frequent clinical expression in women suggest that endogenous sex steroid hormones are important. Luteal phase attacks are probably due to progesterone and its metabolites, which are potent inducers of hepatic ALAS1, whereas estrogens are not. Attacks may occur from administration of progestins, although the risk may be lower with newer low-dose progestin-estrogen oral contraceptives. Although pregnancy is usually well-tolerated despite high progesterone levels, some women experience attacks during pregnancy, and hyperemesis gravidarum, reduced calorie intake, and harmful drugs (e.g., metoclo-pramide) may contribute [5].

Cigarette smoke contains chemicals that can induce ALAS1 and may predispose to attacks [13]. These and other unknown exacerbating factors are additive, which may explain why harmful drugs do not always cause attacks. For example, barbitu-rate anesthetics were observed to exacerbate porphyria more often if symptoms were present before anesthetic exposure [14].

Pertinent Laboratory Data

Measurement of urinary porphobilinogen (PBG) is especially important for initial diagnosis of acute porphyria [1, 5]. The porphyrin precursors ALA and PBG and the porphyrinogens are colorless and nonfluorescent. However, porphyrinogens undergo auto-oxidation outside cells and are excreted primarily as the corresponding por-phyrins, which are reddish and fluoresce on exposure to long-wave ultraviolet light. ALA and PBG are excreted mostly in urine, as are the highly carboxylated porphy-rins, namely, uroporphyrin (octacarboxylporphyrin), heptacarboxylporphyrin, hexacarboxylporphyrin, and pentacarboxylporphyrin. Coproporphyrin (tetracar-boxylporphyrin) is excreted in both urine and bile. Harderoporphyrin and protopor-phyrin, which are tricarboxylic and dicarboxylic porphyrins, are excreted in the bile and feces.

Other laboratory abnormalities may be few. Anemia is absent, since the marrow is not affected significantly in these hepatic porphyrias. Leukocytosis is absent or mild, since there is little inflammation. Hyponatremia and other electrolyte abnor-malities may be present. Chronic hepatic abnormalities including low-grade trans-aminase elevations are common. It is not known whether underlying liver disease is significant and can progress to cirrhosis. However, the risk of liver cancer is increased [15, 16]. AIP may predispose to chronic hypertension and significant renal impairment that may require chronic hemodialysis or renal transplantation [5].

Diagnosis: Key Tests

Acute porphyria should be suspected in any patient with abdominal pain or symp-toms of these diseases when an initial workup for more common conditions does not provide a diagnosis. *A marked increase in urinary PBG excretion, which is characteristic of AIP, HCP, and VP, does not occur in other medical conditions and*

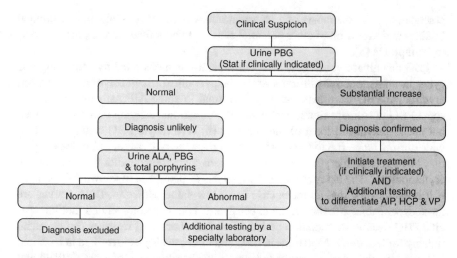

Fig. 20.2 Approach to the diagnosis of acute porphyria in patients with current symptoms that suggest these disorders. A rapid test for elevated urine porphobilinogen will almost always establish or exclude this diagnosis in the acutely ill patient. If a marked porphobilinogen elevation is found, further testing is initiated to establish the type of acute porphyria, but treatment can begin before the laboratory reports those results

is therefore a highly specific and diagnostic finding for acute porphyria. During attacks of AIP, PBG excretion is generally in the range of approximately 50 to 200 mg/day (reference range, 0 to 4 mg/day), and ALA excretion is approximately 20 to 100 mg/day (reference range, 0 to 7 mg/day) but may be somewhat lower and decrease more rapidly in HCP and VP. In ADP, excretion of ALA is markedly increased, and PBG is normal or only slightly increased [4]. Treatment is most effective if implemented early. A diagnostic flow chart for use when acute porphyria is suspected is presented in Fig. 20.2. When acute porphyria is suspected, a spot urine should be obtained for rapid screening for elevated PBG. It is recommended that a kit be available in all medical centers for rapid detection of elevated PBG using a random urine sample [5, 17].

Demonstration of a substantial elevation in urinary PBG is a specific finding that establishes a diagnosis of acute porphyria. Treatment should be started promptly, and additional blood and fecal samples will differentiate HCP and VP from AIP. The urine sample is processed to confirm the elevated PBG by a quantitative method and to measure ALA and porphyrins. The blood sample is used to measure plasma porphyrins (elevated in VP with a distinctive fluorescence peak at neutral pH) [18, 19] and erythrocyte PBG deaminase (usually decreased in AIP). The fecal sample is used to measure porphyrins (elevated in HCP and VP). Samples collected after treatment is started are less useful because levels of ALA, PBG, and porphyrins may decrease, especially after treatment with hemin [5].

Urinary PBG and porphyrin levels may decrease but often remain elevated between attacks of AIP. Although some have proposed that acute attacks must be proven by documenting a particular level of increase in PBG [20], this is not practical, and the diagnosis of a recurrent attack is based on evaluation of clinical findings and exclusion of other potential causes of abdominal pain or other presenting symptoms [5].

PBG deaminase deficiency, most conveniently demonstrated by measuring this cytosolic enzyme activity in erythrocytes, helps confirm a diagnosis of AIP. However, erythrocyte PBG deaminase activity is normal in some AIP patients because (a) some PBG deaminase mutations reduce the ubiquitous enzyme found in the liver, but not the erythroid form of the enzyme; (b) erythrocyte PBG deaminase has a wide normal range (up to threefold) that overlaps the AIP range; and c) the enzyme may be increased in erythrocytes by inapparent concurrent conditions that stimulate erythropoiesis. The assay is useful for analysis of pedigrees of known AIP patients if it is established that an index case has a low value. However, DNA studies are more dependable, although more expensive. It is now recommended that the specific PBG deaminase mutation be identified for a family so relatives can be tested reliably for latent AIP. Mutations in CPO and PPO can also be identified in HCP and VP, respectively; enzyme assays for these mitochondrial enzymes are difficult and not generally available. Importantly, DNA studies and measurement of erythrocyte PBG deaminase are not useful in acutely ill patients because an abnormal finding does not distinguish between active and latent stages of acute porphyrias. Therefore, it remains important to document the diagnosis in active cases of acute porphyrias by measuring PBG, ALA, and total porphyrins in urine. These can be measured in serum in patients with renal insufficiency [5, 21].

Treatment

Attacks may resolve spontaneously. For example, attacks during the luteal phase of the menstrual cycle usually resolve with onset of menses. However, most attacks should be treated with hemin [5, 22, 23]. Effective treatment requires an accurate diagnosis and, in a patient not previously known to have porphyria, a prompt demonstration of a substantial elevation in PBG. Severe attacks may become life-threatening with progression to quadriplegia and respiratory impairment without treatment with hemin. Complete recovery of axonal degeneration can occur even with advanced motor weakness but may require 1–2 years. Residual weakness sometimes affects distal extremities. Hospitalization is usually required for the intravenous administration of glucose and hemin and for monitoring and treatment of symptoms and complications. Precipitating factors, which are often multiple, should be identified and removed whenever possible. Narcotic analgesics are usually required for pain and small or moderate doses of a phenothiazine for nausea, vomiting, anxiety, and restlessness. Bladder distention may require catheterization [5].

Hemin therapy and carbohydrate loading are considered specific therapies because they repress hepatic ALAS1. Hemin 3–4 mg per kilogram body weight infused intravenously once daily for 4 days is most effective. A longer course of treatment may be necessary if treatment is not started soon after onset of symptoms or if neuronal damage is already advanced. Hemin is an approved product in the United States as lyophilized hematin (hydroxyheme, Panhematin®, Recordati®) and should be reconstituted with human albumin [24]. Hemin is available as heme arginate (Normosang®, Orphan Europe) in Europe and South Africa. Availability in other countries is less dependable. Hemin has been administered safely during pregnancy [5, 22, 23, 25, 26].

Carbohydrate loading may suffice for mild attacks (e.g., pain not requiring narcotics and without paresis, seizures, or hyponatremia) and can be given orally as sucrose, glucose polymers, or carbohydrate-rich foods. If oral intake is poorly tolerated or contraindicated by distention and ileus, intravenous administration of glucose (at least 300 g daily) is usually indicated, although larger amounts may be more effective. However, this may entail administration of a large volume of fluids and increase the risk of hyponatremia. A central venous line facilitates more complete parenteral nutrition support and avoids excess fluid volumes [5]. The effect of glucose is mediated in part by elevation of insulin, which reduces expression of PGC-1α in the liver [12].

Treatment of seizures is problematic because many antiseizure drugs can exacerbate AIP. Bromides, gabapentin, and vigabatrin can be given safely. β-Adrenergic blocking agents may control tachycardia and hypertension in acute attacks of porphyria, but they may be hazardous in patients with hypovolemia, in whom increased catecholamine secretion may be an important compensatory mechanism. Cimetidine has been reported to be beneficial, but controlled studies are lacking, and should not be used in place of hemin. Numerous other therapies have been tried in this disease but have not been consistently useful [1, 2, 6].

Hemin infusions can also prevent recurrent attacks but may need to be given as often as weekly [27]. Givosiran (Givlaari®, Alnylam), an interfering RNA therapeutic administered monthly subcutaneously, was recently approved by the FDA as a prophylactic therapy for patients experiencing frequent attacks (>3–4 attacks/year) [28]. Frequent cyclic attacks can be prevented by treatment with a GnRH analogue [29]. Liver transplantation can be curative for patients with repeated disabling attacks that are refractory to medical therapy, which is a strong evidence that the liver is responsible for the neuropathic manifestations of the acute porphyrias [30].

Hemin has few adverse effects. However, hematin is unstable when reconstituted with sterile water, and when infused degradation products adhere to endothelial cells, platelets, and coagulation factors, causing a transient anticoagulant effect and frequently a phlebitis at the site of infusion. Reconstitution with human albumin enhances the stability of hematin and prevents these side effects [24]. Uncommon side effects include fever, aching, malaise, hemolysis, anaphylaxis, and circulatory collapse [31, 32]. Family members should be screened, preferably by DNA methods, to detect latent cases. Potentially harmful drugs and "crash diets" for weight loss should be avoided.

Erythropoietic Protoporphyria "Hepatic Crisis"

Erythropoietic protoporphyria (EPP) causes lifelong photosensitivity due to high levels of protoporphyrin, initially in marrow reticulocytes and then in plasma and circulating erythrocytes [1]. Protoporphyrin is excited by light, generating free radicals and singlet oxygen, leading to skin damage [33]. Factors that increase circulating levels of the hormone erythropoietin and stimulate erythropoiesis may increase protoporphyrin production in the marrow and worsen the disease. Protoporphyrin is water insoluble and is excreted only by the liver into the bile and may form gallstones.

Protoporphyrin is hepatotoxic and can cause significant liver disease in 5% of cases. Liver disease complicating EPP is referred to as protoporphyric hepatopathy. It is also termed EPP crisis when it presents with jaundice, rapidly progressive liver decompensation, and severe right-upper quadrant pain [34, 35].

Clinical Presentation

EPP is the most common porphyria in children and the third most common in adults and is greatly underdiagnosed [36]. Photo-cutaneous symptoms usually begin in childhood. Acute burning, itching, erythema, and swelling can occur within minutes of sun exposure, and the diffuse edema of sun-exposed areas may resemble angioneurotic edema. Chronic skin changes are subtle, with little or no blisters, crusting, or scarring. Mild anemia with hypochromia, microcytosis, and low serum ferritin is common [37]. Protoporphyric hepatopathy may present as a cause of previously unexplained abnormalities in liver function tests, particularly elevated serum transaminases, in a patient with long-standing, previously unexplained photosensitivity.

Pertinent History

There is often no family history of EPP or photosensitivity. In most families, EPP is an autosomal recessive disease due to an inherited deficiency of ferrochelatase (FECH), the final enzyme in the heme biosynthetic pathway [38]. The enzyme activity is less than 30% of normal in affected individuals; in most families a severe *FECH* mutation is inherited from one parent, and a hypomorphic low-expression *FECH* allele is from the other parent [39]. This hypomorphic allele, identified as IVS3-48 T>C, is found in about 10% of Caucasians and by itself has no phenotype even when homozygous. Multiple different *FECH* mutations have been identified in different families [40]. EPP occurs in all races, but the frequency of the hypomorphic *FECH* allele in different populations determines the differences in prevalence of EPP. The hypomorphic allele and EPP are rare in Africa and more common in China, Japan, Europe, and North America. Rarely, a severe *FECH* mutation is inherited from each parent [40, 41]. EPP can also develop late in life in the setting of a myeloproliferative or myelodysplastic disorder due to expansion of a clone of hematopoietic cells with a *FECH* mutation [42–44]. A second form of protoporphyria without *FECH* mutations and a sex-linked inheritance pattern was found to be due to gain-of-function mutations of ALAS2 (the only heme pathway enzyme found on the X chromosome) [45]. This condition, termed X-linked protoporphyria (XLP), comprises up to ~5% of cases of protoporphyria. The clinical phenotype is the same as in EPP but with possibly greater risks for liver disease.

A long history of non-blistering photosensitivity in a patient presenting with acute or chronic liver disease strongly suggests protoporphyric hepatopathy. Patients who present with acutely decompensated liver disease usually have underlying cirrhosis. Rapid progression of liver disease often ensues due to an increasing level of protoporphyrin in plasma, which results from impaired hepatobiliary excretion [34, 35]. Gallstones are commonly present, and acute cholecystitis and common bile duct obstruction must be excluded by imaging. Hepatopathy is sometimes precipitated by another cause of liver dysfunction such as viral or alcoholic hepatitis, which impairs hepatic uptake of protoporphyrin and causes plasma porphyrins to increase further and cause hepatotoxicity [46]. Protoporphyrin can form crystalline structures in hepatocytes, impair mitochondrial function, and damage cholangiocytes, leading to decreased hepatic bile formation and flow [34, 47].

Pertinent Physical Findings

Chronic skin changes such as blistering, milia, scarring, and hypertrichosis, as seen in other cutaneous porphyrias, are not common in EPP. Findings such as lichenification, leathery pseudovesicles, labial grooving, and nail changes may be difficult to recognize. There is no fluorescence of the teeth, and neuropathic manifestations occur only with advanced liver disease [48]. Patients who present acutely with protoporphyric hepatopathy are often jaundiced and have right-upper quadrant tenderness that may suggest cholecystitis or biliary obstruction. They may develop a severe motor neuropathy similar to that seen in the acute porphyrias and manifest initially by proximal muscle weakness that is difficult to detect by physical examination in its early stages and may involve the respiratory muscles [48].

Pertinent Laboratory Data

EPP is associated with marked elevation of metal-free protoporphyrin in erythrocytes. Plasma porphyrins are less elevated than in other cutaneous porphyrias and may be normal in mild cases. Fecal porphyrins are normal or modestly elevated and consist mostly of protoporphyrin. Urine porphyrins are normal in uncomplicated EPP, since protoporphyrin is not excreted in urine.

The diagnosis requires measurement of erythrocyte protoporphyrin and demonstrating that the elevation is predominantly metal-free protoporphyrin rather than zinc protoporphyrin. Zinc protoporphyrin is increased in many other medical conditions such as homozygous porphyrias (including mild cases of CEP), iron deficiency, lead poisoning, anemia of chronic disease [49], hemolytic conditions, and many other erythrocyte disorders [50]. Unfortunately, there is considerable confusion regarding measurement and reporting of erythrocyte protoporphyrin levels [51]. Plasma porphyrins are less increased in EPP and are particularly subject to photodegradation from light exposure during sample processing [52]. *Therefore, measurement of erythrocyte rather than plasma porphyrins should be the primary screening test for EPP.*

The diagnosis of protoporphyric hepatopathy is best documented by liver biopsy, which will demonstrate accumulated protoporphyrin that appears as brown pigment in hepatocytes, Kupffer cells, and biliary canaliculi and is doubly refractive with a Maltese cross appearance under polarizing microscopy [53].

Treatment

Avoidance of sunlight is essential to prevent painful photosensitivity in all patients with EPP. This often requires restrictions in lifestyle and employment and significantly impairs quality of life [36]. Occlusive sunblock may be helpful. Oral β-carotene is available without a prescription as Lumitene™, a high-quality nutritional product that may prevent photosensitivity by quenching activated oxygen radicals [54, 55]. A daily dose of 120–180 mg or higher is recommended to achieve a serum β-carotene level of 600 to 800 μg/dl [56]. Oral cysteine may also quench excited oxygen species and increase sunlight tolerance in EPP [57]. Other treatments that aim to either increase skin pigmentation or scavenge activated oxygen species have been reviewed [55, 58]. Afamelanotide (Scenesse®, subcutaneous implant) is an alpha-melanocyte-stimulating hormone analogue that increases skin melanin and can significantly improve sunlight tolerance in EPP [59]. Because patients limit their exposure to sunlight, vitamin D supplementation is recommended. Hepatitis A and B vaccination and yearly monitoring of liver function tests and erythrocyte and plasma porphyrin levels are also recommended [35].

Protoporphyric hepatopathy may resolve if another reversible cause of liver dysfunction, such as viral hepatitis or alcohol, is contributing [46]. Medical treatment can bridge patients to liver transplantation and sometimes leads to resolution of an acute episode. Plasmapheresis and hemin can lower plasma porphyrin levels [60], and red blood cell transfusions are used to correct anemia [61] and reduce marrow protoporphyrin production. Cholestyramine [34, 62, 63], ursodeoxycholic acid [64], and vitamin E are also recommended [35].

Liver transplantation is as successful in protoporphyric hepatopathy as in other liver diseases, even though the disease may recur in the new liver [65–67]. Because impaired liver function further elevates plasma protoporphyrin levels, these patients are subject to severe phototoxic damage to the exposed skin and visceral surfaces from operating room lights, which can be ameliorated with special filter membranes [68]. Bone marrow transplantation can achieve remission in human EPP [69, 70] as well as in murine models of protoporphyria [71] . Sequential liver and bone marrow transplantation can prevent recurrence of liver disease [72]. But it is not yet possible to predict which patients would benefit from marrow transplantation to prevent hepatopathy. If hepatopathy responds adequately to medical treatment, marrow transplantation to prevent recurrence can be considered [73]. Studies in mice suggest a future role for gene therapy in human EPP [74, 75].

References

1. Phillips JD, Anderson KE. The porphyrias (Chapter 58). In: Kaushansky K, Lichtman MA, Prchal JT, et al., editors. Williams hematology. 9th ed. New York: McGraw-Hill; 2016. p. 839–63.
2. Elder GH. Porphyria cutanea tarda and related disorders (Chapter 88). In: Kadish KM, Smith K, Guilard R, editors. Porphyrin handbook, Part II. San Diego: Academic Press; 2003. p. 67–92.
3. Jalil S, Grady JJ, Lee C, Anderson KE. Associations among behavior-related susceptibility factors in porphyria cutanea tarda. Clin Gastroenterol Hepatol. 2010;8(3):297–302.
4. Lahiji AP, Anderson KE, Chan A, Simon A, Desnick RJ, Ramanujam VMS. 5-Aminolevulinate dehydratase porphyria: update on hepatic 5-aminolevulinic acid synthase induction and long-term response to hemin. Mol Genet Metab. 2020;131(4):418–23.
5. Anderson KE, Bloomer JR, Bonkovsky HL, Kushner JP, Pierach CA, Pimstone NR, et al. Recommendations for the diagnosis and treatment of the acute porphyrias. Ann Intern Med. 2005;142(6):439–50.
6. Eales L, Dowdle EB, Sweeney GD. The electrolyte disorder of the acute porphyric attack and the possible role of delta-aminolaevulic acid. S Afr J Lab Clin Med (Special Issue). 1971;17:89–97.
7. Stein JA, Curl FD, Valsamis M, Tschudy DP. Abnormal iron and water metabolism in acute intermittent porphyria with new morphologic findings. Am J Med. 1972;53:784–9.
8. Tschudy DP, Lamon JM. Porphyrin metabolism and the porphyrias. In: Bondy PK, Rosenberg LE, editors. Duncan's diseases of metabolism. 8th ed. Philadelphia: W.B. Saunders Co; 1980. p. 939–1007.
9. Balwani M, Wang B, Anderson KE, Bloomer JR, Bissell DM, Bonkovsky HL, et al. Acute hepatic porphyrias: recommendations for evaluation and long-term management. Hepatology. 2017;66(4):1314–22.
10. Podvinec M, Handschin C, Looser R, Meyer UA. Identification of the xenosensors regulating human 5-aminolevulinate synthase. Proc Natl Acad Sci U S A. 2004;101(24):9127–32.
11. Frank J, Poh-Fitzpatrick MB, King LE Jr, Christiano AM. The genetic basis of "Scarsdale gourmet diet" variegate porphyria: a missense mutation in the protoporphyrinogen oxidase gene. Arch Dermatol Res. 1998;290(8):441–5.
12. Handschin C, Lin J, Rhee J, Peyer AK, Chin S, Wu PH, et al. Nutritional regulation of hepatic heme biosynthesis and porphyria through PGC-1alpha. Cell. 2005;122(4):505–15.
13. Lip GYH, McColl KEL, Goldberg A, Moore MR. Smoking and recurrent attacks of acute intermittent porphyria. Br Med J. 1991;302:507.
14. Mustajoki P, Heinonen J. General anesthesia in "inducible" porphyrias. Anesthesiology. 1980;53:15–20.
15. Andant C, Puy H, Bogard C, Faivre J, Soule JC, Nordmann Y, et al. Hepatocellular carcinoma in patients with acute hepatic porphyria: frequency of occurrence and related factors. J Hepatol. 2000;32(6):933–9.

16. Saberi B, Naik H, Overbey JR, Erwin AL, Anderson KE, Bissell DM, et al. Hepatocellular carcinoma in acute hepatic Porphyrias: results from the longitudinal study of the U.S. Porphyrias consortium. Hepatology. 2020. https://doi.org/10.1002/hep.31460. Epub ahead of print. PMID: 32681675.
17. Deacon AC, Peters TJ. Identification of acute porphyria: evaluation of a commercial screening test for urinary porphobilinogen. Ann Clin Biochem. 1998;35(Pt 6):726–32.
18. Poh-Fitzpatrick MB, Lamola AA. Direct spectrofluorometry of diluted erythrocytes and plasma: a rapid diagnostic method in primary and secondary porphyrinemias. J Lab Clin Med. 1976;87(2):362–70.
19. Poh-Fitzpatrick MB. A plasma porphyrin fluorescence marker for variegate porphyria. Arch Dermatol. 1980;116:543–7.
20. Schoenfeld N, Mamet R. Individualized workup: a new approach to the biochemical diagnosis of acute attacks of neuroporphyria. Physiol Res. 2006;55(Suppl 2):S103–8.
21. Sardh E, Harper P, Andersson DE, Floderus Y. Plasma porphobilinogen as a sensitive biomarker to monitor the clinical and therapeutic course of acute intermittent porphyria attacks. Eur J Intern Med. 2009;20(2):201–7.
22. Puy H, Gouya L, Deybach JC. Porphyrias. Lancet. 2010;375(9718):924–37.
23. Harper P, Wahlin S. Treatment options in acute porphyria, porphyria cutanea tarda, and erythropoietic protoporphyria. Curr Treat Options Gastroenterol. 2007;10(6):444–55.
24. Anderson KE, Bonkovsky HL, Bloomer JR, Shedlofsky SI. Reconstitution of hematin for intravenous infusion. Ann Intern Med. 2006;144(7):537–8.
25. Mustajoki P, Nordmann Y. Early administration of heme arginate for acute porphyric attacks. Arch Int Med. 1993;153:2004–8.
26. Tenhunen R, Mustajoki P. Acute porphyria: treatment with heme. Semin Liver Dis. 1998;18(1):53–5.
27. Marsden JT, Guppy S, Stein P, Cox TM, Badminton M, Gardiner T, et al. Audit of the use of regular haem arginate infusions in patients with acute porphyria to prevent recurrent symptoms. JIMD Rep. 2015;22:57–65.
28. Balwani M, Sardh E, Ventura P, Peiro PA, Rees DC, Stolzel U, et al. Phase 3 trial of RNAi therapeutic Givosiran for acute intermittent Porphyria. N Engl J Med. 2020;382(24):2289–301.
29. Anderson KE, Spitz IM, Bardin CW, Kappas AA. GnRH analogue prevents cyclical attacks of porphyria. Arch Int Med. 1990;150:1469–74.
30. Lissing M, Nowak G, Adam R, Karam V, Boyd A, Gouya L, et al. Liver Transplantation for Acute Intermittent Porphyria. Liver Transpl. 2020. https://doi.org/10.1002/lt.25959. Epub ahead of print. PMID: 33259654.
31. Daimon M, Susa S, Igarashi M, Kato T, Kameda W. Administration of heme arginate, but not hematin, caused anaphylactic shock. Am J Med. 2001;110(3):240.
32. Khanderia U. Circulatory collapse associated with hemin therapy for acute intermittent porphyria. Clin Pharm. 1986;5:690–2.
33. Sarkany RP. Making sense of the porphyrias. Photodermatol Photoimmunol Photomed. 2008;24(2):102–8.
34. Bloomer JR. The liver in protoporphyria. Hepatology. 1988;8:402–7.
35. Anstey AV, Hift RJ. Liver disease in erythropoietic protoporphyria: insights and implications for management. Postgrad Med J. 2007;83(986):739–48.
36. Holme SA, Anstey AV, Finlay AY, Elder GH, Badminton MN. Erythropoietic protoporphyria in the U.K.: clinical features and effect on quality of life. Br J Dermatol. 2006;155(3):574–81.
37. Bossi K, Lee J, Schmeltzer P, Holburton E, Groseclose G, Besur S, et al. Homeostasis of iron and hepcidin in erythropoietic protoporphyria. Eur J Clin Investig. 2015;45(10):1032–41.
38. Bottomley SS, Tanaka M, Everett MA. Diminished erythroid ferrochelatase activity in protoporphyria. J Lab Clin Med. 1975;86:126–31.
39. Gouya L, Puy H, Robreau AM, Bourgeois M, Lamoril J, Da Silva V, et al. The penetrance of dominant erythropoietic protoporphyria is modulated by expression of wildtype FECH. Nat Genet. 2002;30(1):27–8.
40. Whatley SD, Mason NG, Holme SA, Anstey AV, Elder GH, Badminton MN. Molecular epidemiology of erythropoietic protoporphyria in the United Kingdom. Br J Dermatol. 2010;162(3):642–6.

41. Holme SA, Whatley SD, Roberts AG, Anstey AV, Elder GH, Ead RD, et al. Seasonal palmar keratoderma in erythropoietic protoporphyria indicates autosomal recessive inheritance. J Invest Dermatol. 2009;129(3):599–605.
42. Aplin C, Whatley SD, Thompson P, Hoy T, Fisher P, Singer C, et al. Late-onset erythropoietic porphyria caused by a chromosome 18q deletion in erythroid cells. J Invest Dermatol. 2001;117(6):1647–9.
43. Shirota T, Yamamoto H, Hayashi S, Fujimoto H, Harada Y, Hayashi T. Myelodysplastic syndrome terminating in erythropoietic protoporphyria after 15 years of aplastic anemia. Int J Hematol. 2000;72(1):44–7.
44. Goodwin RG, Kell WJ, Laidler P, Long CC, Whatley SD, McKinley M, et al. Photosensitivity and acute liver injury in myeloproliferative disorder secondary to late-onset protoporphyria caused by deletion of a ferrochelatase gene in hematopoietic cells. Blood. 2006;107(1):60–2.
45. Whatley SD, Ducamp S, Gouya L, Grandchamp B, Beaumont C, Badminton MN, et al. C-terminal deletions in the ALAS2 gene lead to gain of function and cause X-linked dominant protoporphyria without anemia or iron overload. Am J Hum Genet. 2008;83(3):408–14.
46. Bonkovsky HL, Schned AR. Fatal liver failure in protoporphyria: synergism between ethanol excess and the genetic defect. Gastroenterology. 1986;90:191–201.
47. Berenson MM, Kimura R, Samowitz W, Bjorkman D. Protoporphyrin overload in unrestrained rats: biochemical and histopathologic characterization of a new model of protoporphyric hepatopathy. Int J Exp Pathol. 1992;73:665–73.
48. Muley SA, Midani HA, Rank JM, Carithers R, Parry GJ. Neuropathy in erythropoietic protoporphyrias. Neurology. 1998;51(1):262–5.
49. Hastka J, Lasserre JJ, Schwarzbeck A, Strauch M, Hehlmann R. Zinc protoporphyrin in anemia of chronic disorders. Blood. 1993;81:1200–4.
50. Anderson KE, Sassa S, Peterson CM, Kappas A. Increased erythrocyte uroporphyrinogen-I-synthetase, δ-aminolevulinic acid dehydratase and protoporphyrin in hemolytic anemias. Am J Med. 1977;63:359–64.
51. Gou EW, Balwani M, Bissell DM, Bloomer JR, Bonkovsky HL, Desnick RJ, et al. Pitfalls in erythrocyte protoporphyrin measurement for diagnosis and monitoring of protoporphyrias. Clin Chem. 2015;61(12):1453–6.
52. Poh-Fitzpatrick MB, DeLeo VA. Rates of plasma porphyrin disappearance in fluorescent vs. red incandescent light exposure. J Invest Dermatol. 1977;69(6):510–2.
53. Bloomer JR, Enriquez R. Evidence that hepatic crystalline deposits in a patient with protoporphyria are composed of photoporphyrin. Gastroenterology. 1982;82:569–72.
54. Mathews-Roth MM, Pathak MA, Fitzpatrick TB, Harber LH, Kass EH. Beta carotene therapy for erythropoietic protoporphyria and other photosensitivity diseases. Arch Dermatol. 1977;113:1229–332.
55. Minder EI, Schneider-Yin X, Steurer J, Bachmann LM. A systematic review of treatment options for dermal photosensitivity in erythropoietic protoporphyria. Cell Mol Biol (Noisy-le-Grand). 2009;55(1):84–97.
56. Mathews-Roth MM. Systemic photoprotection. Dermatol Clin. 1986;4(2):335–9.
57. Mathews-Roth MM, Rosner B. Long-term treatment of erythropoietic protoporphyria with cysteine. Photodermatol Photoimmunol Photomed. 2002;18(6):307–9.
58. Warren LJ, George S. Erythropoietic protoporphyria treated with narrow-band (TL-01) UVB phototherapy. Australas J Dermatol. 1998;39(3):179–82.
59. Langendonk JG, Balwani M, Anderson KE, Bonkovsky HL, Anstey AV, Bissell DM, et al. Afamelanotide for erythropoietic protoporphyria. N Engl J Med. 2015;373(1):48–59.
60. Lamon JM, Poh-Fitzpatrick MB, Lamola AA. Hepatic protoporphyrin production in human protoporphyria. Effects of intravenous hematin and analysis of erythrocyte protoporphyrin distribution. Gastroenterology. 1980;79(1):115–25.
61. Bechtel MA, Bertolone SJ, Hodge SJ. Transfusion therapy in a patient with erythropoietic protoporphyria. Arch Dermatol. 1981;117:99–101.
62. Bloomer JR. Pathogenesis and therapy of liver disease in protoporphyria. Yale J Biol Med. 1979;52:39–28.
63. Kniffen JC. Protoporphyrin removal in intrahepatic porphyrastasis. Gastroenterology. 1970;58:1027.

64. Gross U, Frank M, Doss MO. Hepatic complications of erythropoietic protoporphyria. Photodermatol Photoimmunol Photomed. 1998;14(2):52–7.
65. McGuire BM, Bonkovsky HL, Carithers RL Jr, Chung RT, Goldstein LI, Lake JR, et al. Liver transplantation for erythropoietic protoporphyria liver disease. Liver Transpl. 2005;11(12):1590–6.
66. Wahlin S, Stal P, Adam R, Karam V, Porte R, Seehofer D, et al. Liver transplantation for erythropoietic protoporphyria in Europe. Liver Transpl. 2011;17(9):1021–6.
67. Dowman JK, Gunson BK, Mirza DF, Badminton MN, Newsome PN. UK experience of liver transplantation for erythropoietic protoporphyria. J Inherit Metab Dis. 2011;34(2):539–45.
68. Wahlin S, Srikanthan N, Hamre B, Harper P, Brun A. Protection from phototoxic injury during surgery and endoscopy in erythropoietic protoporphyria. Liver Transpl. 2008;14(9):1340–6.
69. Poh-Fitzpatrick MB, Wang X, Anderson KE, Bloomer JR, Bolwell B, Lichtin AE. Erythropoietic protoporphyria: altered phenotype after bone marrow transplantation for myelogenous leukemia in a patient heteroallelic for ferrochelatase gene mutations. J Am Acad Dermatol. 2002;46(6):861–6.
70. Wahlin S, Harper P. The role for BMT in erythropoietic protoporphyria. Bone Marrow Transplant. 2010;45(2):393–4.
71. Fontanellas A, Mazurier F, Landry M, Taine L, Morel C, Larou M, et al. Reversion of hepatobiliary alterations by bone marrow transplantation in a murine model of erythropoietic protoporphyria. Hepatology. 2000;32(1):73–81.
72. Rand EB, Bunin N, Cochran W, Ruchelli E, Olthoff KM, Bloomer JR. Sequential liver and bone marrow transplantation for treatment of erythropoietic protoporphyria. Pediatrics. 2006;118(6):e1896–9.
73. Wahlin S, Aschan J, Bjornstedt M, Broome U, Harper P. Curative bone marrow transplantation in erythropoietic protoporphyria after reversal of severe cholestasis. J Hepatol. 2007;46(1):174–9.
74. Pawliuk R, Tighe R, Wise RJ, Mathews-Roth MM, Leboulch P. Prevention of murine erythropoietic protoporphyria-associated skin photosensitivity and liver disease by dermal and hepatic ferrochelatase. J Invest Dermatol. 2005;124(1):256–62.
75. Richard E, Robert E, Cario-Andre M, Ged C, Geronimi F, Gerson SL, et al. Hematopoietic stem cell gene therapy of murine protoporphyria by methylguanine-DNA-methyltransferase-mediated in vivo drug selection. Gene Ther. 2004;11(22):1638–47.
76. Anderson KE. The porphyrias (Chapter 217). In: Goldman L, Schafer AI, editors. Goldman's Cecil medicine. 24th ed. Philadelphia: Elsevier Saunders; 2012. p. 1363–71.

Chapter 21
Acute Pancreatitis Due to Hyperchylomicronemia

P. Barton Duell

Précis

1. Clinical setting: Severe abdominal pain, nausea, and emesis.
2. Diagnosis:

   (a) History: Usually recent onset of severe abdominal pain, often after a period of increased intake of dietary fat and/or alcohol or uncontrolled diabetes. Episodes also can be provoked by the recent addition of triglyceride-raising medications such as oral estrogen therapy, beta-adrenergic blockers, or corticosteroids in patients with baseline hypertriglyceridemia. Some patients may have a history of recurrent bouts of abdominal pain and/or transient outbreaks of small pimple-like lesions (i.e., eruptive xanthomas) on their trunk and extremities.

   (b) Physical Examination: Abdominal tenderness often with peritoneal signs, eruptive xanthomas (sometimes present only on the buttocks), and lipemia retinalis. Blood may appear lipemic ex vivo. Fever, diaphoresis, and hypotension may be present depending on the severity of illness.

   (c) Laboratory values: Plasma triglyceride concentrations >2500–3000 mg/dl are usually required to cause acute pancreatitis, but the triglyceride concentration can drop by more than 1000 mg/dl per day if the patient is NPO with nausea and emesis for 1–2 days prior to presentation. Whole blood will appear lipemic like tomato soup; plasma or serum will have the appearance of whole milk or cream depending on the severity of hypertriglyceridemia. Pseudohyponatremia and pseudohyperbilirubinemia due to inaccurate laboratory diagnostics may be found during chylomicronemia. Clarification of

P. B. Duell (✉)
Division of Endocrinology, Diabetes, and Clinical Nutrition, Oregon Health and Science University, Portland, OR, USA
e-mail: duellb@ohsu.edu

© Springer Nature Switzerland AG 2021   257
L. Loriaux, C. Vanek (eds.), *Endocrine Emergencies*, Contemporary Endocrinology,
https://doi.org/10.1007/978-3-030-67455-7_21

plasma or serum by ultracentrifugation will correct lab abnormalities. Hyperglycemia and hypothyroidism need to be identified and treated. Laboratory abnormalities related to complications of pancreatitis are often seen (e.g., hypocalcemia, hypoalbuminemia, anemia).

(d) Imaging: Abdominal CT imaging is useful for diagnosis and staging of pancreatitis regardless of the etiology.

3. Treatment: The primary treatment for chylomicronemia-induced pancreatitis involves making the patient NPO, giving fluid resuscitation and analgesia as needed, and waiting for plasma chylomicrons to be cleared by zero-order kinetics. Intravenous fat emulsions should be avoided. If hyperglycemia is present, an insulin drip is indicated to reduce free fatty acid release from tissues, decrease glucose substrate for hepatic triglyceride synthesis, and restore lipoprotein lipase activity. Patients with hypothyroidism need to receive thyroid hormone replacement. Nonfat or very low-fat foods ($\leq 10\%$ of energy from fat) should be provided when the patient begins oral nutrient intake. Lipid-lowering medications normally do not serve a role in the acute management of pancreatitis and may have increased toxicity in acutely ill patients, but are often required in the long-term management of this condition. Treatment of complications of pancreatitis, such as pancreatic hemorrhage or pseudocyst formation, is the same as in other forms of pancreatitis.

Pancreatitis is a life-threatening complication of severe hypertriglyceridemia, usually associated with plasma triglyceride concentrations >2500–3000 mg/dl. Hypertriglyceridemia is the third most common cause of pancreatitis, following gallstones and alcohol [1, 2], but alcohol intake is often a contributor to hypertriglyceridemia and may precipitate pancreatitis through direct toxicity and indirectly through aggravation of hypertriglyceridemia. Rapid diagnosis and treatment of triglyceride-induced pancreatitis are important to improve patient survival and avoid complications.

Most patients who develop triglyceride-induced pancreatitis have an underlying genetic disorder of triglyceride metabolism that is aggravated by other factors, resulting in severe hypertriglyceridemia. Under optimal conditions, the genetically susceptible patient may have fasting triglyceride concentrations as low as 150–500 mg/dl, which are insufficient to cause pancreatitis. When additional aggravating factors are superimposed on the platform of baseline hypertriglyceridemia, the ensuing progressive accumulation of chylomicrons in plasma can lead to triglyceride concentrations sufficient to cause pancreatitis. In contrast, an individual with normal triglyceride metabolism may experience modest hypertriglyceridemia in response to the superimposition of factors that aggravate hypertriglyceridemia but very rarely will achieve plasma triglyceride concentrations >600–800 mg/dl. Accordingly, the identification of triglyceride-induced pancreatitis is usually a marker for an underlying genetic predisposition for hypertriglyceridemia in combination with one or more aggravating factors responsible for secondary hypertriglyceridemia. It is important for the clinician to carefully scrutinize the patient history so they can identify and treat all of the precipitating factors that may be operative in patients with triglyceride-induced pancreatitis.

Triglyceride Metabolism

Triglycerides consist of a glycerol backbone covalently bound to three triglyceride molecules. They are an important form of energy storage as well as a source of fatty acids for synthetic function and energy production. Being insoluble in aqueous solutions, triglycerides are packaged with phospholipids, cholesteryl esters, cholesterol, and apoproteins in lipoprotein particles for transport in plasma. Chylomicrons and very-low-density lipoproteins (VLDL) carry the majority of triglycerides in plasma. Chylomicrons are produced from dietary fat and cholesterol via the exogenous pathway, and VLDL are secreted by the liver via the endogenous pathway. Both deliver fatty acids to peripheral tissues as well as transport other cargos such as some fat-soluble vitamins and other lipid and apoprotein moieties.

Although all of us undergo transient periods of chylomicronemia after ingestion of dietary fat, the term chylomicronemia usually refers to the presence of chylomicrons in plasma or serum after fasting for more than 10–12 hours. Hyperchylomicronemia may be a more precise term for pathological chylomicronemia, but the term chylomicronemia is often sufficient because chylomicrons are normally absent from plasma after fasting overnight. The half-life of chylomicrons in plasma is normally minutes, but the slow intestinal uptake of dietary triglycerides and secretion of chylomicrons into the circulation via the thoracic duct produces peak postprandial triglyceride concentrations after 3–4 hours in normal individuals with a return to baseline after 6–8 hours (Fig. 21.1). The amount of fat ingested is an important determinant of postprandial excursions in plasma triglyceride concentrations (Fig. 21.1), as is the fasting plasma triglyceride concentration. Among patients with disorders of triglyceride clearance, the peak in postprandial plasma triglyceride concentrations may be delayed to 6–8 hours, and baseline levels may not be reached for 8–12 hours or longer, as shown in Fig. 21.2. These individuals also experience a more dramatic rise in peak postprandial triglyceride levels and a greater area under the curve in response to a high-fat dietary load (Fig. 21.2), which emphasizes the need for restriction of dietary fat intake in these individuals. Chylomicrons are almost always present in plasma when the fasting plasma triglyceride concentration is >1000 mg/dl and usually absent when the fasting triglyceride concentration is below 800–900 mg/dl [3].

Chylomicrons are large triglyceride-rich lipoprotein particles that have a diameter of 80 to 500 nm, a composition that is about 85% triglycerides, a single molecule of apo-B-48 (the truncated form of apo-B containing 48% of the sequence of apo-B-100), and variable amounts of apo-A-I, apo-A-II, apo-A-IV, apo-C-I, apo-C-II, apo-C-III, apo-E, and other apoproteins [4]. During dietary fat absorption, triglycerides are hydrolyzed in the intestinal lumen to facilitate uptake of fatty acids by enterocytes. The enterocyte subsequently re-esterifies the intracellular fatty acids to form triglycerides, which are packaged with apo-B-48, phospholipids, cholesteryl esters, and cholesterol to form chylomicrons. Chylomicrons are slowly released into circulation via the thoracic duct, making them available for utilization by various tissues. After secretion into the blood, chylomicrons acquire

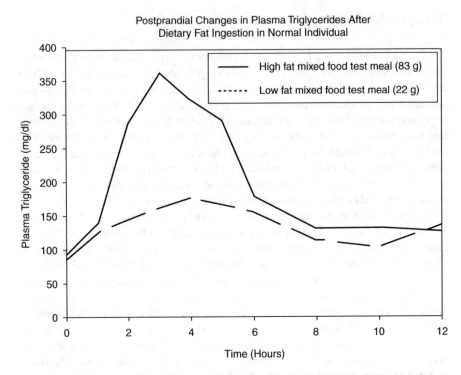

Fig. 21.1 Postprandial changes in plasma triglycerides in a normal individual. The high-fat test meal providing 83 grams of fat caused a tripling in the plasma triglyceride concentration at 3 hours, whereas the low-fat meal providing only 22 grams of fat caused a minimal excursion in the plasma triglyceride concentration. This demonstrates the significant impact of dietary fat ingestion on plasma triglyceride concentrations

apo-C-II primarily from high-density lipoprotein (HDL) particles. The acquired apo-C-II is a cofactor for lipoprotein lipase (LPL), a key triglyceride-hydrolyzing enzyme that is present on the luminal plasma membrane of vascular endothelial cells and is essential for triglyceride clearance. LPL interacts with chylomicrons and very-low-density lipoprotein (VLDL) particles on the surface of endothelial cells through interactions with proteoglycans and glycosylphosphatidylinositol-anchored high-density lipoprotein-binding protein 1 (GPIHBP1), thereby catalyzing the release of fatty acids for uptake by adjacent cells [5]. The heart, skeletal muscle, and adipose tissue are the primary sites of lipoprotein-derived triglyceride hydrolysis and uptake of released fatty acids. The resulting chylomicron and VLDL remnants that remain after partial triglyceride depletion are cleared by the liver, but a proportion of chylomicron and VLDL remnants can be deposited in the artery wall, leading to atherosclerotic plaque formation. Accumulation of elevated concentrations of remnant lipoproteins in plasma is a risk factor for atherosclerotic vascular disease.

Genetic or primary causes of hypertriglyceridemia are shown in Table 21.1. Familial combined hyperlipidemia is one of the more common causes of primary

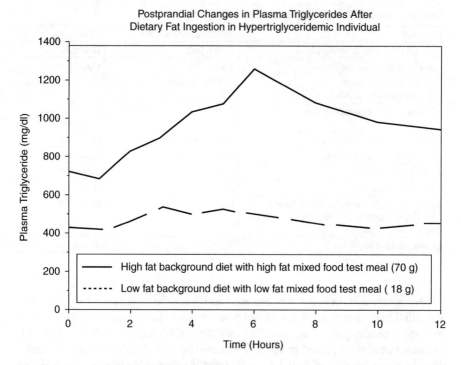

Fig. 21.2 Postprandial changes in plasma triglycerides in a typical hypertriglyceridemic individual. In contrast to the data shown in Fig. 21.1, hypertriglyceridemic individuals have higher-fasting plasma triglyceride concentrations, a greater postprandial increase in the plasma triglyceride concentration, a delay in reaching the postprandial peak, and prolongation of the time to return to baseline levels. The incremental area under the curve for the high-fat meal is about fourfold higher than the area under the curve shown in Fig. 21.1. Consumption of the low-fat background diet for 7 weeks was associated with a 40% reduction in the fasting plasma triglyceride concentration as a consequence of decreased input of chylomicrons. The low-fat test meal caused a minimal excursion in the plasma triglyceride concentration. This demonstrates the benefit of chronic restriction of dietary fat intake in patients with marked hypertriglyceridemia

hypertriglyceridemia, occurring in about 1 in 100 individuals and typically being associated with overproduction of apo-B and VLDL and commonly associated with elevated LDL-C [4, 6]. Monogenic polymorphisms in a variety of genes (e.g., LPL [2–20%], LDLR, FCHL1 [upstream stimulatory factor 1 (USF1)], FCHL2, others) can cause a clinical phenotype consistent with familial combined hyperlipidemia, but the majority of patients with this condition have polygenic dyslipidemia. Familial hypertriglyceridemia is also relatively common. Type III hyperlipidemia, also known as dysbetalipoproteinemia, is seen in only 1 in 5000–10,000 individuals and is usually associated with homozygosity for apo-E2, a ligand that has reduced receptor affinity, resulting in accumulation of remnant lipoproteins in plasma. Apo-E2 homozygosity alone does not cause hyperlipidemia, but the addition of a disorder of VLDL and triglyceride overproduction causes the dyslipidemia to be manifested.

Table 21.1 Genetic causes of hypertriglyceridemia

Disorder	Estimated Prevalence	Inheritance
Familial combined hyperlipidemia	1:100–200	Dominant
Familial hypertriglyceridemia	1:200–500	Dominant
Type III hyperlipidemia (dysbetalipoproteinemia)	1:5000–10,000	Usually recessive
Multifactorial chylomicronemia	1:600	Polygenic and acquired
Polygenic chylomicronemia	1:10,000–20,000	Polygenic
Lipoprotein lipase deficiency	$1:10^6$	Recessive
Apo CII deficiency	Rare	Recessive
Apo-A-V deficiency	Rare	Recessive
Glycosylphosphatidylinositol-anchored high-density lipoprotein binding protein-1 (GPI-HBP-1) deficiency	Rare	Recessive
Lipase maturation factor 1	Rare	Recessive

Monogenic LPL deficiency is a rare recessive condition occurring in about 1 in 10^6 individuals that is often associated with recurrent pancreatitis in about half of patients, typically presenting initially in childhood. Monogenic deficiency of LPL function can also be caused in 10–20% of cases by loss of function biallelic mutations in genes for one of four LPL-associated proteins, resulting in deficiency of apolipoprotein CII, apolipoprotein AV, glycosylphosphatidylinositol-anchored high-density lipoprotein-binding protein 1 (GPI-HBP-1), or lipase maturation factor 1 (LMF-1). Monogenic LPL deficiency or loss of function is also known as familial chylomicronemia syndrome (FCS) and accounts for about 1% of cases of chylomicronemia [7]. This condition in the context of normal or increased dietary fat intake is sufficient to produce severe hypertriglyceridemia and pancreatitis. Restriction of dietary fat intake is the primary and essential intervention because the central defect is an inability to clear triglycerides from plasma due to LPL deficiency or impaired LPL function.

Polygenic chylomicronemia is about two orders of magnitude more common than monogenic LPL deficiency, occurring in about 1;10,000–20,000 individuals [7, 8]. This condition results from small effect changes in numerous genes related to triglyceride metabolism that in combination produce major perturbations in triglyceride metabolism substantial enough to mimic the clinical phenotype of monogenic LPL deficiency. Polygenic chylomicronemia is a subset of multifactorial chylomicronemia, a condition that results from the combined effects of acquired and polygenic defects in triglyceride metabolism and occurs in about 1:600 individuals.

Chylomicronemia is a highly dynamic process that can change in severity over hours to days in response to external or internal aggravating factors superimposed on a genetic or acquired susceptibility to hypertriglyceridemia. These aggravating factors are causes of secondary hypertriglyceridemia (Table 21.2) that influence the

Table 21.2 Causes of secondary hypertriglyceridemia

Category	Condition
Dietary (especially excess dietary fat)	Excess calories
Endocrine	Insulin deficiency (relative or absolute)
	Hyperglycemia (diabetes and impaired glucose tolerance) Hypothyroidism Obesity (can be more severe during weight gain) Lipodystrophy Cushing syndrome Acromegaly Some glycogen storage diseases
Drugs	Alcohol
	Glucocorticoids Oral estrogen and estrogen analogues/SERMs Older beta-adrenergic blockers Thiazides Retinoic acid derivatives Newer antipsychotic medications (e.g., risperidone) Protease inhibitors and HAART regimens for HIV Immunosuppressants (e.g., sirolimus) Bile acid sequestrants
Others	Renal insufficiency/failure
	Proteinuria/nephrotic syndrome Pregnancy

production of triglycerides and triglyceride-rich lipoproteins, the catabolism of lipoproteins and clearance of triglycerides, or both production and clearance of triglycerides. As noted above, one or more aggravating factors often are required in addition to underlying genetic susceptibility to produce severe hypertriglyceridemia and chylomicronemia. Conditions such as diabetes or hypothyroidism tend to cause more chronic increases in plasma triglyceride concentrations, but other factors such as acute increases in intake of dietary fat and/or alcohol can lead to severe hypertriglyceridemia and precipitation of pancreatitis over a period of days. Similarly, acute decompensation of glycemic control can produce severe hypertriglyceridemia during a relatively short time span, but not all patients with uncontrolled diabetes develop severe hypertriglyceridemia. The addition of triglyceride-raising medications such as prednisone or oral estrogen can potentially precipitate severe hypertriglyceridemia and pancreatitis over a period of days to weeks. The most common aggravating factors are increases in intake of alcohol and fat, particularly in combination with hyperglycemia and relative or absolute insulin deficiency.

Uncontrolled diabetes causes hypertriglyceridemia through several mechanisms that are relevant to the therapeutic interventions required for treatment of triglyceride-induced pancreatitis [9]. First, glucose is a substrate for triglyceride synthesis in the liver, so hyperglycemia drives hepatic triglyceride overproduction. Second, deficient insulin action in the adipocyte allows excess lipolysis of stored triglycerides, resulting in increased flux of free fatty acids to the liver and stimulation of hepatic triglyceride overproduction. Third, insulin is needed for maintenance of full LPL activity on the endothelial surface, so absolute or relative insulin deficiency is associated with a reduction in LPL activity, thereby diminishing the capacity for triglyceride clearance. The combination of these factors results in overproduction and decreased clearance of triglycerides, but these adverse conditions can be ameliorated by insulin administration and correction of hyperglycemia. Alcohol intake also drives triglyceride overproduction and impairs triglyceride catabolism.

Mechanism of Chylomicron-Induced Pancreatitis

The mechanism by which chylomicronemia causes pancreatitis is unclear, but it is believed to be related to pancreatic cytotoxicity mediated by free fatty acids and lysolecithin that are produced by pancreatic lipases from excess amounts of chylomicrons in pancreatic capillaries [10]. Hyperviscosity due to hyperchylomicronemia has also been proposed. Surprisingly, not all patients with severe hypertriglyceridemia develop pancreatitis, with some patients remaining completely asymptomatic despite plasma triglyceride concentrations as high as 15,000–20,000 mg/dl. This suggests that there are genetic factors or other variables that influence the susceptibility to chylomicron-induced pancreatitis. Several genetic factors have been identified that are associated with the increased risk of pancreatitis in patients without hypertriglyceridemia, such as gain-of-function polymorphisms in the cationic trypsinogen gene (PRSS1) or loss-of-function polymorphisms in the genes for protective anionic trypsinogen (PRSS2), cystic fibrosis transmembrane regulator (CFTR), and serine protease inhibitor kazal type 1 (SPINK1) encoding pancreatic secretory trypsin inhibitor (PST1) [11, 12], all of which are associated with increased trypsin activity. It is plausible that these factors may also synergistically influence the susceptibility of patients to triglyceride-induced pancreatitis. Loss-of-function polymorphisms in the PRSS1 gene may protect against pancreatitis. Miniature Schnauzer dogs are an animal model that is predisposed to develop hypertriglyceridemia and pancreatitis, the latter of which may be related to an increased prevalence of homozygosity for mutations in SPINK1 [13]. In a Chinese population, a mutation in the gene for CFTR and polymorphisms in the tumor necrosis factor (TNF) promoter were both associated with the risk of triglyceride-induced pancreatitis [14]. The results of more recent analyses verified that mutations in SPINK1 and CFTR are important causes of hereditary pancreatitis but also showed associations with polymorphisms in genes for cytokines (such as interleukin 1-beta (Il1-beta), interleukin 6 (Il6), and interleukin 18 (Il18)), mitochondrial aldehyde dehydrogenase (ALDH2), and redox enzymes (such as glutathione S-transferase) [15, 16].

Clinical Presentation

Patients with triglyceride-induced pancreatitis often present with the same symptoms and signs as patients with other etiologies of pancreatitis [2], but there may be additional history and physical findings that suggest the diagnosis of chylomicronemia. Symptoms of pancreatitis typically involve an acute onset of sharp abdominal pain with possible radiation to the back, nausea, and emesis. Some patients may have indolent symptoms with recurrent episodes of abdominal pain and nausea over months prior to presenting with acute illness. Since the nausea and abdominal pain can lead to decreased oral intake of calories and fat, the change in dietary habits can be sufficient to temporarily reduce the severity of hypertriglyceridemia and result in resolution of symptoms, averting the development of overt pancreatitis. Specific questioning may yield a history of increased intake of fatty foods and alcohol during the days prior to presentation. An example of this that may be seen during summer months is a high intake of hotdogs, hamburgers, potato chips, and potato salad (all high in fat) in combination with excess beer at weekend picnics. Patients also need to be questioned about all medications with a focus on agents that may aggravate hypertriglyceridemia. Some patients may forget to mention, for example, a recent prescription for a short course of prednisone. Diabetic patients may report a recent exacerbation of hyperglycemia, possibly related to infection, changes in dietary habits, or changes in diabetes medications. Uncontrolled diabetes and alcohol intake may account for 50–75% of cases of triglyceride-induced pancreatitis in some settings [17]. Patients with chylomicronemia may also have symptoms of dyspnea, paresthesia of the hands, peripheral neuropathy, and reversible memory impairment and cognitive dysfunction.

Physical findings in patients with all etiologies of pancreatitis who seek emergency care typically include tachycardia, possible hypotension, and abdominal pain with rebound tenderness. Lipemia retinalis, the presence of retinal blood vessels with a milky discoloration instead of the usual dark red appearance (Fig. 21.3), is a definitive evidence of chylomicronemia, but the retina is often not examined in acutely ill patients. This physical finding is often identified retrospectively after the diagnosis of chylomicronemia has been made. An alternative assessment is a visual inspection of the patients' plasma after centrifugation or sitting for 20–60 minutes. Because of their large size, chylomicrons in plasma cause light scattering producing the appearance of turbidity. Plasma with a triglyceride concentration of 500 mg/dl will usually appear turbid, and plasma with a triglyceride concentration of 1000 mg/dl (1% fat content) will have an appearance similar to skim milk. At a triglyceride concentration of 2000 mg/dl, the plasma will appear more latescent, and at levels >4000–5000 mg/d, the plasma will appear creamy (Fig. 21.4). Accordingly, the visual identification of creamy plasma or serum is sufficient to make the diagnosis of severe hypertriglyceridemia prior to the availability laboratory results. With experience, the plasma triglyceride concentration can be estimated on the basis of appearance (Fig. 21.5). It can be beneficial to show patients their lactescent plasma, since the visualization of cream in their blood can be therapeutically motivating.

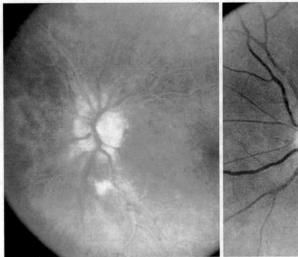
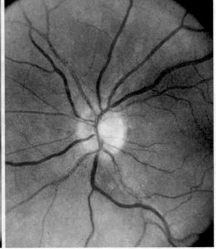

Baseline Plasma Triglyceride
Concentration> 5000 mg/dl

Post-Treatment Plasma Triglyceride
Corcentration < 200 mg/dl

Fig. 21.3 Lipemia retinalis before and after treatment of chylomicronemia

Fig. 21.4 Appearance
of normal and
chylomicronemia plasma
after blood standing for
60 minutes without
centrifugation. The plasma
on the left has a normal
triglyceride concentration
<150 mg/dl, and the
plasma on the right has a
triglyceride concentration
of 5600 mg/dl

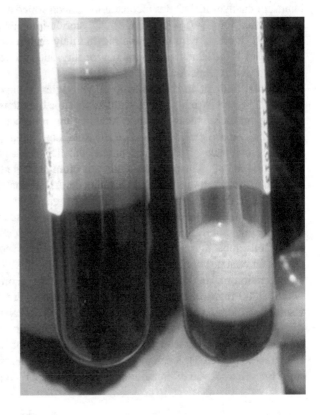

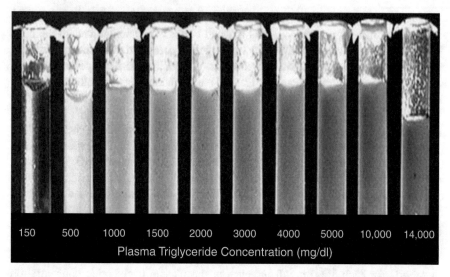

Fig. 21.5 Visual assessment of plasma triglyceride concentrations. The range of turbidity, left to right, is indicative of plasma triglyceride concentrations from <150 mg/dl to >14,000 mg/dl

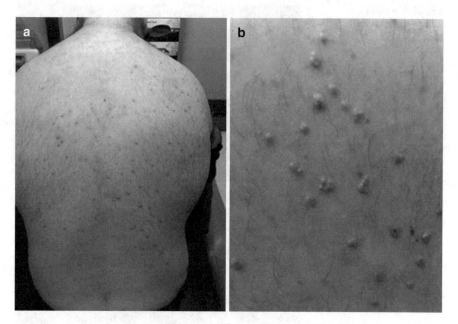

Fig. 21.6 (**a**) Eruptive xanthomas on the back of a patient; (**b**) Close-up view of eruptive xanthomas

Patients with chylomicronemia may have additional physical findings of eruptive xanthomas (Fig. 21.6), hepatomegaly resulting from hepatic steatosis, and possible splenomegaly or splenic firmness. Eruptive xanthomas are cutaneous accumulations of triglyceride-laden macrophages and extracellular lipids that have the appearance of small painless raised pimples, sometimes with an erythematous base. They occur most commonly on the back and buttocks and sometimes on the neck and other extensor surfaces but rarely on the palms, soles, or face. Patients with type III hyperlipidemia may have palmar xanthomas, which consist of a yellowish waxy coloration of the palmar creases (Fig. 21.7) and tuberoeruptive xanthomas, which occur on the elbows and extensor surfaces and consist of bulbous tuberous xanthomas surrounded by eruptive xanthomas (Fig. 21.8) [18].

Routine diagnostic testing in the setting of pancreatitis includes a chemistry battery, lipase and possibly amylase, and complete blood count. Abdominal ultrasonography or CT imaging also may be performed, as well as an ECG. Laboratory testing specifically should include measurements of plasma triglycerides and cholesterol, plasma glucose, HgbA1c, TSH, free T4, and urinalysis for detection of proteinuria. Measurements of low-density lipoprotein (LDL) cholesterol are unimportant in the acute setting and typically are very low because of the derangement of lipid metabolism and impaired conversion of VLDL to LDL. The sodium concentration in non-clarified plasma may artifactually drop (pseudohyponatremia) by 2 to 4 mEq/L for each 1000 mg/dl increase in the plasma triglyceride concentration because of the volume of plasma displaced by chylomicrons [19].

Fig. 21.7 Palmar xanthomas in type III hyperlipidemia

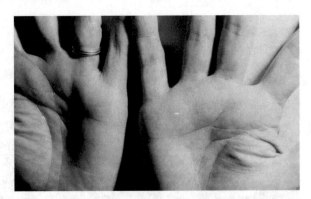

Fig. 21.8 Tuberoeruptive xanthomas on the Elbows

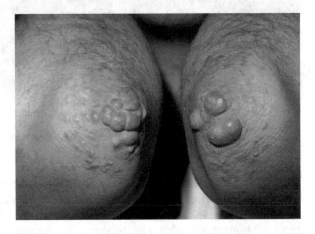

Occasionally, patients with pancreatitis will have plasma triglyceride concentrations less than the 2000–2500 mg/dl threshold that is generally thought to be required to precipitate pancreatitis. In some of these cases, the self-imposed starvation and cessation of dietary fat intake resulting from nausea and emesis may have been sufficient to reduce the plasma triglyceride concentration from higher levels to <2000 mg/dl prior to admission.

Treatment

In the acute phase, most aspects of treatment are the same as for other forms of pancreatitis. Acutely ill patients are typically admitted to the intensive care unit for close monitoring for complications. Patients are made NPO, IV hydration is provided, appropriate analgesia is administered, and precipitating factors are identified and corrected. Imaging of the abdomen, commonly by computed tomography, is indicated for evaluation of possible hemorrhagic pancreatitis and/or pseudocyst formation.

Additional measures are required for patients with chylomicronemia-induced pancreatitis. If hyperglycemia is present, initiation of an insulin drip is indicated to help restore euglycemia, suppress lipolysis in adipocytes, and facilitate restoration of LPL activity. The effects of insulin on lipolysis take longer to accrue than the glucose-lowering effects of insulin, so co-administration of a glucose infusion can be initiated to allow continuation of the insulin drip after glucose levels approach normal. The improvement in LPL activity can take weeks to occur in response to long-term insulin therapy. Administration of insulin probably has minimal benefit in patients who do not have hyperglycemia or insulin insufficiency, so treatment with insulin is not indicated in this setting.

The cessation of fat intake during the acute phase of treatment also needs to include avoidance of intravenous fat emulsions because these preparations are cleared from plasma similarly to chylomicrons. Triglyceride-lowering medications are often unnecessary because the plasma triglyceride concentration can decrease by 1000–2000 mg/dl daily in response to being NPO with no fat intake in combination with insulin treatment in hyperglycemic individuals (Fig. 21.9). Since triglyceride clearance pathways are saturated in the setting of chylomicronemia, and triglyceride-lowering medications suppress triglyceride production more than they increase triglyceride clearance [20], administration of triglyceride-lowering medications may not significantly accelerate the resolution of chylomicronemia. Moreover, medications such as fibrates and niacin can cause hepatotoxicity and muscle toxicity, effects that are more frequent in the acutely ill patient, so we prefer to delay initiating these medications until after the acute illness resolves.

It has been proposed that plasmapheresis may be helpful in the management of chylomicron-induced pancreatitis [2]. This is a logical consideration because plasmapheresis can rapidly clear chylomicrons from plasma, thereby reducing the mass

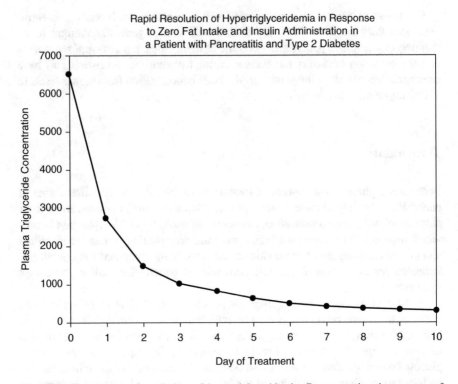

Fig. 21.9 Time course of resolution of hypertriglyceridemia. Representative time course of changes in plasma triglycerides over time showing rapid resolution of hypertriglyceridemia in response to zero-fat intake and treatment of hyperglycemia with insulin in a patient with chylomicronemia-induced pancreatitis and uncontrolled diabetes

of pancreatitis-causing chylomicrons, but the results of clinical trial data have not demonstrated a clear benefit of this intervention, and the procedure is not risk-free. The primary support comes from case reports and uncontrolled case series, which are insufficient to demonstrate benefit from plasmapheresis. The results of one large case series compared the outcomes of hypertriglyceridemic pancreatitis in 34 patients treated prior to the availability of plasmapheresis at their hospital versus 20 patients treated after plasmapheresis became available [21]. The results showed no differences in complications or mortality between the two groups, suggesting that plasmapheresis did not provide clinical benefit [21]. In another trial, sixty-six patients were prospectively randomized to receive high-volume hemofiltration versus low-molecular-weight heparin plus insulin, but no difference in clinical outcomes was identified [22]. The requirement for dual venous access and an extracorporeal blood volume of several hundreds of milliliters, as well as possible risks of bleeding and citrate-induced hypocalcemia, can add risk in an acutely ill patient. At this time, it is unclear whether plasmapheresis actually improves patient outcomes.

Although heparin was recognized long ago as a plasma-clearing factor in hyper-triglyceridemic patients [23], the administration of heparin during acute pancreatitis may not appreciably increase LPL activity, and it can significantly increase the risk of hemorrhagic complications. Therefore, heparin is not indicated in the acute treatment of triglyceride-induced pancreatitis.

The chronic phase of treatment requires major lifestyle modifications by the patient. As the patient begins to recover and food intake is initiated, dietary fat intake should be restricted to <10% of energy intake, which is easy to regulate in the hospital. As the patient prepares for discharge, it may be possible to liberalize the dietary fat intake, but the goal of <10–20% of energy should be emphasized. Although the low-fat diet may initially be unpleasant or difficult for the patient, many acclimate well to low-fat eating over time, particularly when they understand the importance of this intervention in avoiding recurrent pancreatitis. Alcohol intake also needs to be restricted or eliminated. Regular exercise is an important component of the outpatient treatment regimen, which helps reduce hyperglycemia, improves insulin sensitivity, lowers plasma triglycerides, and can facilitate weight loss. Efforts to achieve sustainable weight loss are indicated in overweight and obese patients, but weight regain needs to be avoided because it can cause rebound hypertriglyceridemia. Lifestyle modification is the cornerstone for weight loss, but pharmacologic treatment can be considered for patients with BMI > 27–30 kg/m^2, and bariatric surgery is a consideration for patients with BMI > 35–40 kg/m^2. Evaluation and counseling by a dietitian are invaluable in this endeavor. Patients are usually highly motivated to make changes immediately after hospitalization for acute pancreatitis, so the opportunity should be seized to maximize patient education and implementation of essential lifestyle changes. Unfortunately, motivation and compliance tend to wane during the months after discharge, so close follow-up of the patient with repeated reinforcement of positive lifestyle habits helps the patient to persevere in the difficult task of maintaining healthy lifestyle attributes.

Pharmacologic treatment of the hypertriglyceridemia and associated conditions is often also needed in addition to lifestyle modification [6]. An exception to this is the rare condition of LPL deficiency (and related conditions with loss of LPL activity) in which avoidance of dietary fat is the key intervention and triglyceride-lowering medications provide only minimal efficacy [24]. In response to lifestyle changes, the fasting plasma triglyceride concentration may decrease to 200–800 mg/dl. Rarely, patients may achieve a normal triglyceride concentration < 150 mg/dl, but persistent hypertriglyceridemia is the norm. Identification and correction of secondary hyperlipidemia is an important first step (Table 21.2). Attention should include a focus on control of hyperglycemia in diabetic patients and titration of thyroid hormone replacement to achieve euthyroidism in hypothyroid patients.

Several medications are helpful in the treatment of hypertriglyceridemia [24] (Table 21.3). Fibrates are PPAR-alpha agonists that reduce triglyceride synthesis and can help increase LPL activity. Gemfibrozil is the oldest fibrate that is currently available and has been shown to prevent CHD events in the Helsinki Heart Study [25] and the VA-HIT study [26]. Fenofibrate is a newer fibrate that showed a reduction in CHD events in the FIELD trial but only after adjusting for the important

Table 21.3 Medications for treatment of hypertriglyceridemia

Fibrates	Fenofibrate/Gemfibrozil/Fenofibric acid
Niacin	OTC nicotinic acid
	OTC slow or intermediate release nicotinic acid Prescription intermediate release nicotinic acid (Niaspan)
Fish oil	OTC fish oil
Prescription concentrated distilled ethyl esters of EPA + DHA	Purified EPA (Vascepa)/Lovaza

confounding effect of statin use in the placebo arm [27]. Fenofibrate was associated with cardiovascular benefit compared to placebo when added to statin therapy in the subgroup with elevated triglycerides ≥204 mg/dl and low HDL-C ≤ 34 mg/dl in the ACCORD trial [28]. Gemfibrozil and fenofibrate are useful for the treatment of hypertriglyceridemia, but fenofibrate has fewer drug-drug interactions, particularly in combination with statins [20].

Niacin is the best all-around lipid-altering medication, but side effects such as flushing and aggravation of hyperglycemia or gout can be limiting factors. Niacin is the best agent for raising HDL cholesterol levels, moderately efficacious for lowering lipoprotein(a), and moderately effective for lowering triglycerides and LDL-C. Niacin reduced the risk of myocardial infarction in the Coronary Drug Project, one of the first tests of the cholesterol hypothesis [29].

Fish oil in its various forms can be useful in the treatment of hypertriglyceridemia and is often underutilized. Eicosapentaenoic acid (EPA) and docosahexaenoic acid (DHA) are the active ingredients responsible for triglyceride lowering, but EPA alone may be advantageous. A minimum triglyceride-lowering dose of EPA and DHA is about 2 grams daily. Proper dosing is confounded by variability in the EPA and DHA content of various over-the-counter (OTC) preparations, but 6 grams of typical OTC fish oil containing 30% EPA + DHA will provide 1.8 grams of EPA + DHA, which is a starting dose. Branded Lovaza™ (and generic equivalents) is a prescription preparation of distilled, purified, and concentrated ethyl esters of EPA and DHA that comprise 84% of the mass of the product. The FDA-approved dose is 4 grams daily, which provides about 3.4 grams of EPA + DHA. Branded Vascepa™ (icosapent ethyl), a fish oil preparation containing an ethyl ester EPA, without DHA, may have the advantage of avoiding the modest increases in LDL cholesterol that may occur during treatment with the combination of EPA + DHA. In addition, treatment of high-ASCVD-risk patients with plasma triglycerides 150–500 mg/dl with icosapent ethyl 4 grams daily was associated with a 25% reduction in ASCVD events compared to placebo [30].

Statins are second-line drugs for the treatment of hypertriglyceridemia because they may lower the triglyceride concentration by only 25–35%, which is less than the 30–50% reduction that can be achieved with the other medications. Combination therapy with two or more drugs may be required for patients who have severe residual hypertriglyceridemia.

Promising experimental treatments are in development for patients with familial chylomicronemia syndrome include volanesorsen, an antisense oligonucleotide that binds apo-CIII; and evinacumab (Evkeeza™), a monoclonal antibody that binds ANGPTL3 was FDA approved in the United States in February 2021. Gene therapy for LPL gene replacement, Glybera™ (alipogene tiparvovec), was developed and approved in the European Commission, but it was not widely used clinically for a variety of reasons including high cost, need for up to 60 intramuscular injections under anesthesia, and a requirement for temporary immunosuppression [7].

Summary

In summary, chylomicronemia-induced pancreatitis is a potentially life-threatening condition that warrants emergency treatment. Most patients with this problem have an underlying genetic disorder of triglyceride metabolism on which is superimposed one or more forms of secondary hypertriglyceridemia, commonly related to uncontrolled diabetes, alcohol intake, and excess dietary fat intake. Patients with chylomicronemia-induced pancreatitis present with symptoms and signs that are similar to other patients with pancreatitis, but they also can have hepatosplenomegaly related to hepatic steatosis and eruptive xanthomas or tuberoeruptive xanthomas. Lipemic plasma is the hallmark of chylomicronemia that can be visualized as lipemia retinalis or ex vivo in plasma or serum. Treatment of chylomicronemia-induced pancreatitis is focused on correction of the chylomicronemia as well as reversal of the factors that may be aggravating hypertriglyceridemia. Long-term therapy requires extensive lifestyle changes, often with the addition of triglyceride-lowering drugs. A very low-fat diet, avoidance of alcohol, regular exercise, and sustainable weight loss are important components of the intervention. Patients who are compliant with their treatment regimen can often avoid a recurrence of pancreatitis, but recurrent pancreatitis occurs in many patients, including some who are very compliant.

References

1. Pancreatitis. National Institute of Diabetes and Digestive and Kidney Diseases. http://digestive.niddk.nih.gov/ddiseases/pubs/pancreatitis/. Last accessed January 5, 2013.
2. Tsuang W, Navaneethan U, Ruiz L, Palascak JB, Gelrud A. Hypertriglyceridemic pancreatitis: presentation and management. Am J Gastroenterol. 2009;104:984–91.
3. Brunzell JB, Bierman EL. Chylomicronemia syndrome. Med Clin North Amer. 1982;66:455.
4. Duell PB, Roullet JB, Steiner RD. Inborn errors of metabolism: disorders of lipid, lipoprotein, and bile acid metabolism. In: McIntosh N, Helms PJ, Smyth RL, editors. Forfar and Arneils

textbook of pediatrics. 7th ed. Edinburgh: Churchill Livingstone, Elsevier Limited; 2008. p. 1089–101.

5. Beigneux A,. Davies B.S.J, Gin P, Weinstein MM, Farber E, Qiao X, . Peale F, Bunting S, Walzem RL, Wong JS *et al:* Glycosylphosphatidylinositol-anchored high-density lipoprotein-binding protein 1 plays a critical role in the Lipolytic processing of chylomicrons, Cell Metab 2007;5:279–291.

6. Berglsnd L, Brunzell JD, Goldberg AC, Goldberg IJ, Sacks F, Murad MH, Stalenhoef AFH. Evaluation and treatment of hypertriglyceridemia: an endocrine society clinical practice guideline. J Clin Endocrinol Metab. 2012;97:2969–89.

7. Baass A, Paquette M, Bernard S, Hegele RA. Familial chylomicronemia syndrome: an under-recognized cause of severe hypertriglyceridaemia. J Int Med. 2020;287:340–8.

8. Warden BA, Minnier J, Duell PB, Fazio S, Shapiro MD. Chylomicronemia syndrome: familial or not? J Clin Lipidol. 2020;14:201–6.

9. Duell PB. Dyslipidemia in diabetes. In: Betteridge DJ, Illingworth DR, Sheppard J, editors. Lipoproteins in health and disease. London: Edward Arnold; 1999. p. 897–929.

10. Kimura W, Mossner J. Role of hypertriglyceridemia in the pathogenesis of experimental acute pancreatitis in rats. Int J Pancreatol. 1996;20:177.

11. Ellis I. Genetic counseling for hereditary pancreatitis – the role of molecular genetics testing for the cationic trypsinogen gene, cystic fibrosis and serine protease inhibitor Kazal type 1. Gastro Clin North Am. 2004;33:839–54.

12. Mayerle J, Sendler M, Hegyi E, Beyer G, Lerch MM, Sahin-Toth M. Genetics and pathophysiology of pancreatitis. Gastroenterology. 2019;156:1951–68.

13. Bishop MA, Xenoulis PG, Levinski MD, Suchodolski JS, Steiner JM. Identification of variants in the SPINK1 gene and their associations with pancreatitis in Miniature Schnauzers. Am J Veterinary Res. 2010;71:527–3.

14. Chang YT, Chang MC, Su TC, et al. Association of cystic fibrosis transmembrane conductance regulator (CFTR) mutation/variant/haplotype and tumor necrosis factor (TNF) promoter polymorphism in hyperlipidemic pancreatitis. Clin Chem. 2008;54:131–8.

15. van den Berg FF, Kempeneers MA, van Santvoort HC, Zwinderman AH, Issa Y, Boermeester MA. Systematic review: meta-analysis and field synopsis of genetic variants associated with the risk and severity of acute pancreatitis. BJS Open. 2020;4:3–15.

16. Lee PJ, Papachristou GI. New insights into acute pancreatitis. Nat Rev Gastroenterol Hepatol. 2019;16:479–96.

17. Fortson MR, Freedman SN, Webster PDIII. Clinical assessment of hyperlipidemic pancreatitis. Am J Gastroenterol. 1995;90:2134–9.

18. Duell PB. Hypertriglyceridemia - pathophysiology, diagnosis, and treatment. Endocrinologist. 1992;2:321–31.

19. Steffes MW, Freier EF. A simple and precise method of determining true sodium, potasium, and chloride concentrations in hyperlipidemia. J Lab Clin Med. 1876;88:683.

20. Duell PB. Differential pharmacokinetics and adverse effects of gemfibrozil, fenofibrate, and fenofibric acid. Lipid Spin. 2010;8(3):9–12,44.

21. Chen JH, Yeh JH, Lai HW, et al. Therapeutic plasma exchange in patients with hyperlipidemic pancreatitis. World J Gastroenterol. 2004;10:2272–4.

22. He WH, Yu M, Zhu Y, Xia L, Liu P, Zeng H, Zhu Y, Lu NH. Emergent triglyceride-lowering therapy with early high-volume hemofiltration against low-molecular-weight heparin combined with insulin in hypertriglyceridemic pancreatitis: a prospective randomized controlled trial. J Clin Gastroenterol. 2016;50(9):772–8.

23. Korn ED. Clearing factor, a heparin-activated lipoprotein lipase. I. Isolation and characterization of the enzyme from normal rat heart. J Biol Chem. 1955;215:1.

24. Brunzell JD. Hypertriglyceridemia. N Engl J Med. 2007;357:1009–17.

25. Frick MH, Elo O, Haapa OP, et al. Helsinki Heart Study: primary-prevention trial with gemfibrozil in middle-aged men with dyslipidemia. Safety of treatment, changes in risk factors, and incidence of coronary heart disease. N Engl J Med. 1987;317(20):1237–45.

26. Robins SJ, Collins D, Wittes JT, et al. Relation of gemfibrozil treatment and lipid levels with major coronary events: VA-HIT: a randomized controlled trial. JAMA. 2001;285(12):1585–91.
27. The FIELD Study Investigators. Effects of long-term fenofibrate therapy on cardiovascular events in 9795 people with type 2 diabetes mellitus (the FIELD study): randomised controlled trial. Lancet. 2005;366:1849–61.
28. The ACCORD Study Group. Effects of combination lipid therapy in type 2 diabetes mellitus. N Engl J Med. 2010;362:1563–74.
29. Coronary Drug Project Research Group. Clofibrate and niacin in coronary heart disease. JAMA. 1975;231(4):360–81.
30. Bhatt DL, Steg PG, Miller M, Brinton EA, Jacobson TA, et al. Cardiovascular risk reduction with Icosapent ethyl for hypertriglyceridemia. N Engl J Med. 2019;380:11–22.

Index

© Springer Nature Switzerland AG 2021
L. Loriaux, C. Vanek (eds.), *Endocrine Emergencies*, Contemporary Endocrinology,
https://doi.org/10.1007/978-3-030-67455-7

Printed in the United States
by Baker & Taylor Publisher Services